Dr. med. B. Kirschsieper

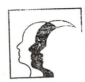

Praxis
Dr. med. Boris Kirschsieper
Facharzt für Nuklearmedizin
Facharzt für Diagnostische Radiologie

Balger Strasse 50   Tel: (07221) 91 27 94
79532 Baden-Baden Fax: (07221) 91 27 98

Web: www.Praxis-Kirschsieper.de
E-Mail: info@Praxis-Kirschsieper.de

D1729392

T. B. Möller · E. Reif

MRI Atlas of the Musculoskeletal System

MRI Atlas of the Musculoskeletal System

TORSTEN B. MÖLLER
Consultant Radiologist
Centre for Radiology and Nuclear Medicine
D-66763 Dillingen, Saar, Germany

EMIL REIF
Consultant in Nuclear Medicine
Centre for Radiology and Nuclear Medicine
D-66763 Dillingen, Saar, Germany

WITH THE COLLABORATION OF

BEATE HILPERT AND

UDO SCHUMACHER

BOSTON
BLACKWELL SCIENTIFIC PUBLICATIONS
OXFORD LONDON EDINBURGH
MELBOURNE PARIS BERLIN VIENNA

© 1993 by
Blackwell Wissenschafts-Verlag GmbH
English language edition
© 1993 by
Blackwell Scientific Publications, Inc.
Editorial Offices:
238 Main Street, Cambridge, Massachusetts 02142, USA
Osney Mead, Oxford OX2 0EL, England
25 John Street, London WC1N 2BL, England
23 Ainslie Place, Edinburgh EH3 6AJ, Scotland
54 University Street, Carlton, Victoria 3053, Australia

Other Editorial Offices:

Librairie Arnette SA
1, rue de Lille
F-75007 Paris
France

Blackwell Wissenschafts-Verlag GmbH
Düsseldorfer Str. 38
D-10707 Berlin
Germany

Blackwell MZV
Feldgasse 13
A-1238 Wien
Austria

All rights reserved. No part of this book may be reproduced in any form or by any electronic or mechanical means, including information storage and retrieval systems, without permission in writing from the publisher, except by a reviewer who may quote brief passages in a review.

First published 1993
This translation published 1993

Cover design: R. Hübler, 12163 Berlin, Germany
Production: Goldener Schnitt · Rainer Kusche, 76547 Sinzheim, Germany
Printed by Druckhaus Beltz, 69502 Hemsbach, Germany
Bound by J. Schäffer, 67261 Grünstadt, Germany

DISTRIBUTORS

USA
Blackwell Scientific Publications, Inc.
238 Main Street
Cambridge, Massachusetts 02142
(*Orders:* Tel: 617 876-7000
            800 759-6102)

Canada
Times Mirror Professional Publishing, Ltd
130 Flaska Drive
Markham, Ontario L6G 1B8
(*Orders:* Tel: 416 470-6739
            800 268-4178)

Australia
Blackwell Scientific Publications Pty Ltd
54 University Street
Carlton, Victoria 3053
(*Orders:* Tel: 03 347-5552)

Outside North America and Australia
Marston Book Services Ltd
PO Box 87
Oxford OX2 0DT
(*Orders:* Tel: 0865 791155
            Fax: 0865 791927
            Telex: 837515)

**Library of Congress
Cataloging-in-Publication Data**
Möller, Torsten B.
  [MR-Atlas des Muskuloskelettalen Systems. English]
  MRI atlas of the musculoskeletal system / Torsten B. Möller, Emil Reif : with the collaboration of Beate Hilpert. — English language ed.
      p.   cm.
    ISBN 0-86542-291-5
    1. Musculoskeletal system—Magnetic resonance imaging—Atlases.
  I. Reif, Emil. II. Hilpert, Beate. III. Title.
    [DNLM: 1. Musculoskeletal System—anatomy & histology—atlases.
    2. Magnetic Resonance Imaging—atlases.   WE 17 M7262m 1993]
RC925.7.M6513   1993
616.7′07548—dc20

Dedication

– to my beloved daughter Nina Maureen. I wish her with all my heart fortune and contentment, health and gladness on her way in life.

Torsten B. Möller

– to my children Jan und Anne

Emil Reif

Abbreviations

A.	= artery	M.	= muscle	post.	= posterior
Aa.	= arteries	Mm.	= muscles	Proc.	= process
ant.	= anterior	med.	= medial	R.	= ramus
Lig.	= ligament	N.	= nerve	V.	= vein
Ligg.	= ligaments	Nn.	= nerves	Vv.	= veins

Preface

MRI is now established as an important tool in the daily routine of radiologists, orthopedists, and rheumatologists in the diagnosis, treatment and monitoring of musculoskeletal disorders. This extends not only to joints but also bone, bone marrow and soft tissues.

The quality and sophistication of the MR image allows much finer discrimination in differential diagnosis, and therefore demands a far greater appreciation of the relevant anatomical detail. Pathological diagnosis is impossible without a detailed knowledge of normal appearances. MRI will become the diagnostic procedure of choice: unlike radiography it is harmless, and its spread will be hastened by the new fast MRI machines, which are small, light, cheap and easy to use.

Existing books normally present MRI scans with accompanying photographs of morbid anatomy. This book takes a new approach; the MRI scans are unlabelled, but are accompanied by line diagrams in the same place, at the same level. These diagrams have been drawn by the authors direct from the scans to prevent transfer errors and to ensure the greatest accuracy. The line diagrams are in colour and the same colours are used to differentiate different tissues throughout the book: bone is beige, gut and viscera are brown, nerves are yellow, veins are dark blue, arteries are bright red. Muscles are differentiated by various colours; every group of muscles has its own colour and each is re-identified on each page. All the images were taken on living patients.

The atlas is divided into two main sections: upper and lower limbs. At the beginning of each, the transverse cuts (the MRI slices) are shown sequentially on a longitudinal line diagram to show the levels at which they were shot.

Both the arm and leg have been pictured as a whole, as described above, and their joints are pictured coronally. The only exception is the shoulder, where the coronal and sagittal planes are oblique, and angled parallel to the supraspinatus muscle; the normal clinical approach.

The sagittal planes of the foot chosen are parallel to the first and third metatarsal bone.

All T-1-weighted images were obtained on a 1.5 Tesla system using commercially available surface and body coils and spin-echo pulse sequences.

Dillingen/Saar, November 1993

Torsten B. Möller · Emil Reif

Acknowledgements

An atlas such as this requires the assistance of many people to whom we are deeply indebted. First we would like to thank our entire staff whose spontaneous and continous help was always encouraging. We would like to acknowledge by name our physician Thomas Recktenwald, our radiologic technologists Monika Baumann, Andrea Britz, Giovanna Vivaqua, Pia Saar, Annika Schmitz and Gisela Wagner.

Our sincere thanks also go to Blackwell and specially to Axel Bedürftig, M.D., whose enthusiasm for this atlas helped to see it through.

Many thanks also go to Thomas Warncke for his advice on how to choose the right colour for the drawings.

We acknowledge with deep appreciation the extraordinary support, assistance and advice of Beate Hilpert, M.D. Her constructive input has helped to improve the final result immensely.

To my wife Barbara with love and sincere thanks whose patience allowed me to spend so many hours with the book instead of with her.

Torsten B. Möller · Emil Reif

Contents

Upper Limbs

Upper Limbs Axial
Shoulder — 5
Upper Arm — 13
Elbow — 19
Forearm — 25
Wrist and Hand — 31

Shoulder
Coronal — 47
Sagittal — 57

Upper Arm
Coronal — 67
Sagittal — 75

Elbow
Coronal — 85
Sagittal — 91

Forearm
Coronal — 99
Sagittal — 107

Wrist and Hand
Coronal — 119
Sagittal — 127

Lower Limbs

Lower Limbs Axial
Hip — 137
Thigh — 147
Knee — 155
Lower Leg — 159
Ankle and Foot — 171

Hip
Coronal — 185
Sagittal — 195

Thigh
Coronal — 205
Sagittal — 219

Knee
Coronal — 229
Sagittal — 241

Lower Leg
Coronal — 255
Sagittal — 265

Ankle and Foot
Coronal — 277
Sagittal — 293

References — 301

Subject Index — 303

Upper Limbs

Upper Limbs Axial

Shoulder

Upper Arm

Elbow

Forearm

Wrist and Hand

Upper Limbs Axial – Shoulder

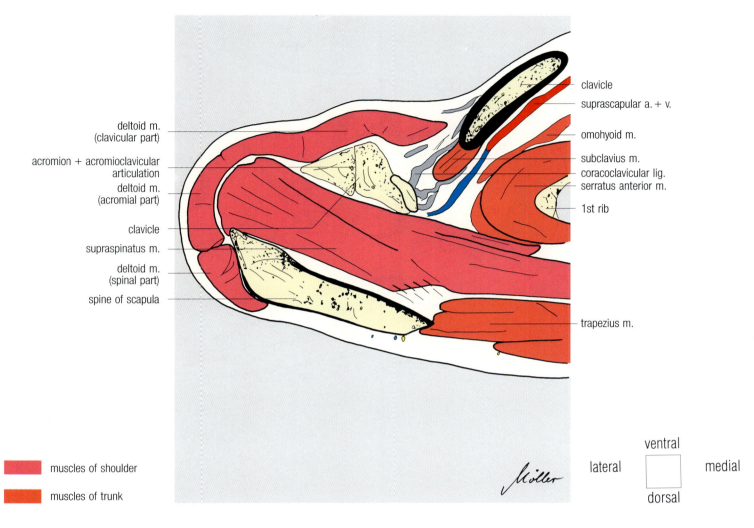

- deltoid m. (clavicular part)
- acromion + acromioclavicular articulation
- deltoid m. (acromial part)
- clavicle
- supraspinatus m.
- deltoid m. (spinal part)
- spine of scapula
- clavicle
- suprascapular a. + v.
- omohyoid m.
- subclavius m.
- coracoclavicular lig.
- serratus anterior m.
- 1st rib
- trapezius m.

muscles of shoulder
muscles of trunk

ventral / lateral / medial / dorsal

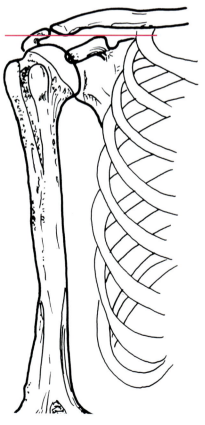

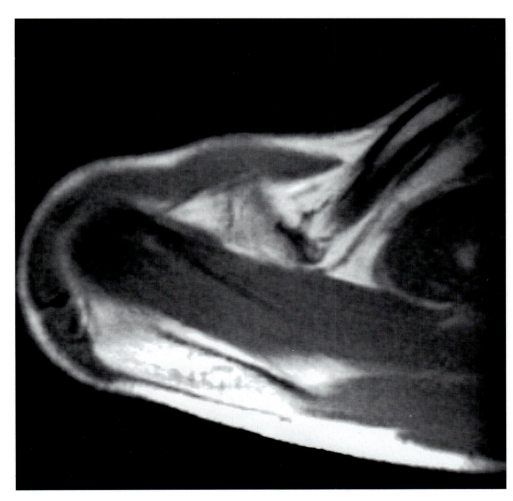

Upper Limbs Axial – Shoulder

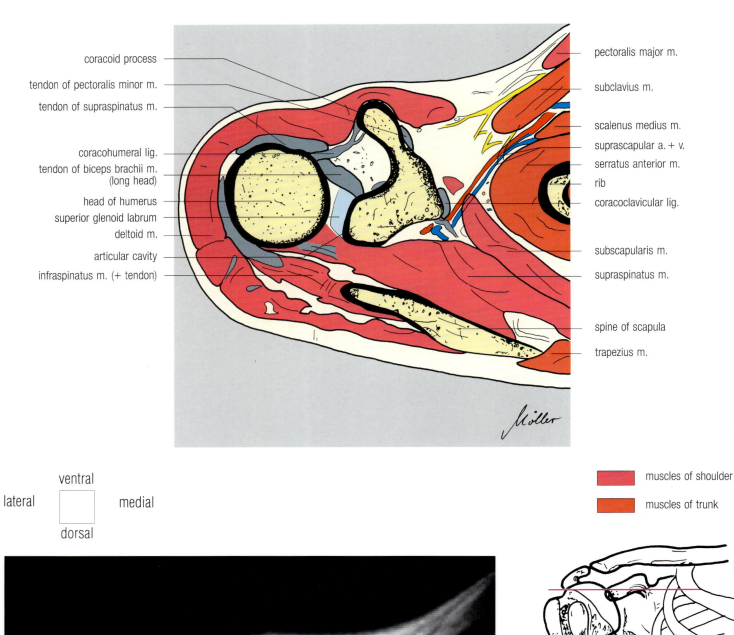

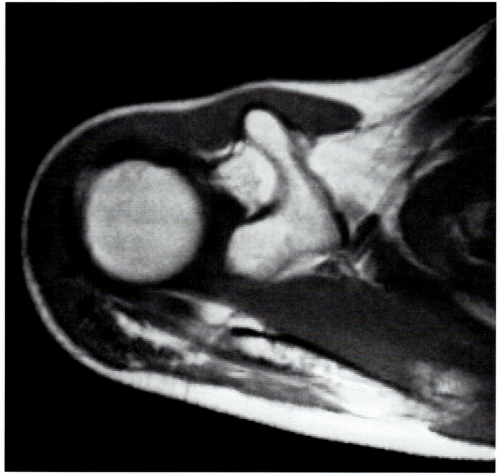

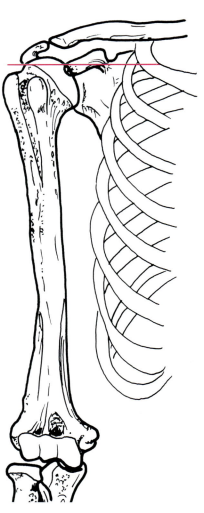

Upper Limbs Axial – Shoulder

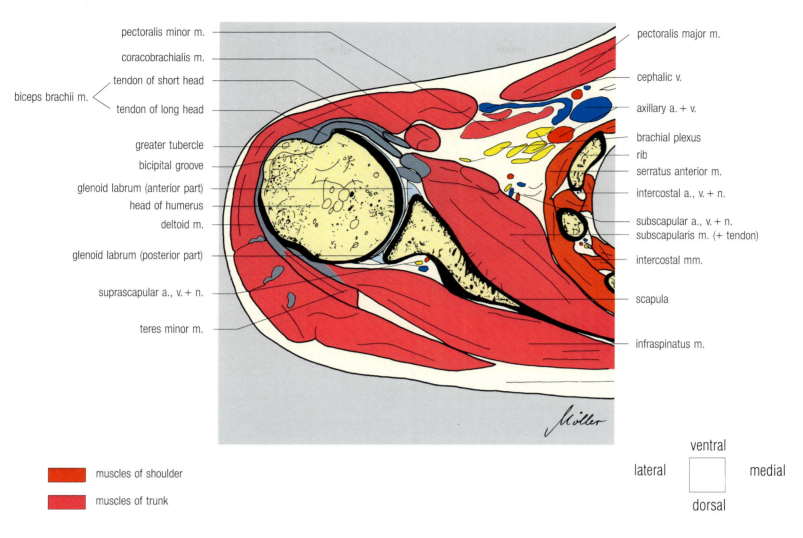

muscles of shoulder
muscles of trunk

ventral
lateral — medial
dorsal

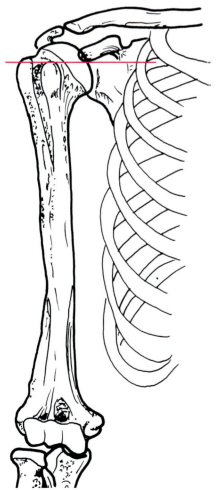
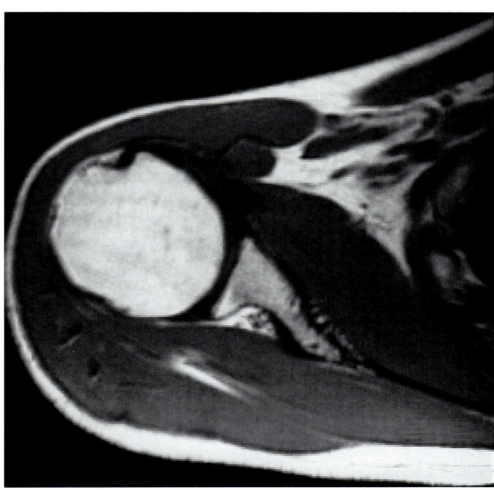

Upper Limbs Axial – Shoulder

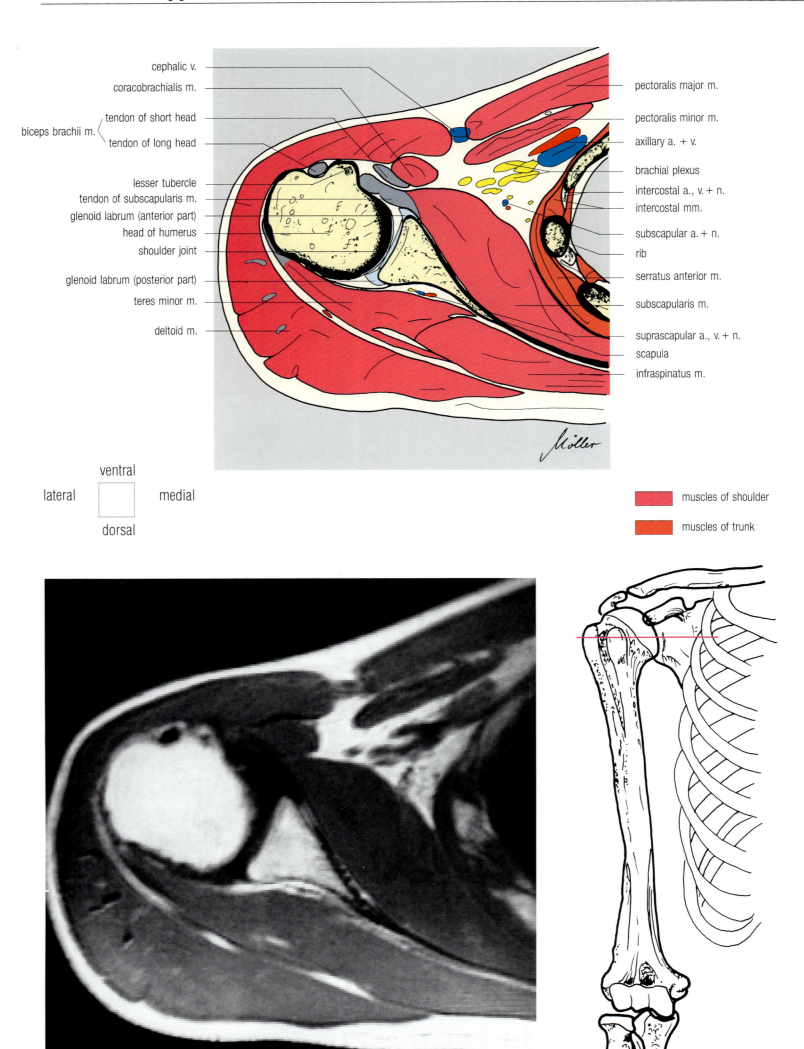

Upper Limbs Axial – Shoulder

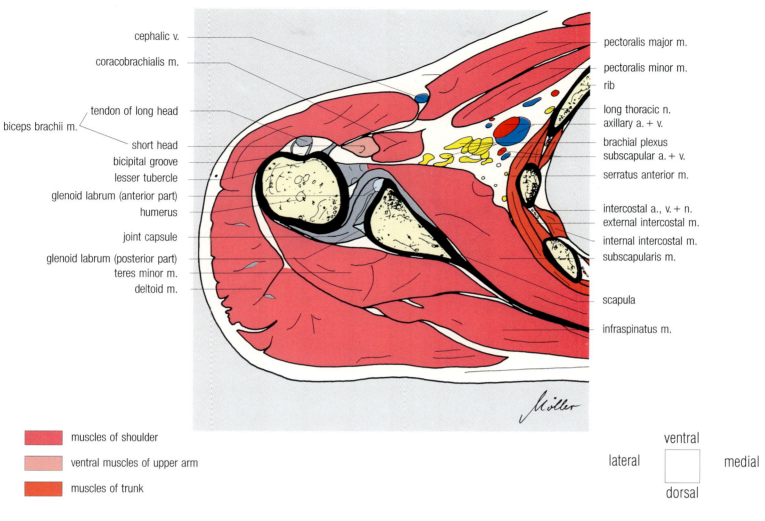

- muscles of shoulder
- ventral muscles of upper arm
- muscles of trunk

lateral — ventral / dorsal — medial

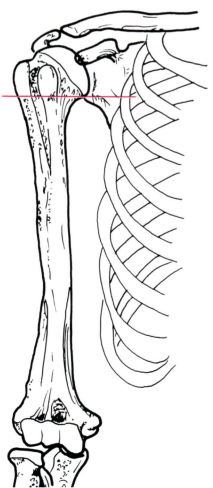
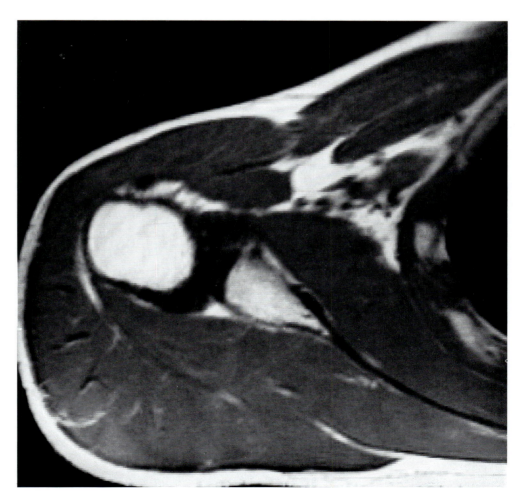

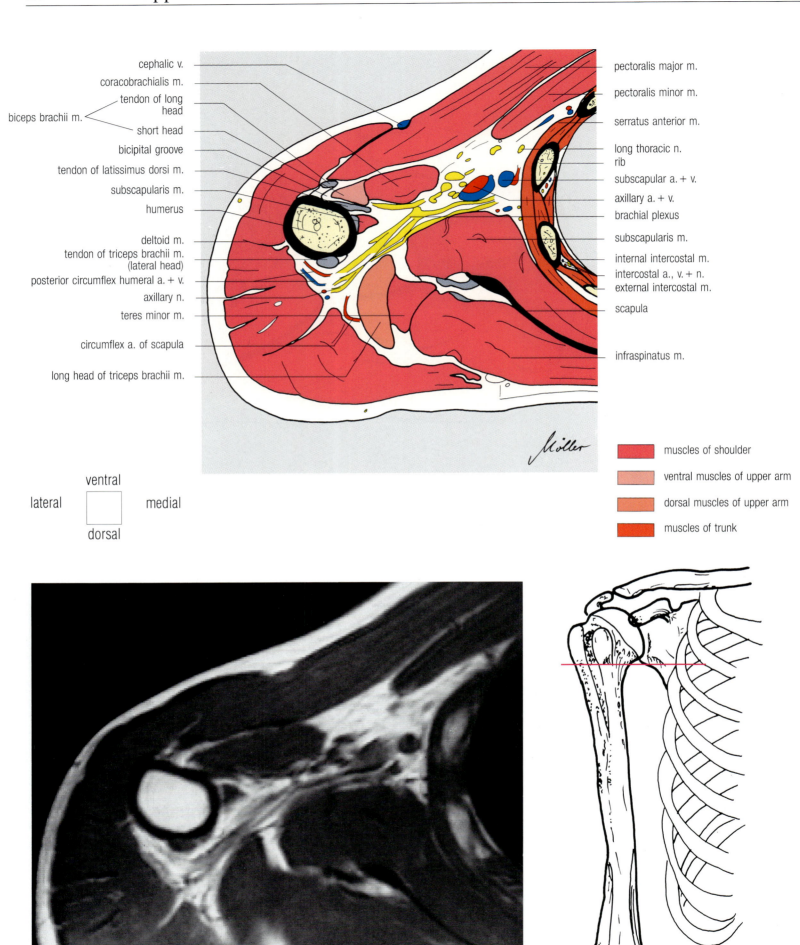

Upper Limbs Axial – Shoulder

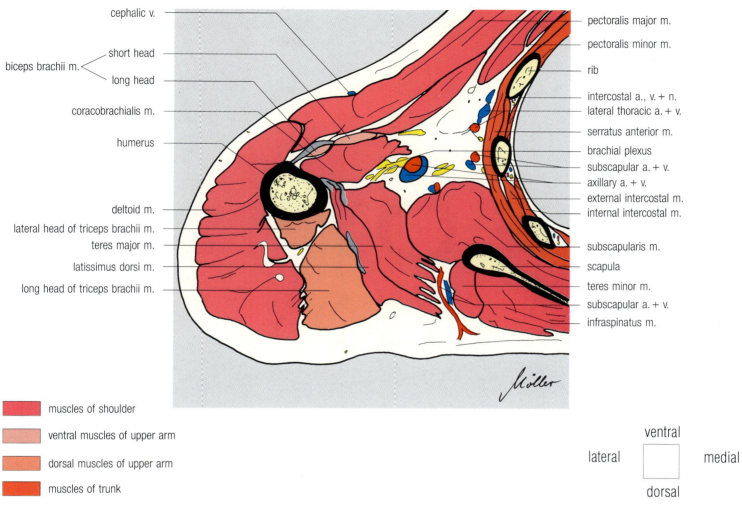

- muscles of shoulder
- ventral muscles of upper arm
- dorsal muscles of upper arm
- muscles of trunk

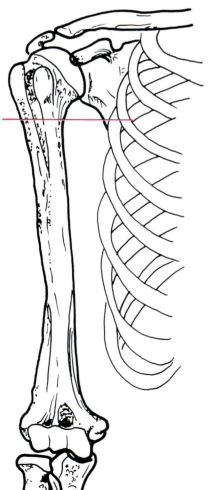

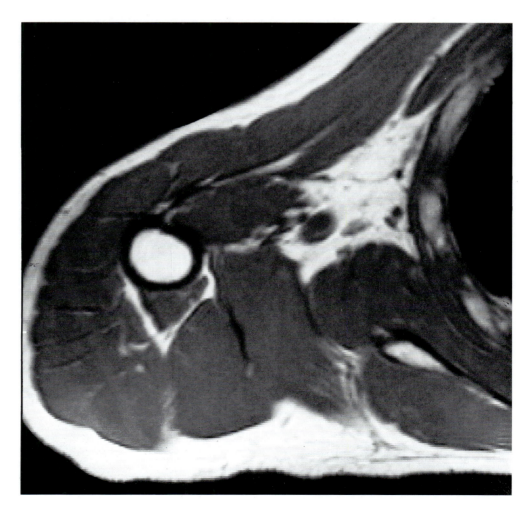

12 Upper Limbs Axial – Shoulder

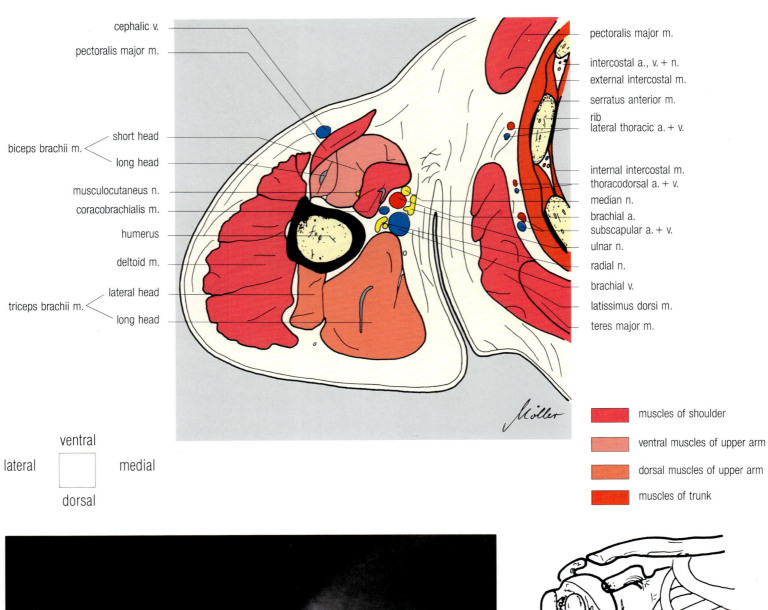

cephalic v.
pectoralis major m.

biceps brachii m. — short head
— long head

musculocutaneus n.
coracobrachialis m.
humerus
deltoid m.

triceps brachii m. — lateral head
— long head

pectoralis major m.
intercostal a., v. + n.
external intercostal m.
serratus anterior m.
rib
lateral thoracic a. + v.
internal intercostal m.
thoracodorsal a. + v.
median n.
brachial a.
subscapular a. + v.
ulnar n.
radial n.
brachial v.
latissimus dorsi m.
teres major m.

ventral
lateral ☐ medial
dorsal

■ muscles of shoulder
■ ventral muscles of upper arm
■ dorsal muscles of upper arm
■ muscles of trunk

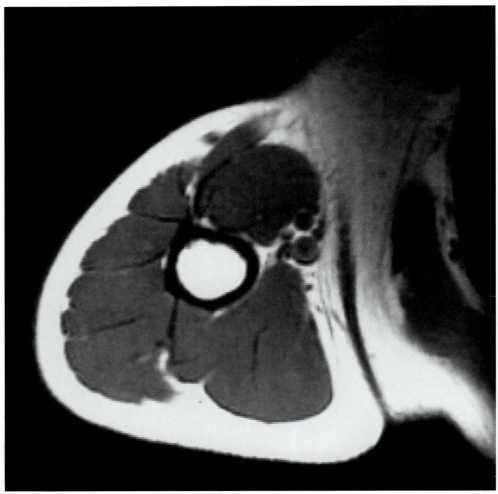
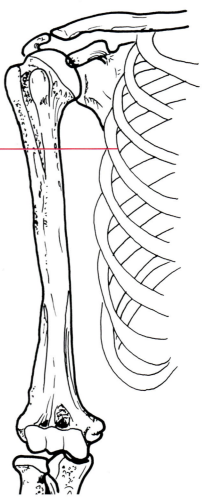

Upper Limbs Axial – Shoulder

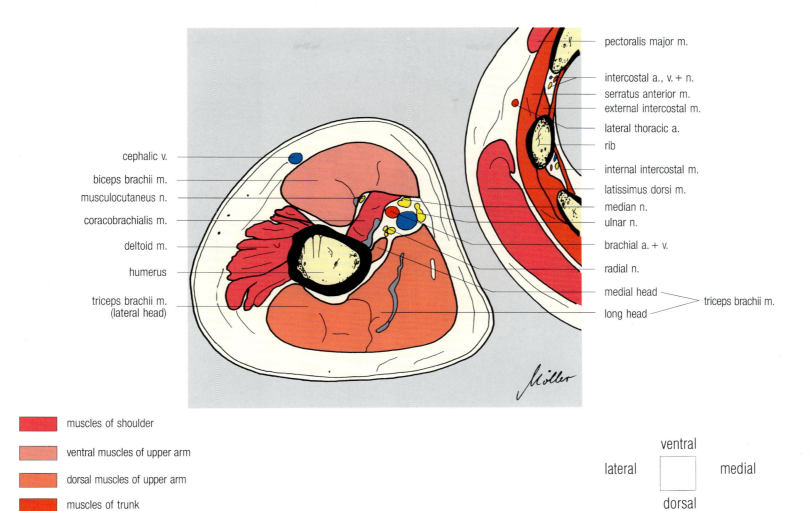

- pectoralis major m.
- intercostal a., v. + n.
- serratus anterior m.
- external intercostal m.
- lateral thoracic a.
- rib
- internal intercostal m.
- latissimus dorsi m.
- median n.
- ulnar n.
- brachial a. + v.
- radial n.
- medial head — triceps brachii m.
- long head

- cephalic v.
- biceps brachii m.
- musculocutaneus n.
- coracobrachialis m.
- deltoid m.
- humerus
- triceps brachii m. (lateral head)

- muscles of shoulder
- ventral muscles of upper arm
- dorsal muscles of upper arm
- muscles of trunk

ventral / lateral / medial / dorsal

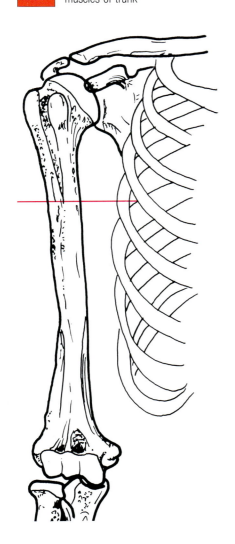
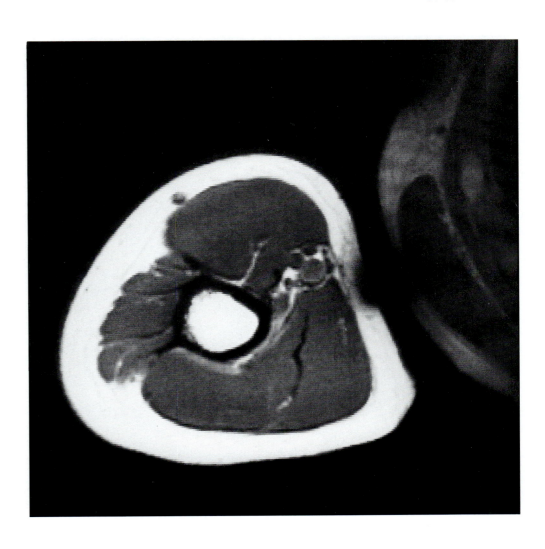

Upper Limbs Axial – Upper Arm

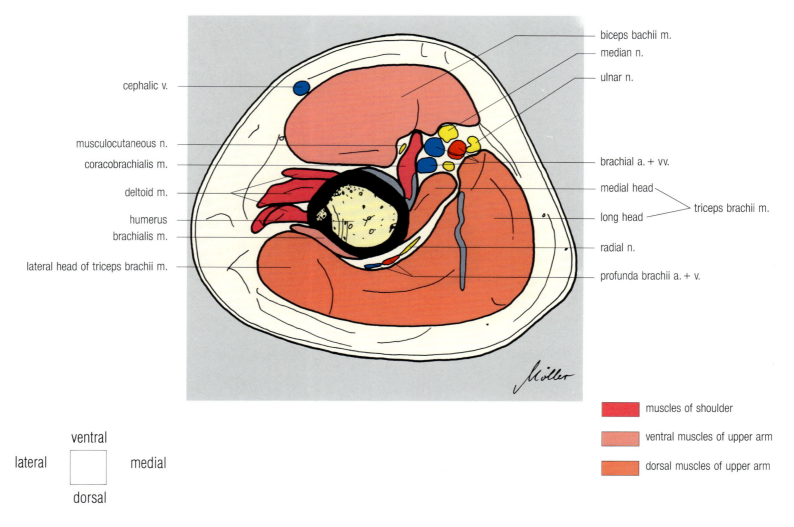

muscles of shoulder
ventral muscles of upper arm
dorsal muscles of upper arm

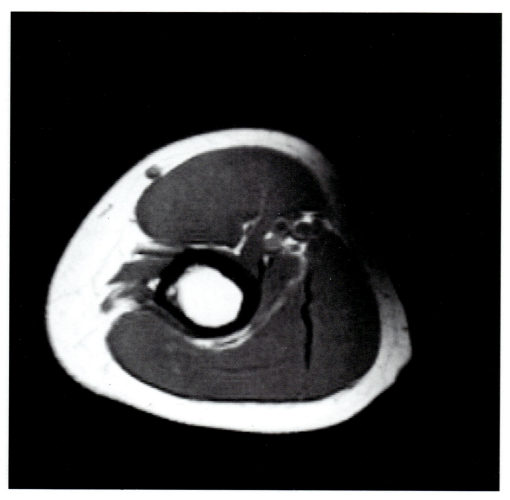

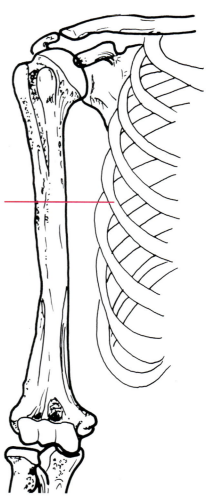

Upper Limbs Axial – Upper Arm

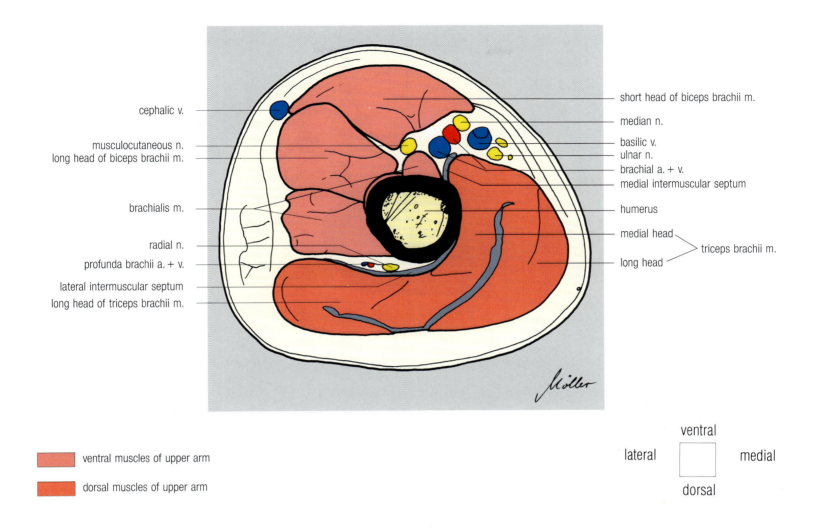

- ventral muscles of upper arm
- dorsal muscles of upper arm

ventral
lateral | | medial
dorsal

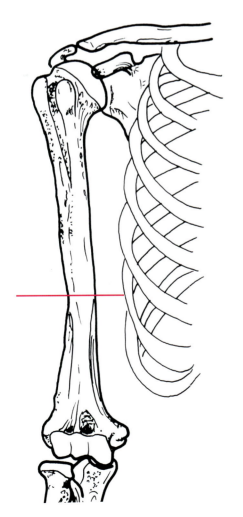

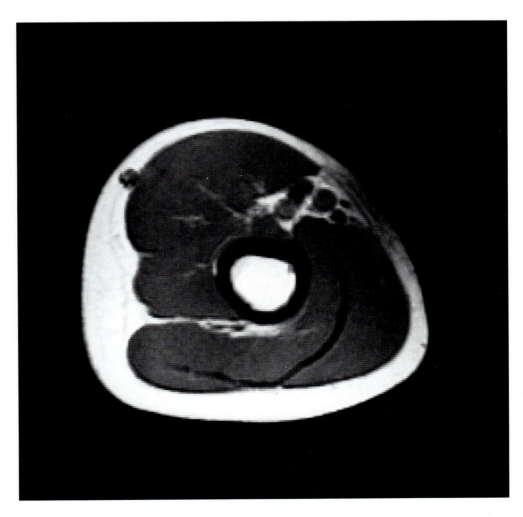

Upper Limbs Axial – Upper Arm

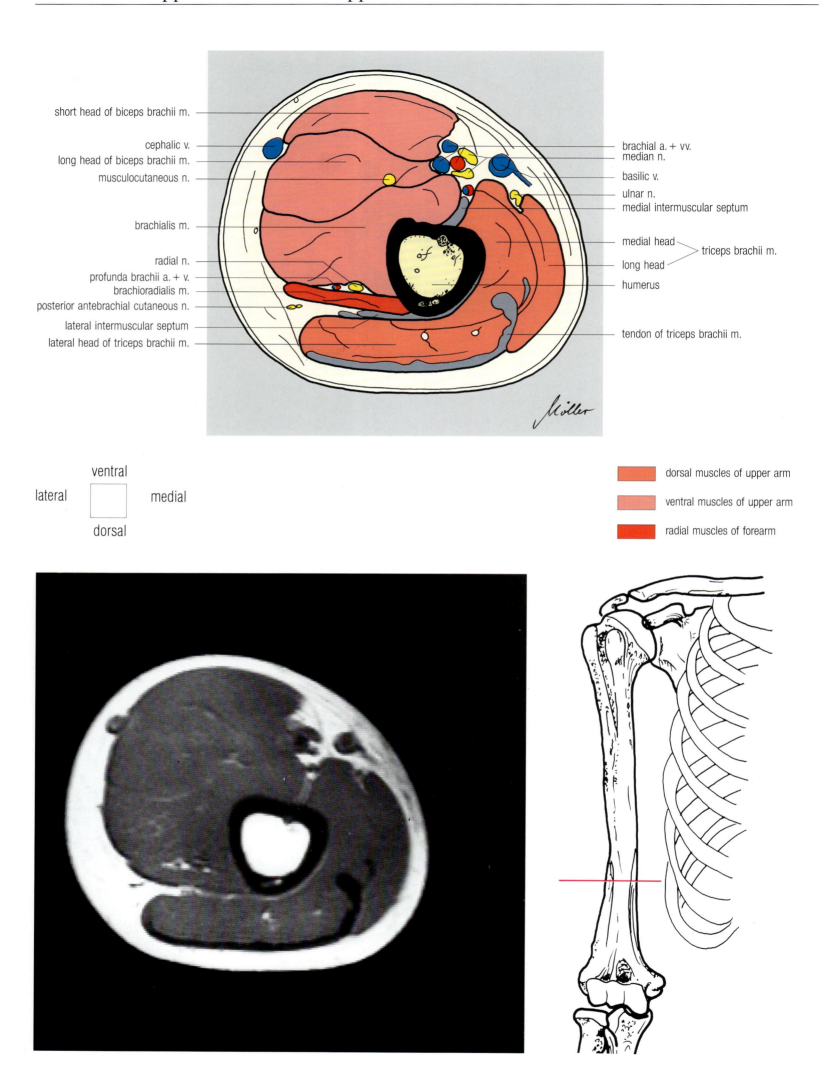

Upper Limbs Axial – Upper Arm 17

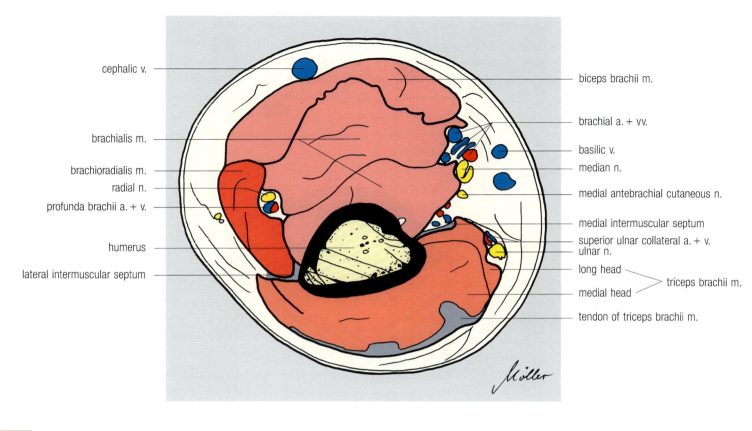

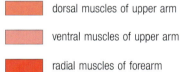

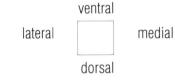

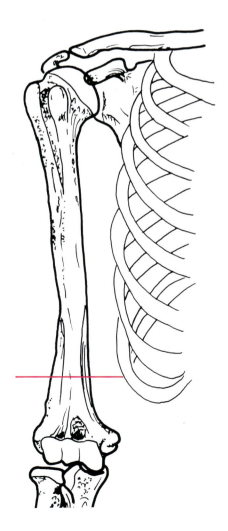

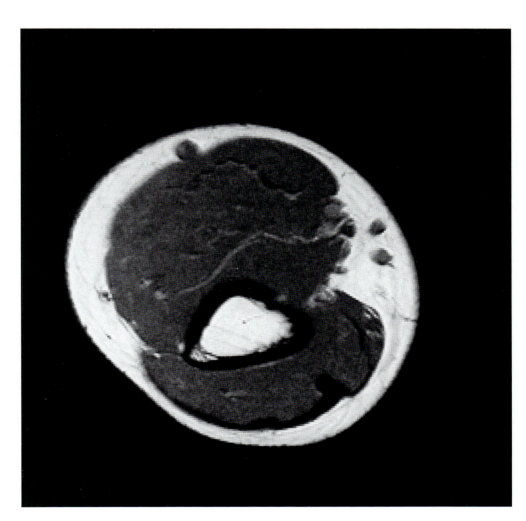

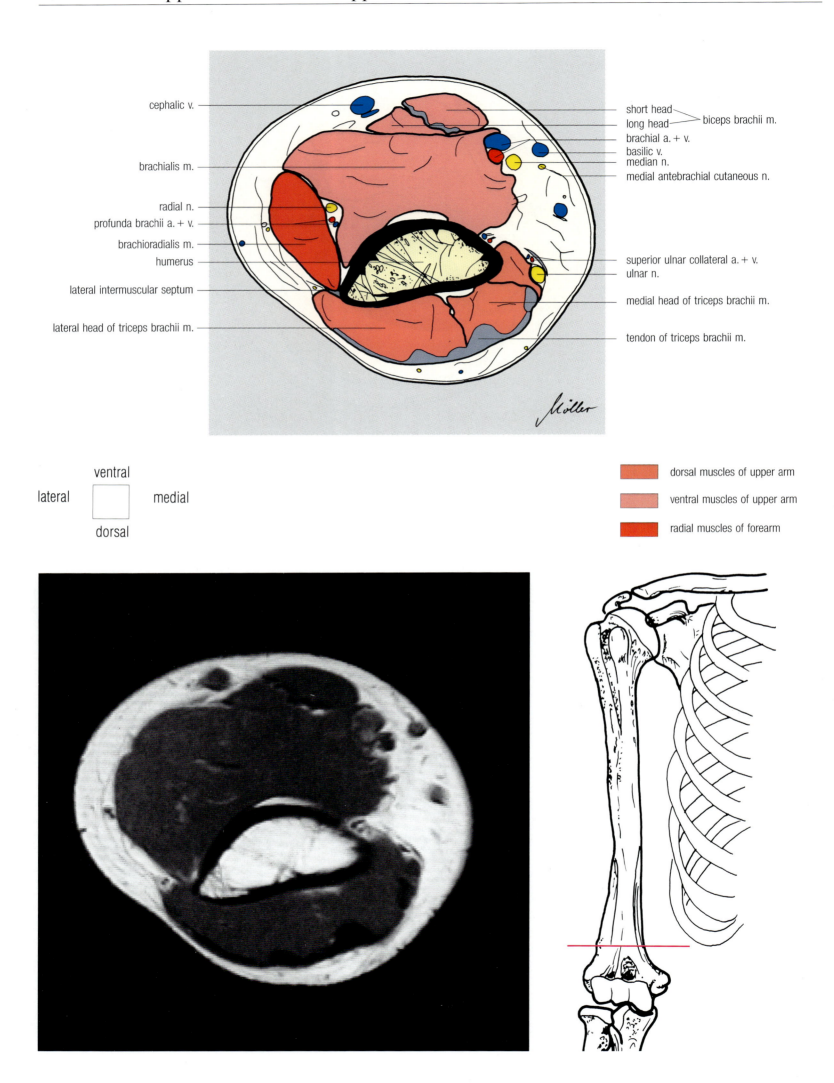

Upper Limbs Axial – Elbow

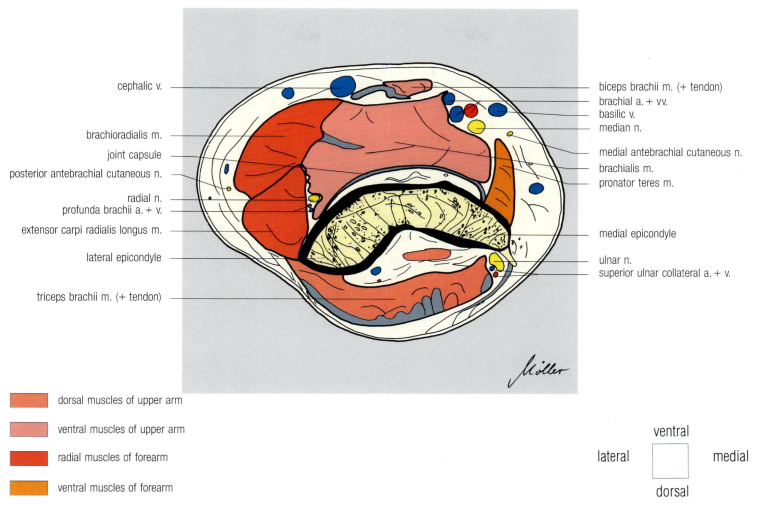

- dorsal muscles of upper arm
- ventral muscles of upper arm
- radial muscles of forearm
- ventral muscles of forearm

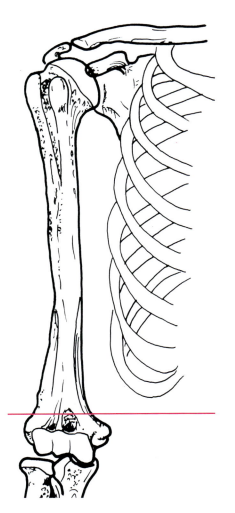

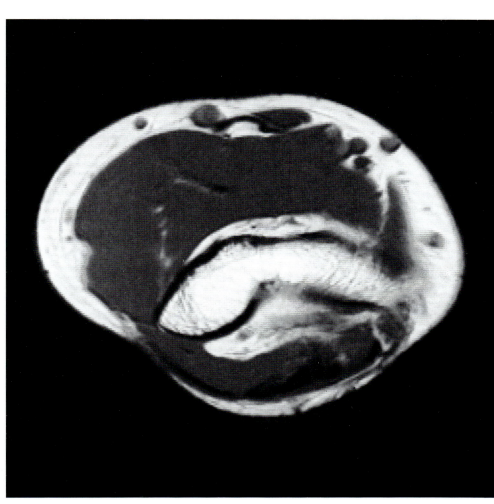

Upper Limbs Axial – Elbow

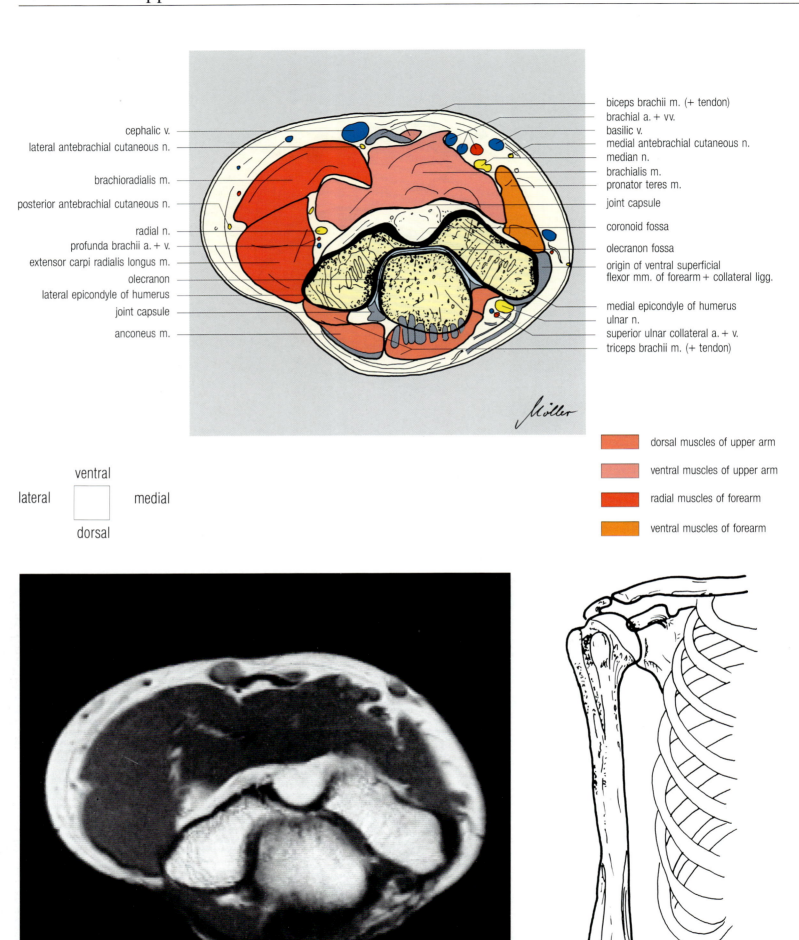

- cephalic v.
- lateral antebrachial cutaneous n.
- brachioradialis m.
- posterior antebrachial cutaneous n.
- radial n.
- profunda brachii a. + v.
- extensor carpi radialis longus m.
- olecranon
- lateral epicondyle of humerus
- joint capsule
- anconeus m.

- biceps brachii m. (+ tendon)
- brachial a. + vv.
- basilic v.
- medial antebrachial cutaneous n.
- median n.
- brachialis m.
- pronator teres m.
- joint capsule
- coronoid fossa
- olecranon fossa
- origin of ventral superficial flexor mm. of forearm + collateral ligg.
- medial epicondyle of humerus
- ulnar n.
- superior ulnar collateral a. + v.
- triceps brachii m. (+ tendon)

ventral
lateral — medial
dorsal

- dorsal muscles of upper arm
- ventral muscles of upper arm
- radial muscles of forearm
- ventral muscles of forearm

Upper Limbs Axial – Elbow

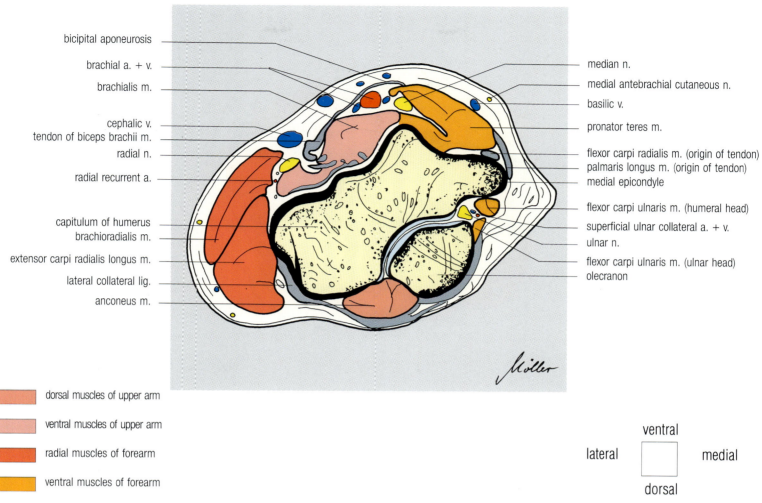

- bicipital aponeurosis
- brachial a. + v.
- brachialis m.
- cephalic v.
- tendon of biceps brachii m.
- radial n.
- radial recurrent a.
- capitulum of humerus
- brachioradialis m.
- extensor carpi radialis longus m.
- lateral collateral lig.
- anconeus m.

- median n.
- medial antebrachial cutaneous n.
- basilic v.
- pronator teres m.
- flexor carpi radialis m. (origin of tendon)
- palmaris longus m. (origin of tendon)
- medial epicondyle
- flexor carpi ulnaris m. (humeral head)
- superficial ulnar collateral a. + v.
- ulnar n.
- flexor carpi ulnaris m. (ulnar head)
- olecranon

- dorsal muscles of upper arm
- ventral muscles of upper arm
- radial muscles of forearm
- ventral muscles of forearm

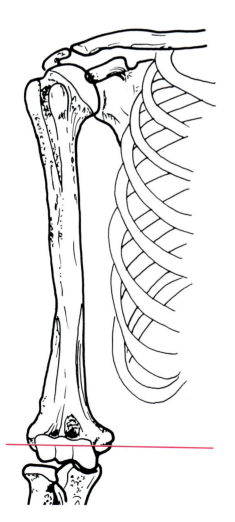

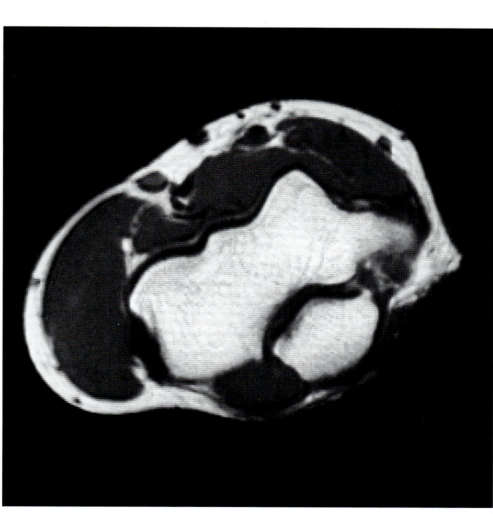

Upper Limbs Axial – Elbow

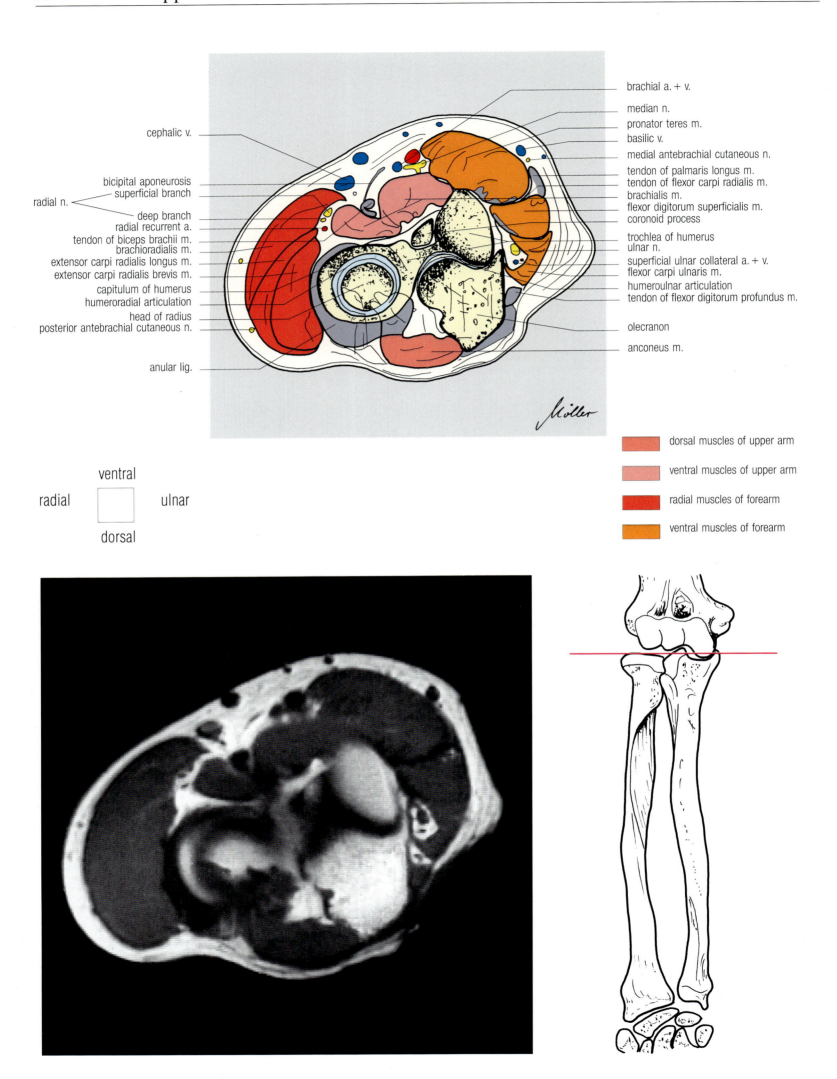

Upper Limbs Axial – Elbow

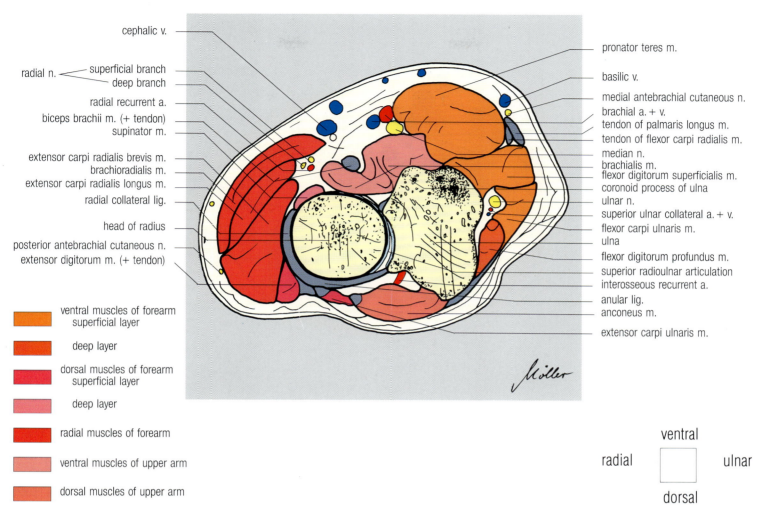

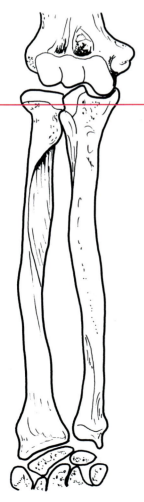
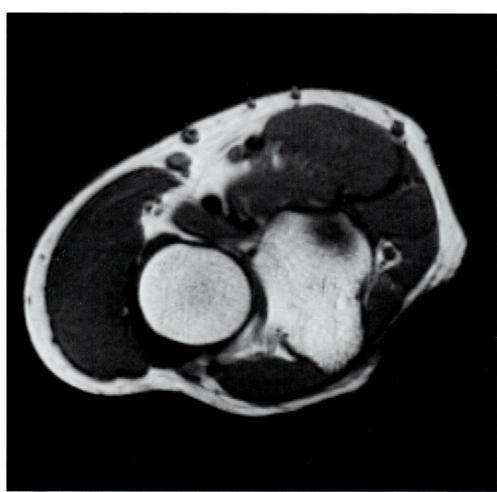

Upper Limbs Axial – Elbow

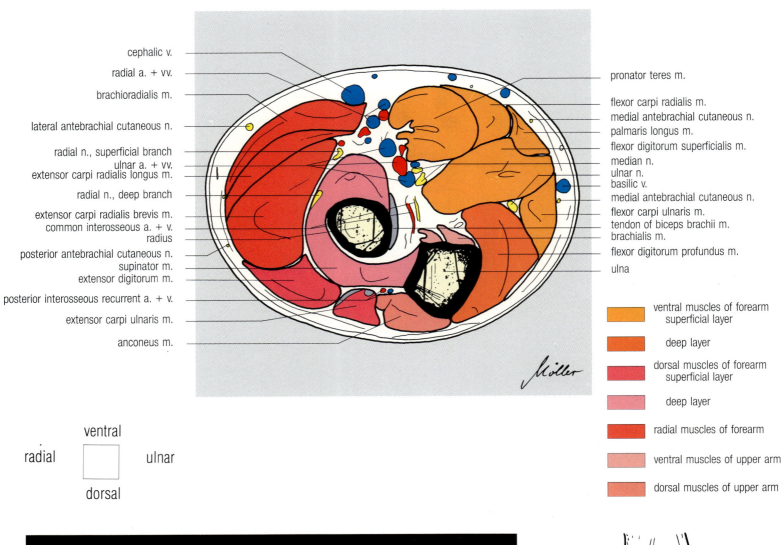

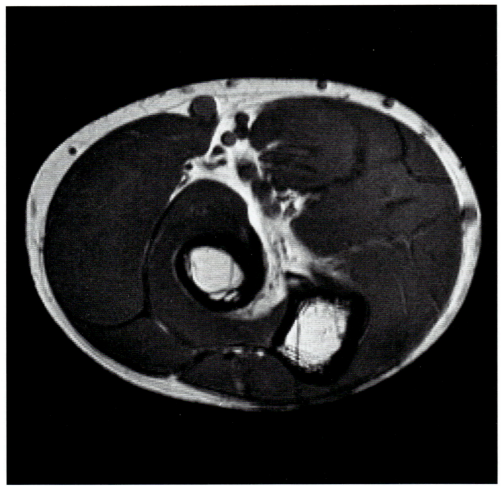 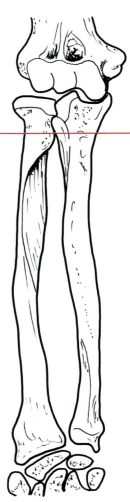

Upper Limbs Axial – Forearm

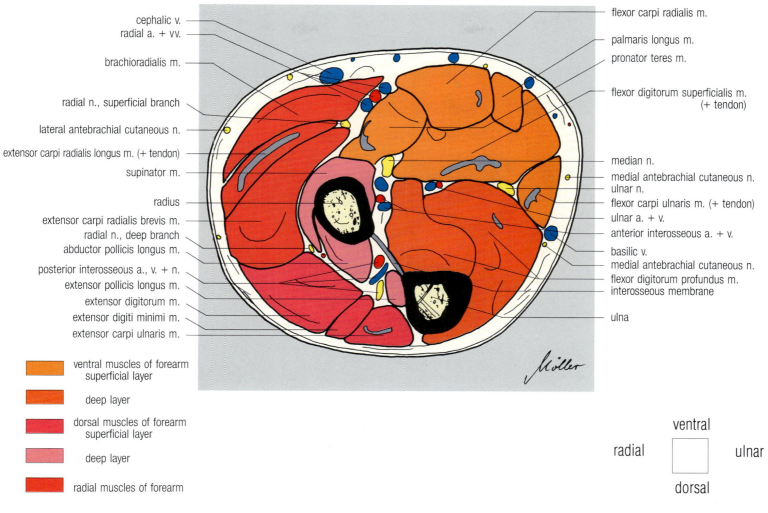

- cephalic v.
- radial a. + vv.
- brachioradialis m.
- radial n., superficial branch
- lateral antebrachial cutaneous n.
- extensor carpi radialis longus m. (+ tendon)
- supinator m.
- radius
- extensor carpi radialis brevis m.
- radial n., deep branch
- abductor pollicis longus m.
- posterior interosseous a., v. + n.
- extensor pollicis longus m.
- extensor digitorum m.
- extensor digiti minimi m.
- extensor carpi ulnaris m.

- flexor carpi radialis m.
- palmaris longus m.
- pronator teres m.
- flexor digitorum superficialis m. (+ tendon)
- median n.
- medial antebrachial cutaneous n.
- ulnar n.
- flexor carpi ulnaris m. (+ tendon)
- ulnar a. + v.
- anterior interosseous a. + v.
- basilic v.
- medial antebrachial cutaneous n.
- flexor digitorum profundus m.
- interosseous membrane
- ulna

	ventral muscles of forearm superficial layer
	deep layer
	dorsal muscles of forearm superficial layer
	deep layer
	radial muscles of forearm

```
        ventral
radial  [    ]  ulnar
        dorsal
```

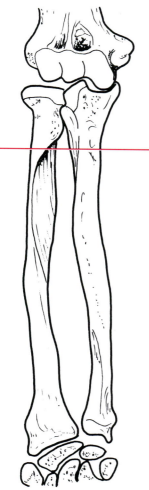

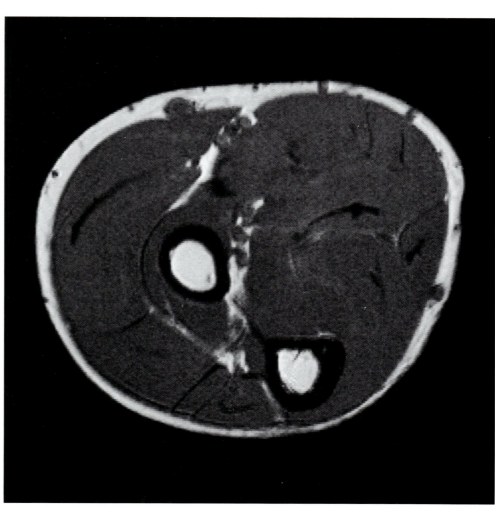

Upper Limbs Axial – Forearm

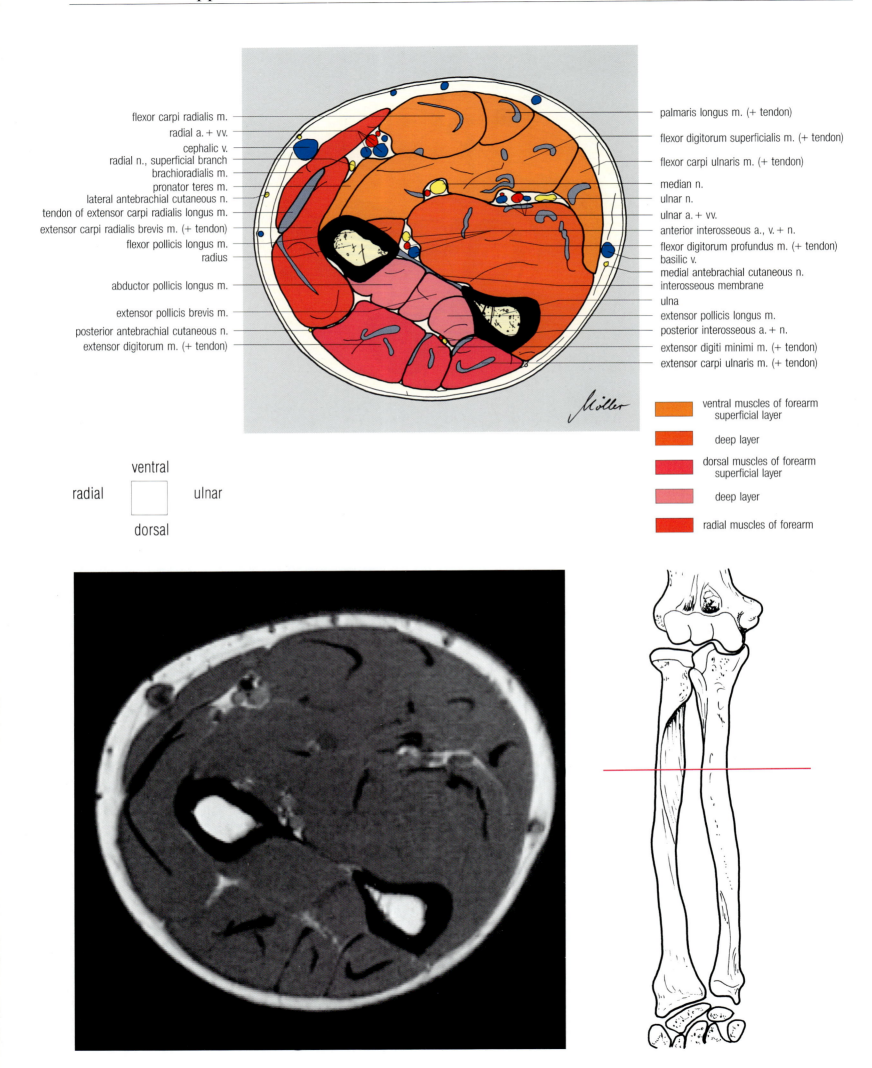

Upper Limbs Axial – Forearm

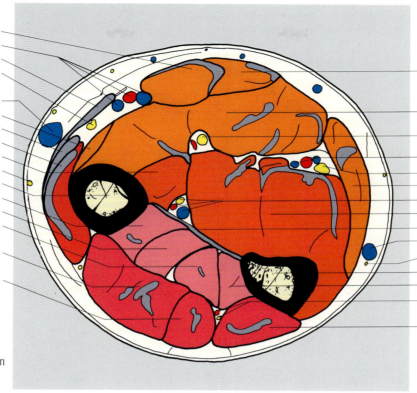

flexor carpi radialis m. (+ tendon)
radial a. + vv.
tendon of brachioradialis m.
radial n., superficial branch
cephalic v.
pronator teres m.
tendon of extensor carpi radialis longus m.
extensor carpi radialis brevis m. (+ tendon)
flexor pollicis longus m.
lateral antebrachial cutaneous n.
radius
abdcutor pollicis longus m.
extensor pollicis brevis m.
extensor pollicis longus m.
extensor digitorum m. (+ tendon)
extensor digiti minimi m. (+ tendon)

palmaris longus m. (+ tendon)
flexor digitorum superficialis m. (+ tendon)
median n.
ulnar a. + vv.
ulnar n.
flexor carpi ulnaris m. (+ tendon)
anterior interosseous a., v. + n.
flexor digitorum profundus m. (+ tendon)
interosseous membrane
basilic v.
medial antebrachial cutaneous n.
ulna
extensor indicis m.
posterior interosseous a. + n.
extensor carpi ulnaris m. (+ tendon)

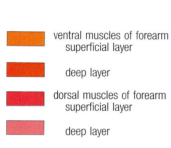

- ventral muscles of forearm superficial layer
- deep layer
- dorsal muscles of forearm superficial layer
- deep layer
- radial muscles of forearm

ventral
radial □ ulnar
dorsal

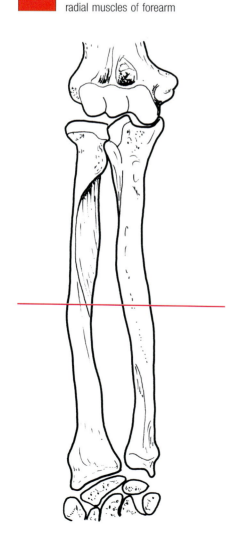

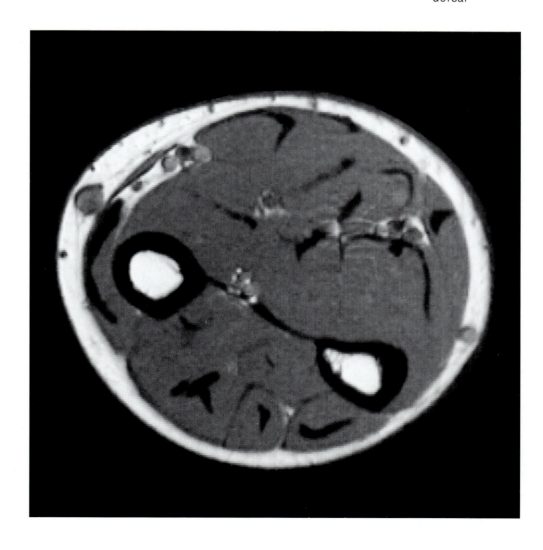

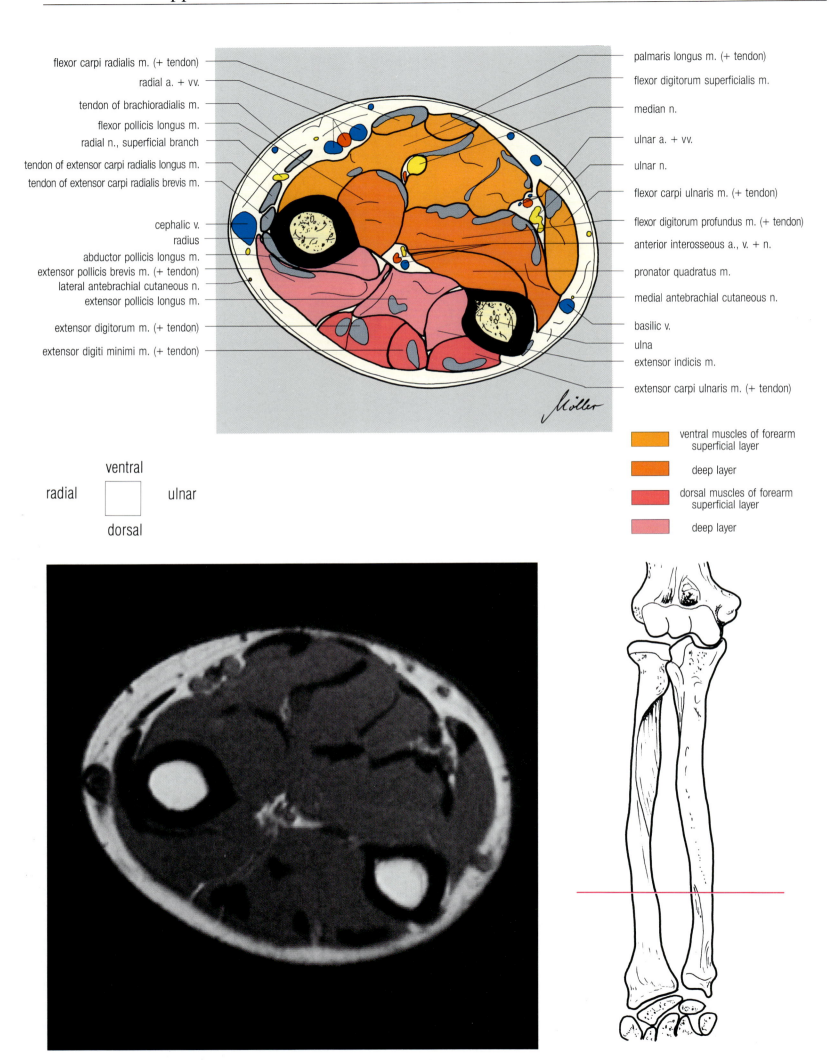

Upper Limbs Axial – Forearm

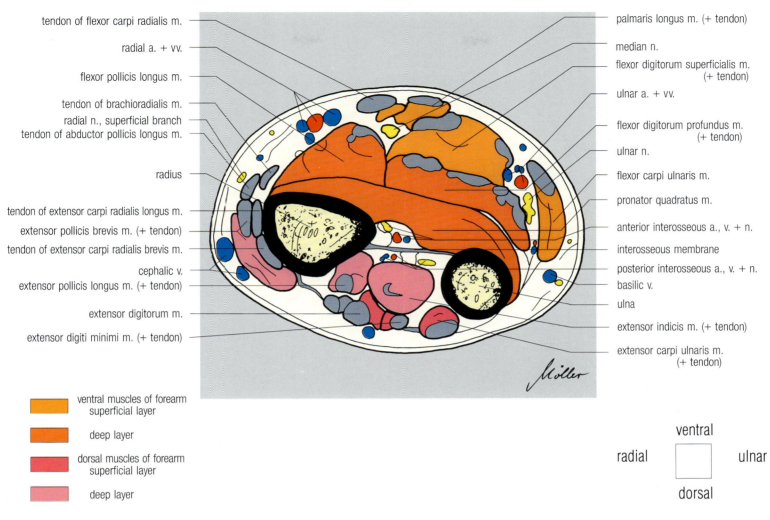

- tendon of flexor carpi radialis m.
- radial a. + vv.
- flexor pollicis longus m.
- tendon of brachioradialis m.
- radial n., superficial branch
- tendon of abductor pollicis longus m.
- radius
- tendon of extensor carpi radialis longus m.
- extensor pollicis brevis m. (+ tendon)
- tendon of extensor carpi radialis brevis m.
- cephalic v.
- extensor pollicis longus m. (+ tendon)
- extensor digitorum m.
- extensor digiti minimi m. (+ tendon)

- palmaris longus m. (+ tendon)
- median n.
- flexor digitorum superficialis m. (+ tendon)
- ulnar a. + vv.
- flexor digitorum profundus m. (+ tendon)
- ulnar n.
- flexor carpi ulnaris m.
- pronator quadratus m.
- anterior interosseous a., v. + n.
- interosseous membrane
- posterior interosseous a., v. + n.
- basilic v.
- ulna
- extensor indicis m. (+ tendon)
- extensor carpi ulnaris m. (+ tendon)

■ ventral muscles of forearm superficial layer
■ deep layer
■ dorsal muscles of forearm superficial layer
■ deep layer

ventral
radial ⬜ ulnar
dorsal

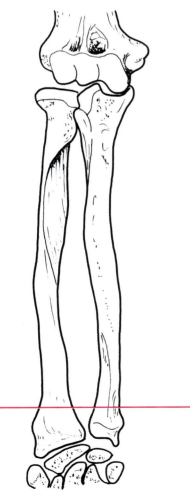
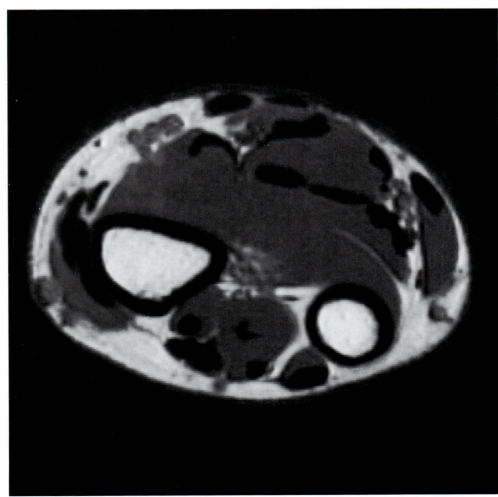

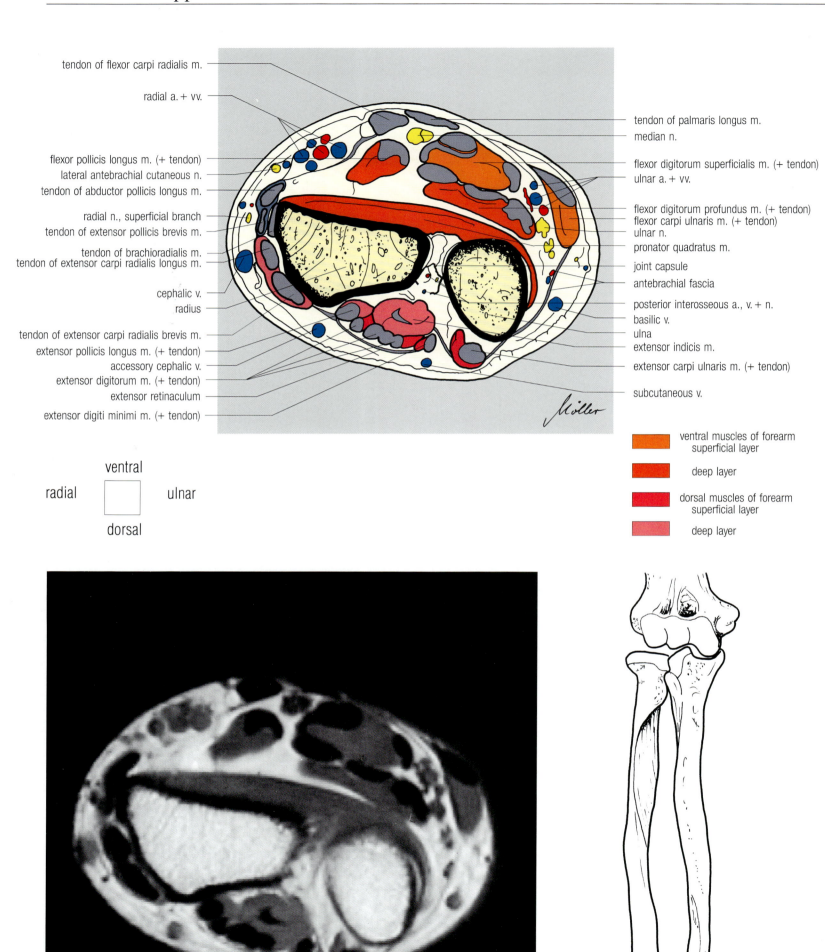

Upper Limbs Axial – Wrist and Hand

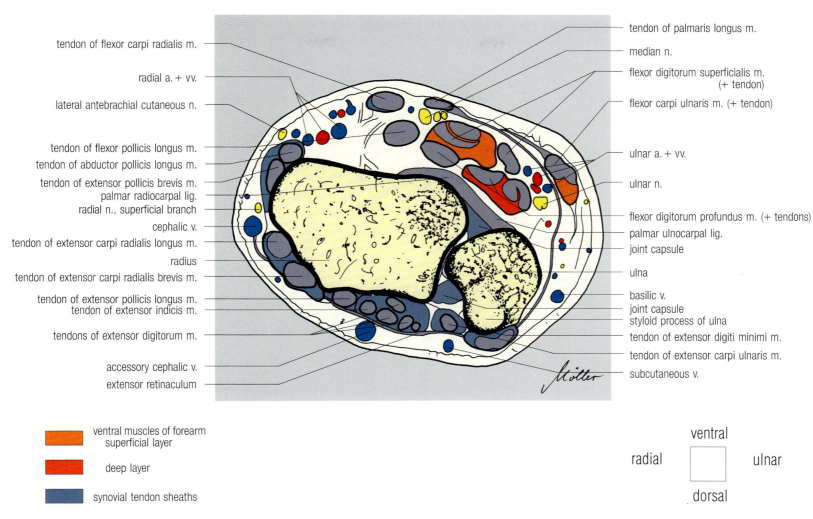

- tendon of flexor carpi radialis m.
- radial a. + vv.
- lateral antebrachial cutaneous n.
- tendon of flexor pollicis longus m.
- tendon of abductor pollicis longus m.
- tendon of extensor pollicis brevis m.
- palmar radiocarpal lig.
- radial n., superficial branch
- cephalic v.
- tendon of extensor carpi radialis longus m.
- radius
- tendon of extensor carpi radialis brevis m.
- tendon of extensor pollicis longus m.
- tendon of extensor indicis m.
- tendons of extensor digitorum m.
- accessory cephalic v.
- extensor retinaculum

- tendon of palmaris longus m.
- median n.
- flexor digitorum superficialis m. (+ tendon)
- flexor carpi ulnaris m. (+ tendon)
- ulnar a. + vv.
- ulnar n.
- flexor digitorum profundus m. (+ tendons)
- palmar ulnocarpal lig.
- joint capsule
- ulna
- basilic v.
- joint capsule
- styloid process of ulna
- tendon of extensor digiti minimi m.
- tendon of extensor carpi ulnaris m.
- subcutaneous v.

- ventral muscles of forearm superficial layer
- deep layer
- synovial tendon sheaths

ventral / radial / ulnar / dorsal

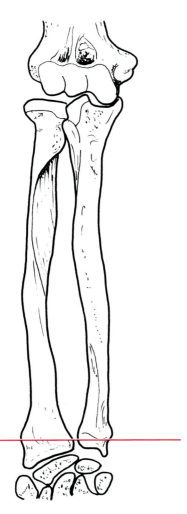

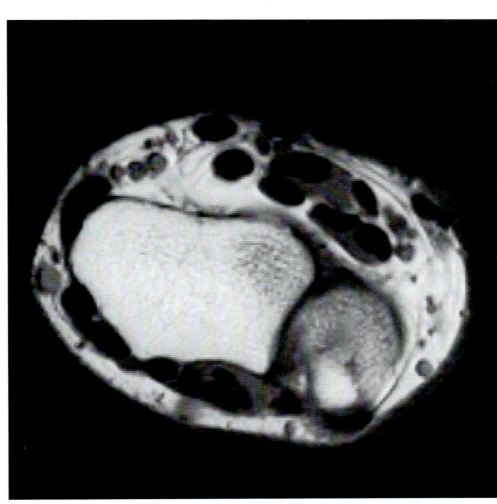

Upper Limbs Axial – Wrist and Hand

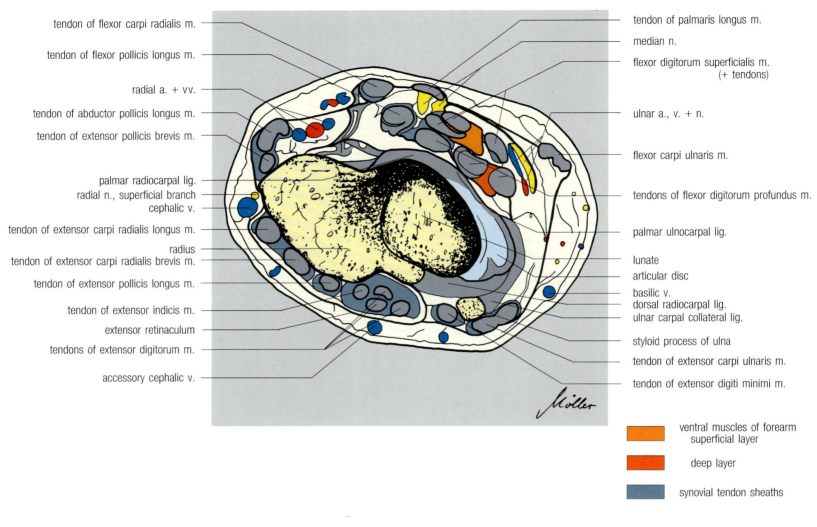

- tendon of flexor carpi radialis m.
- tendon of flexor pollicis longus m.
- radial a. + vv.
- tendon of abductor pollicis longus m.
- tendon of extensor pollicis brevis m.
- palmar radiocarpal lig.
- radial n., superficial branch
- cephalic v.
- tendon of extensor carpi radialis longus m.
- radius
- tendon of extensor carpi radialis brevis m.
- tendon of extensor pollicis longus m.
- tendon of extensor indicis m.
- extensor retinaculum
- tendons of extensor digitorum m.
- accessory cephalic v.

- tendon of palmaris longus m.
- median n.
- flexor digitorum superficialis m. (+ tendons)
- ulnar a., v. + n.
- flexor carpi ulnaris m.
- tendons of flexor digitorum profundus m.
- palmar ulnocarpal lig.
- lunate
- articular disc
- basilic v.
- dorsal radiocarpal lig.
- ulnar carpal collateral lig.
- styloid process of ulna
- tendon of extensor carpi ulnaris m.
- tendon of extensor digiti minimi m.

- ventral muscles of forearm superficial layer
- deep layer
- synovial tendon sheaths

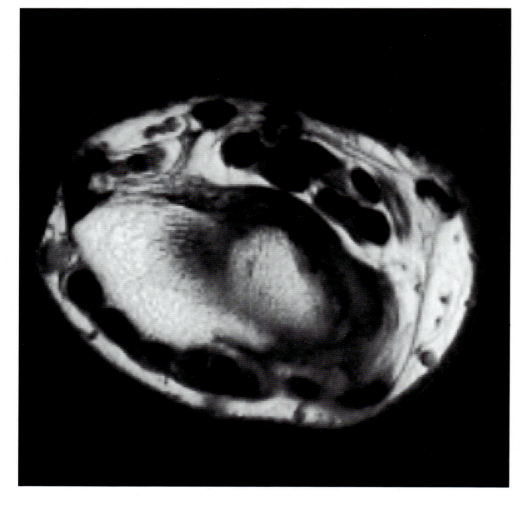

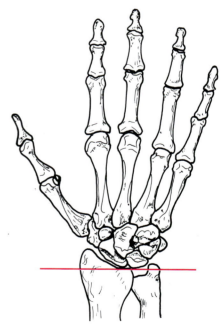

palmar
radial ulnar
dorsal

Upper Limbs Axial – Wrist and Hand

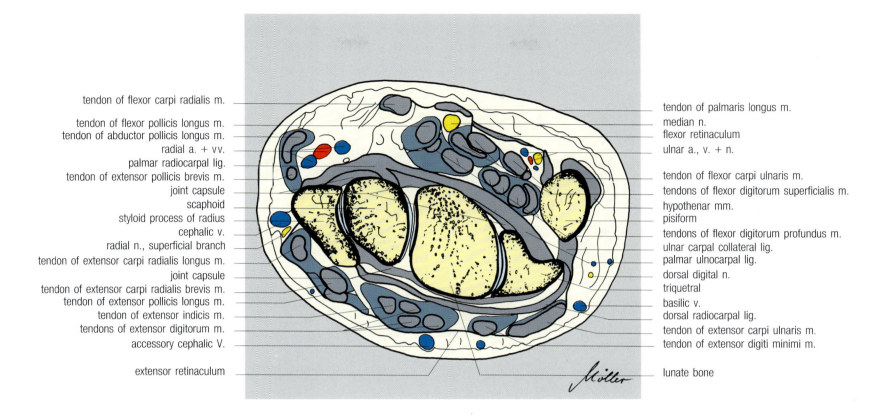

tendon of flexor carpi radialis m.
tendon of flexor pollicis longus m.
tendon of abductor pollicis longus m.
radial a. + vv.
palmar radiocarpal lig.
tendon of extensor pollicis brevis m.
joint capsule
scaphoid
styloid process of radius
cephalic v.
radial n., superficial branch
tendon of extensor carpi radialis longus m.
joint capsule
tendon of extensor carpi radialis brevis m.
tendon of extensor pollicis longus m.
tendon of extensor indicis m.
tendons of extensor digitorum m.
accessory cephalic V.

extensor retinaculum

tendon of palmaris longus m.
median n.
flexor retinaculum
ulnar a., v. + n.
tendon of flexor carpi ulnaris m.
tendons of flexor digitorum superficialis m.
hypothenar mm.
pisiform
tendons of flexor digitorum profundus m.
ulnar carpal collateral lig.
palmar ulnocarpal lig.
dorsal digital n.
triquetral
basilic v.
dorsal radiocarpal lig.
tendon of extensor carpi ulnaris m.
tendon of extensor digiti minimi m.
lunate bone

synovial tendon sheaths

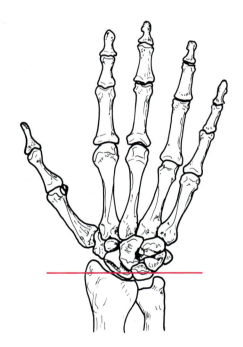

palmar
radial — ulnar
dorsal

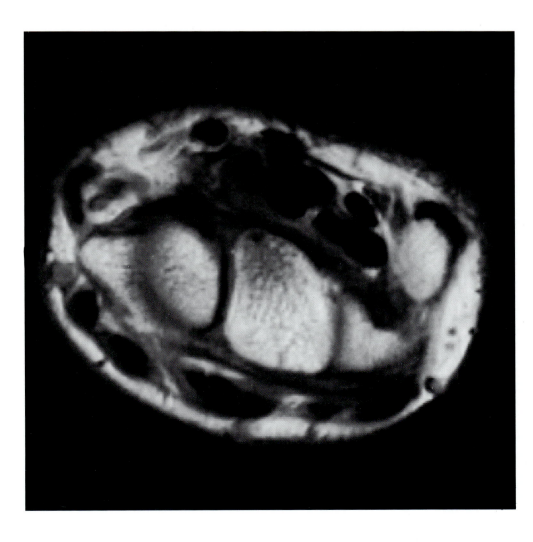

Upper Limbs Axial – Wrist and Hand

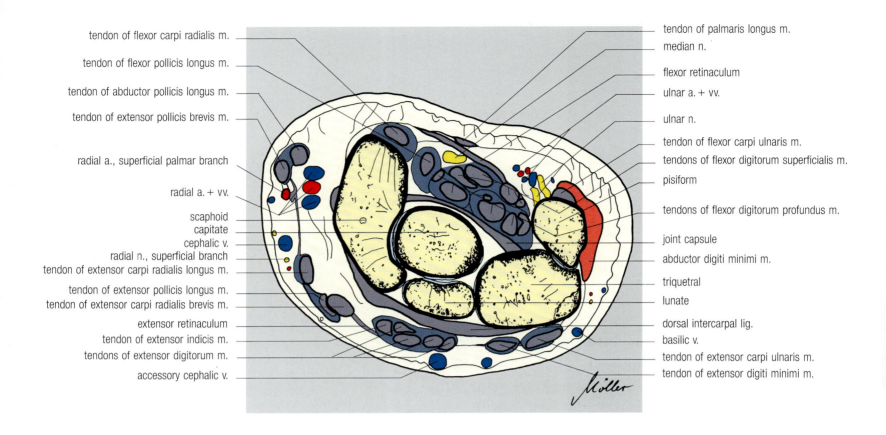

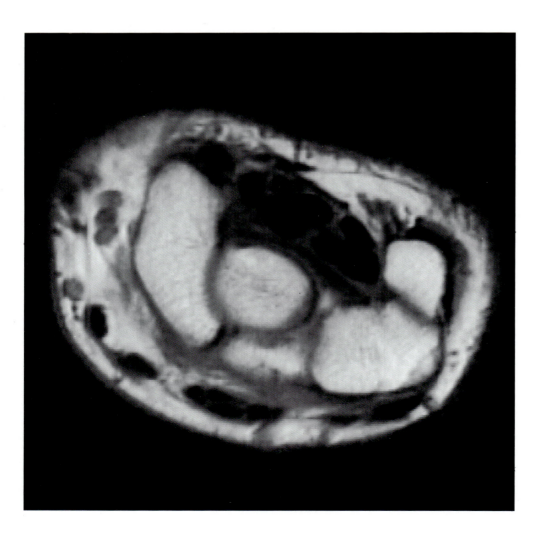

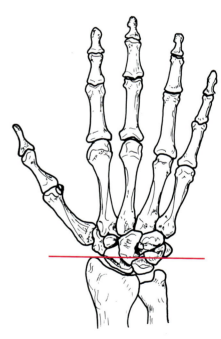

Upper Limbs Axial – Wrist and Hand

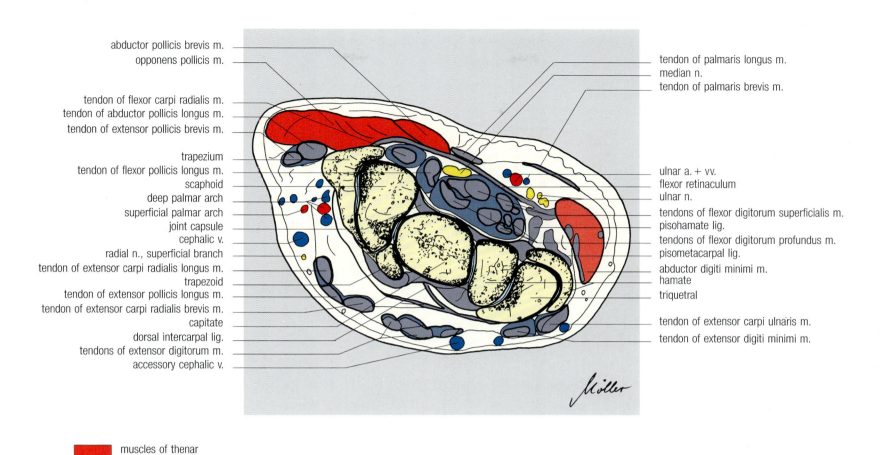

- muscles of thenar
- muscles of hypothenar
- synovial tendon sheaths

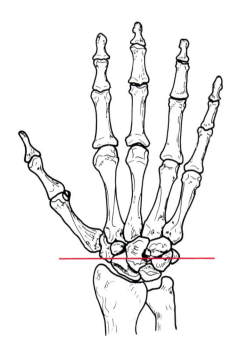

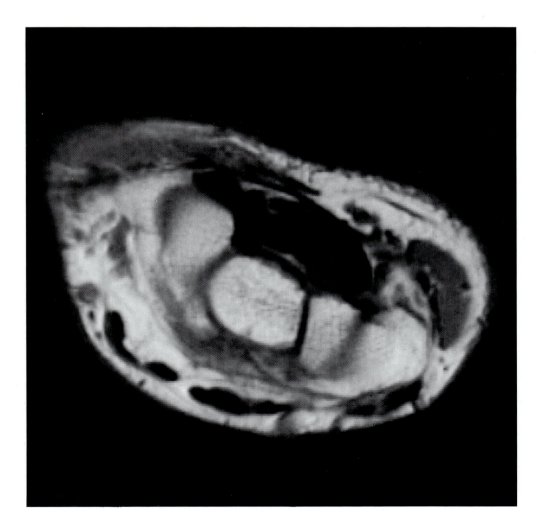

palmar
radial — ulnar
dorsal

Upper Limbs Axial – Wrist and Hand

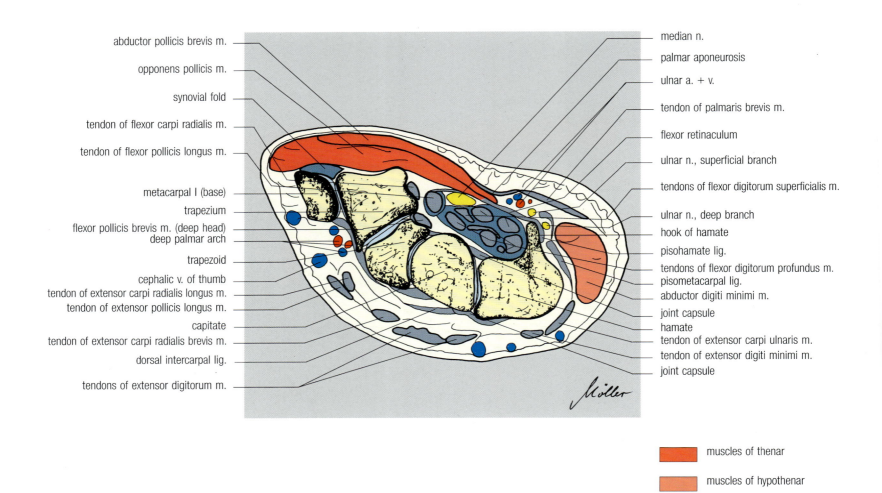

- abductor pollicis brevis m.
- opponens pollicis m.
- synovial fold
- tendon of flexor carpi radialis m.
- tendon of flexor pollicis longus m.
- metacarpal I (base)
- trapezium
- flexor pollicis brevis m. (deep head)
- deep palmar arch
- trapezoid
- cephalic v. of thumb
- tendon of extensor carpi radialis longus m.
- tendon of extensor pollicis longus m.
- capitate
- tendon of extensor carpi radialis brevis m.
- dorsal intercarpal lig.
- tendons of extensor digitorum m.

- median n.
- palmar aponeurosis
- ulnar a. + v.
- tendon of palmaris brevis m.
- flexor retinaculum
- ulnar n., superficial branch
- tendons of flexor digitorum superficialis m.
- ulnar n., deep branch
- hook of hamate
- pisohamate lig.
- tendons of flexor digitorum profundus m.
- pisometacarpal lig.
- abductor digiti minimi m.
- joint capsule
- hamate
- tendon of extensor carpi ulnaris m.
- tendon of extensor digiti minimi m.
- joint capsule

- muscles of thenar
- muscles of hypothenar
- synovial tendon sheaths

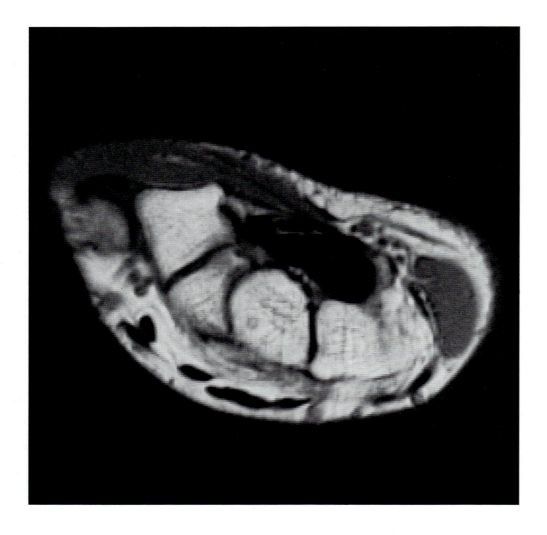

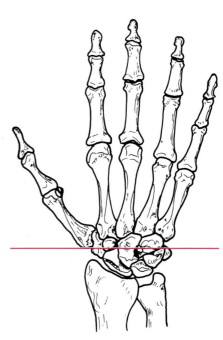

palmar
radial ulnar
dorsal

Upper Limbs Axial – Wrist and Hand

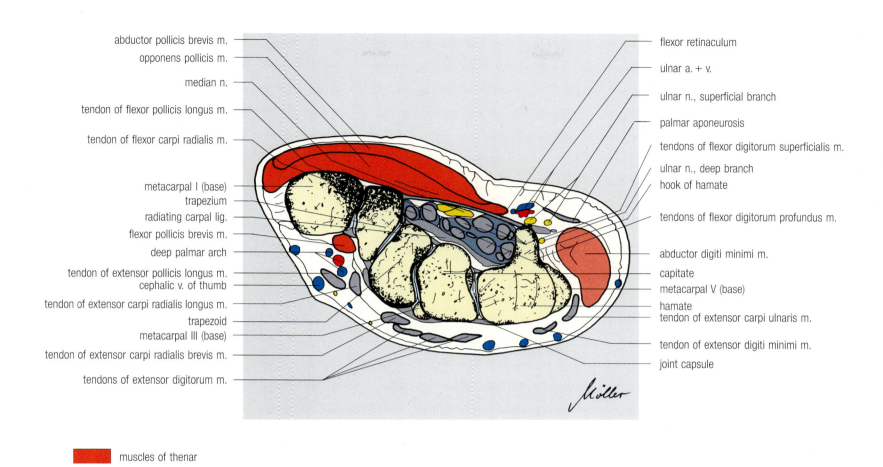

- muscles of thenar
- muscles of hypothenar
- synovial tendon sheaths

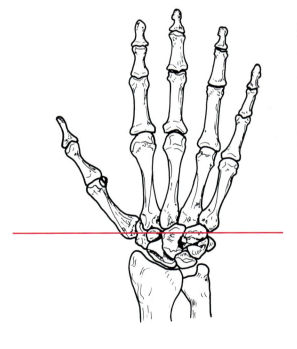

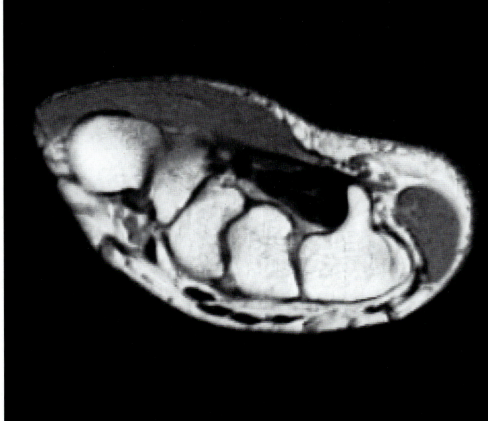

Upper Limbs Axial – Wrist and Hand

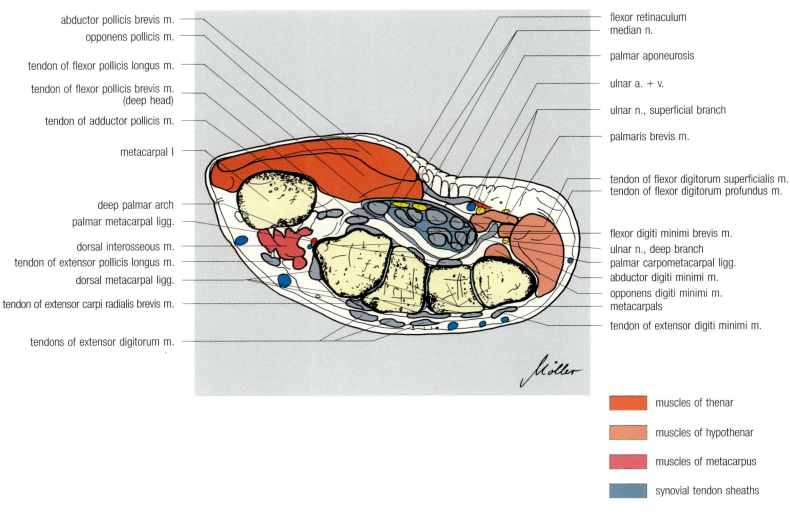

- abductor pollicis brevis m.
- opponens pollicis m.
- tendon of flexor pollicis longus m.
- tendon of flexor pollicis brevis m. (deep head)
- tendon of adductor pollicis m.
- metacarpal I
- deep palmar arch
- palmar metacarpal ligg.
- dorsal interosseous m.
- tendon of extensor pollicis longus m.
- dorsal metacarpal ligg.
- tendon of extensor carpi radialis brevis m.
- tendons of extensor digitorum m.

- flexor retinaculum
- median n.
- palmar aponeurosis
- ulnar a. + v.
- ulnar n., superficial branch
- palmaris brevis m.
- tendon of flexor digitorum superficialis m.
- tendon of flexor digitorum profundus m.
- flexor digiti minimi brevis m.
- ulnar n., deep branch
- palmar carpometacarpal ligg.
- abductor digiti minimi m.
- opponens digiti minimi m.
- metacarpals
- tendon of extensor digiti minimi m.

▪ muscles of thenar
▪ muscles of hypothenar
▪ muscles of metacarpus
▪ synovial tendon sheaths

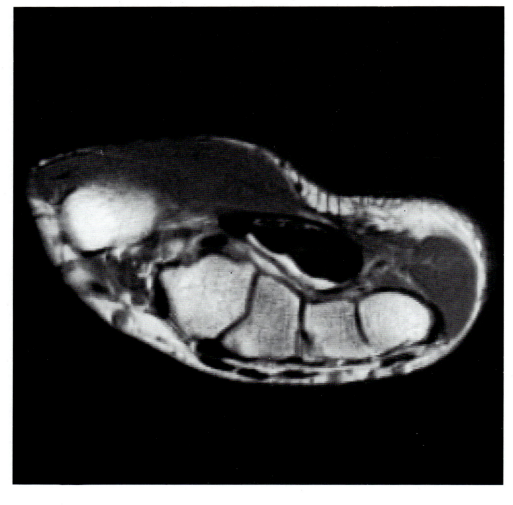

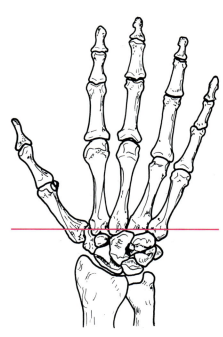

palmar
radial — ulnar
dorsal

Upper Limbs Axial – Wrist and Hand

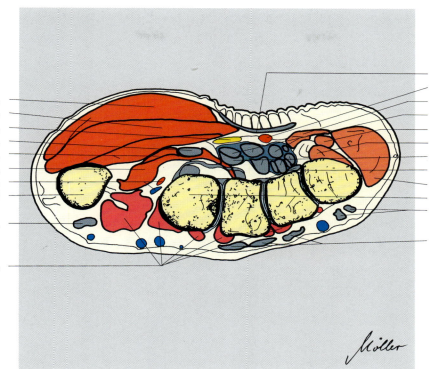

- abductor pollicis brevis m.
- opponens pollicis m.
- median n.
- tendon of flexor pollicis longus m.
- flexor pollicis brevis m.
- adductor pollicis m.
- deep palmar arch
- metacarpal I
- tendon of extensor pollicis longus m.
- dorsal interossei mm.

- palmar aponeurosis
- ulnar a.
- palmaris brevis m.
- tendons of flexor digitorum superficialis m.
- flexor digiti minimi brevis m.
- opponens digiti minimi m.
- tendons of flexor digitorum profundus m.
- palmar metacarpal ligg.
- abductor digiti minimi m.
- metacarpals
- tendons of extensor digiti minimi m.
- tendons of extensor digitorum m.

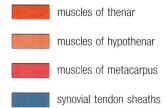

- muscles of thenar
- muscles of hypothenar
- muscles of metacarpus
- synovial tendon sheaths

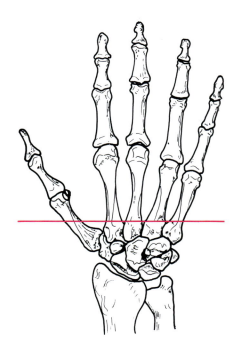

palmar
radial ulnar
dorsal

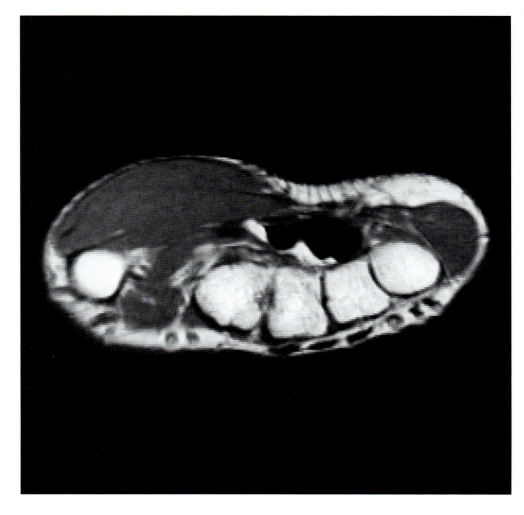

Upper Limbs Axial – Wrist and Hand

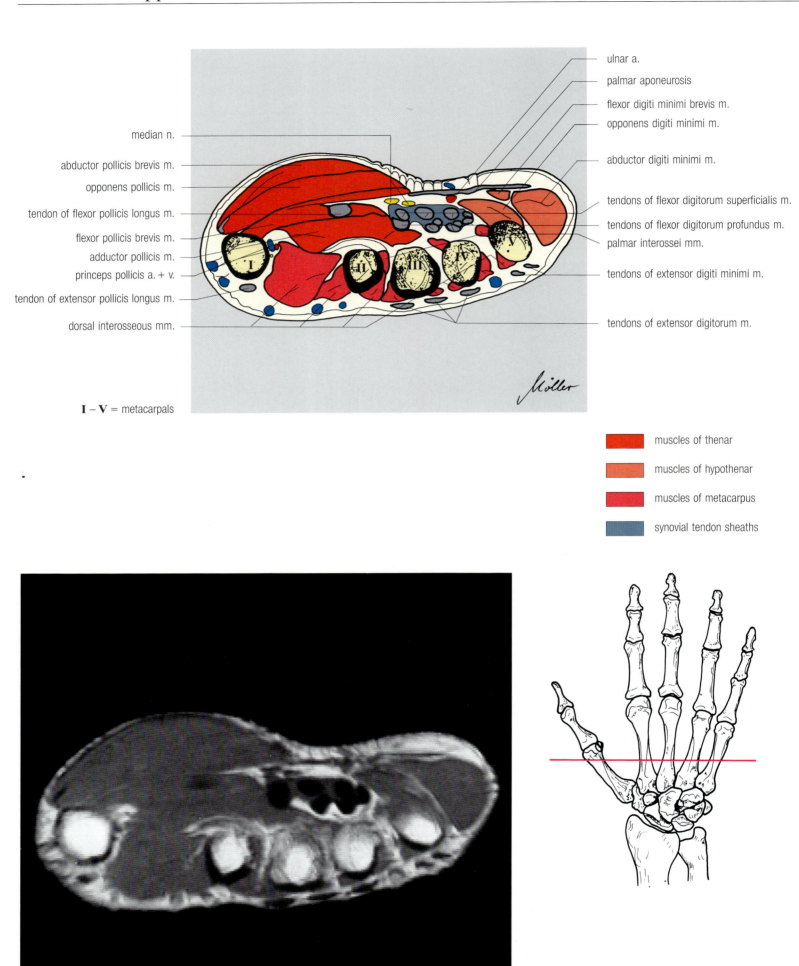

I – V = metacarpals

■ muscles of thenar
■ muscles of hypothenar
■ muscles of metacarpus
■ synovial tendon sheaths

Upper Limbs Axial – Wrist and Hand

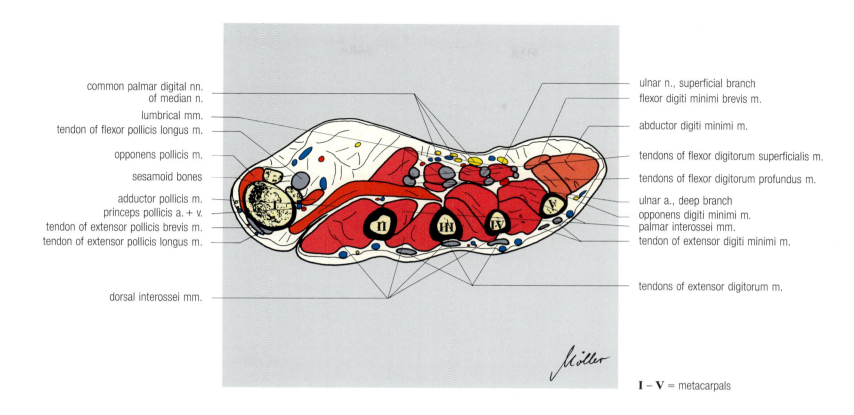

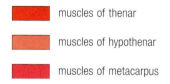

- muscles of thenar
- muscles of hypothenar
- muscles of metacarpus

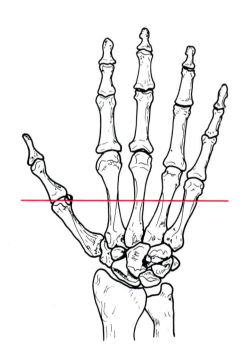

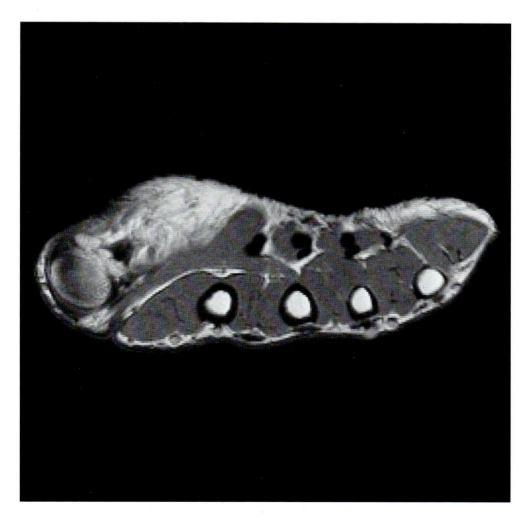

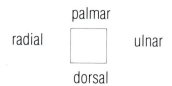

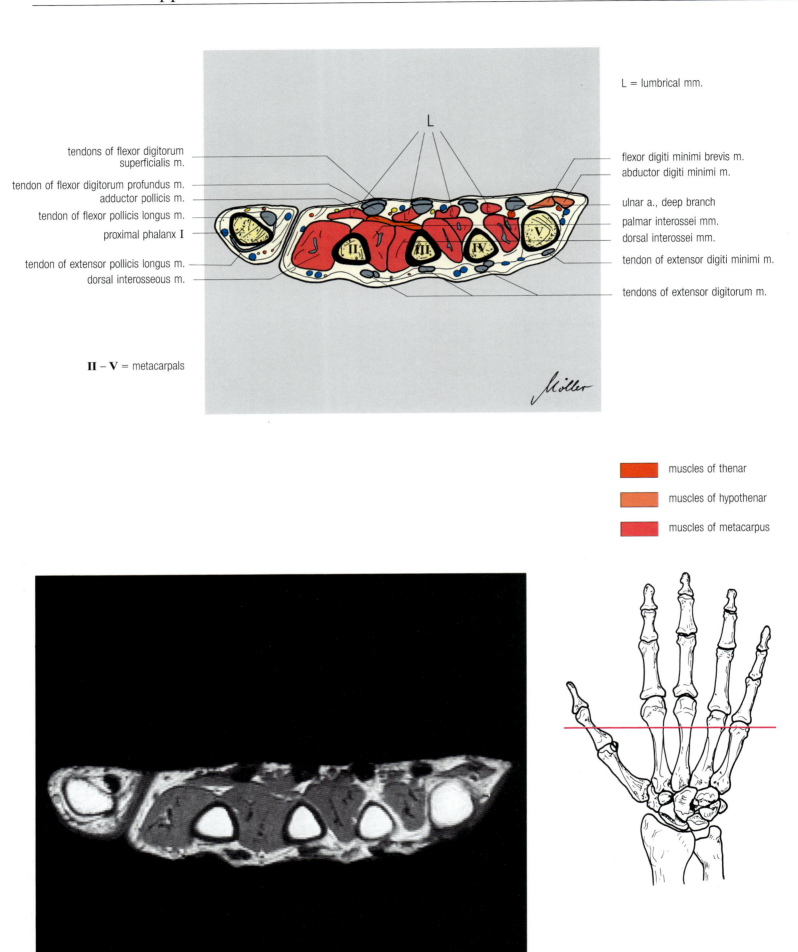

Upper Limbs Axial – Wrist and Hand

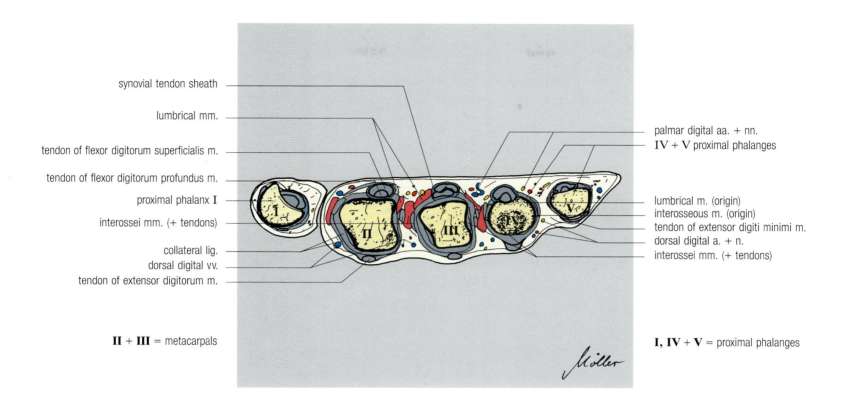

- synovial tendon sheath
- lumbrical mm.
- tendon of flexor digitorum superficialis m.
- tendon of flexor digitorum profundus m.
- proximal phalanx I
- interossei mm. (+ tendons)
- collateral lig.
- dorsal digital vv.
- tendon of extensor digitorum m.

- palmar digital aa. + nn.
- IV + V proximal phalanges
- lumbrical m. (origin)
- interosseous m. (origin)
- tendon of extensor digiti minimi m.
- dorsal digital a. + n.
- interossei mm. (+ tendons)

II + III = metacarpals

I, IV + V = proximal phalanges

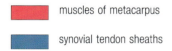

muscles of metacarpus

synovial tendon sheaths

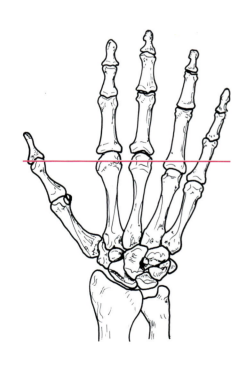

palmar

radial ulnar

dorsal

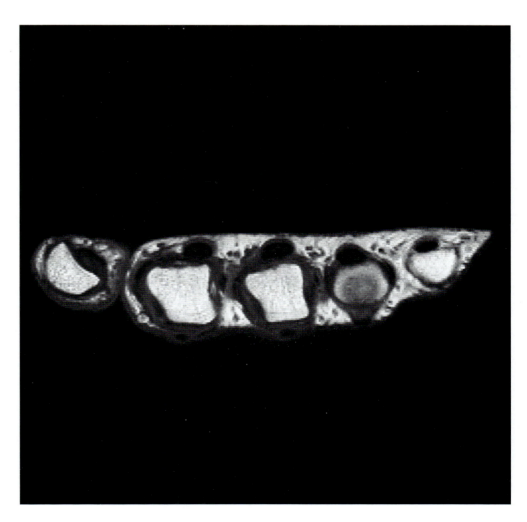

Upper Limbs Axial – Wrist and Hand

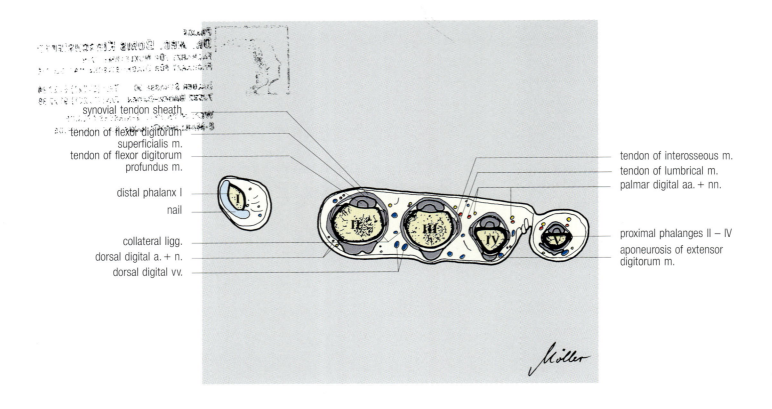

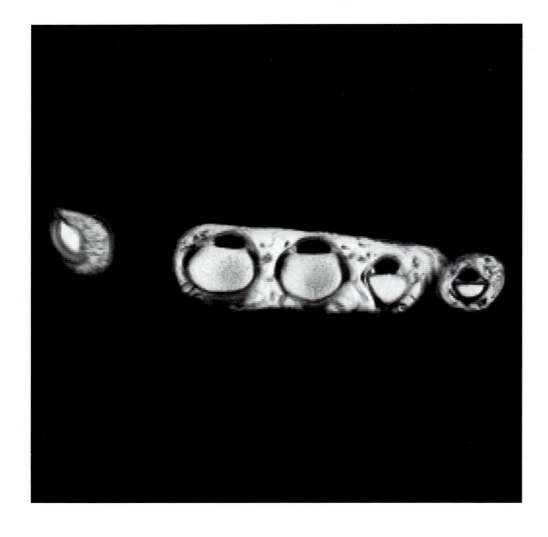

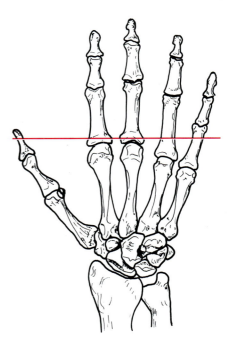

Praxis
DR. MED. BORIS KIRSCHSIEPER
FACHARZT FÜR NUKLEARMEDIZIN
FACHARZT FÜR DIAGNOSTISCHE RADIOLOGIE

BALGER STRASSE 50   TEL: (07221) 91 27 94
76532 BADEN-BADEN   FAX: (07221) 91 27 98

WEB: WWW.PRAXIS-KIRSCHSIEPER.DE
E-MAIL: INFO@PRAXIS-KIRSCHSIEPER.DE

Shoulder

Coronal

Sagittal

Shoulder – Coronal

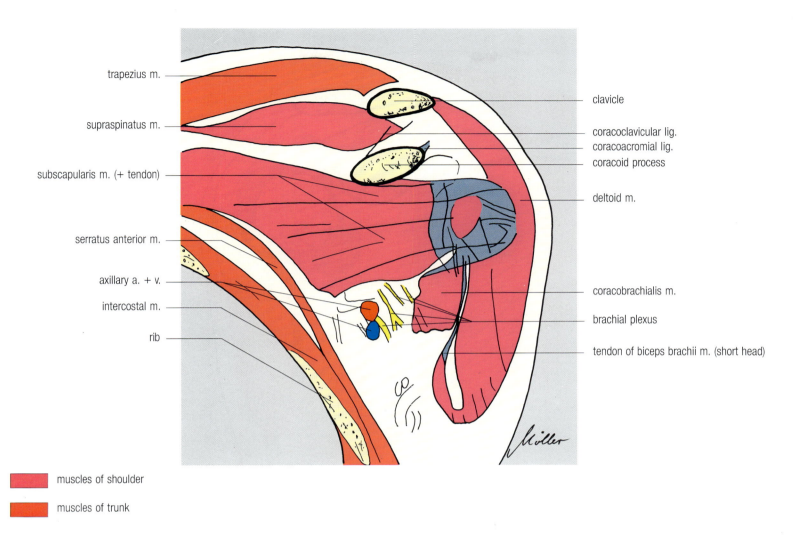

- trapezius m.
- supraspinatus m.
- subscapularis m. (+ tendon)
- serratus anterior m.
- axillary a. + v.
- intercostal m.
- rib
- clavicle
- coracoclavicular lig.
- coracoacromial lig.
- coracoid process
- deltoid m.
- coracobrachialis m.
- brachial plexus
- tendon of biceps brachii m. (short head)

■ muscles of shoulder
■ muscles of trunk

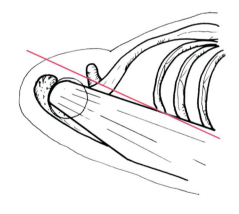

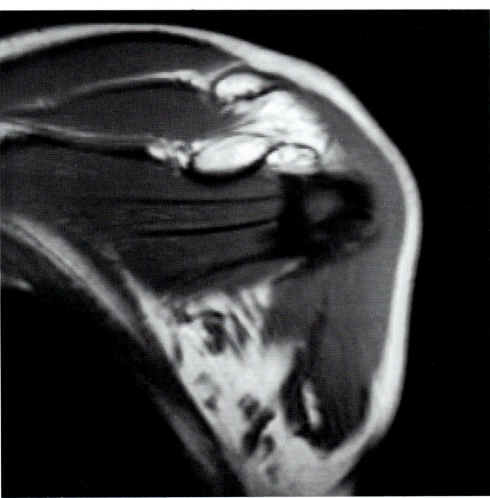

cranial
medial — lateral
caudal

48 Shoulder – Coronal

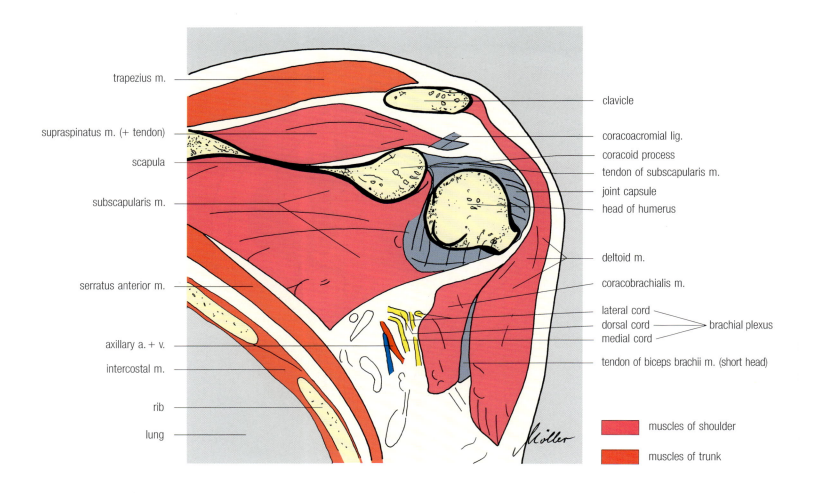

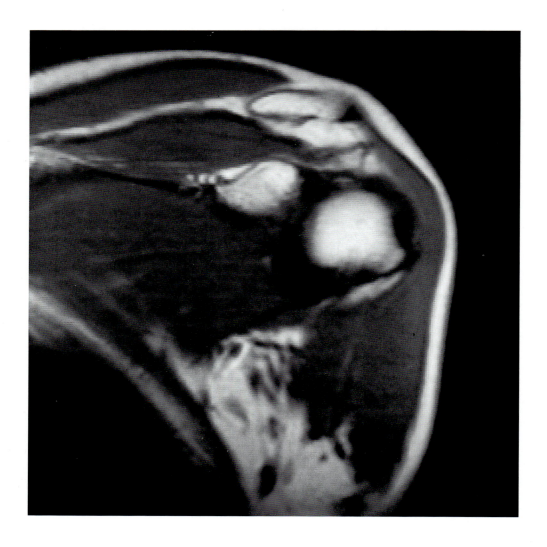

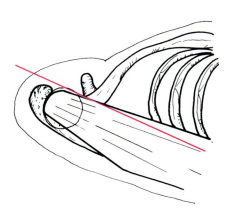

Shoulder – Coronal 49

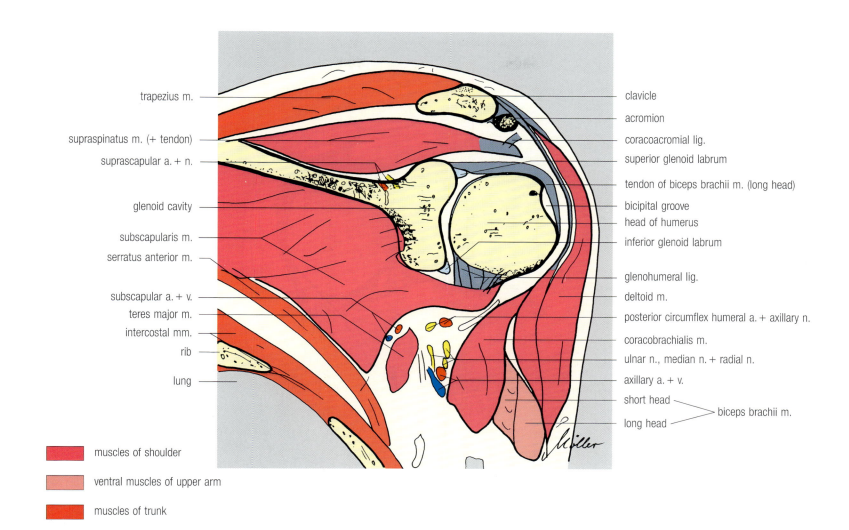

- muscles of shoulder
- ventral muscles of upper arm
- muscles of trunk

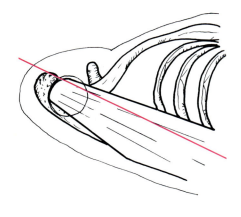

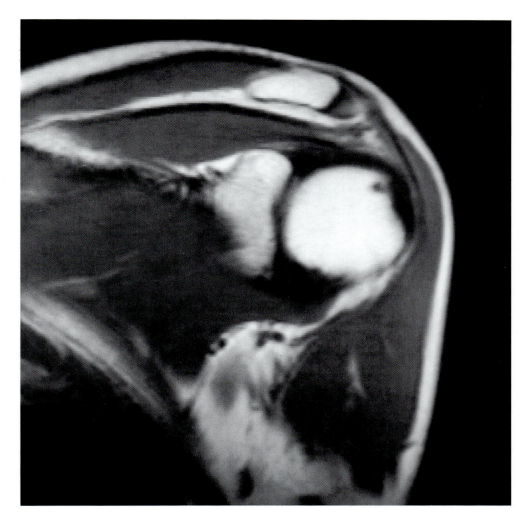

Shoulder – Coronal

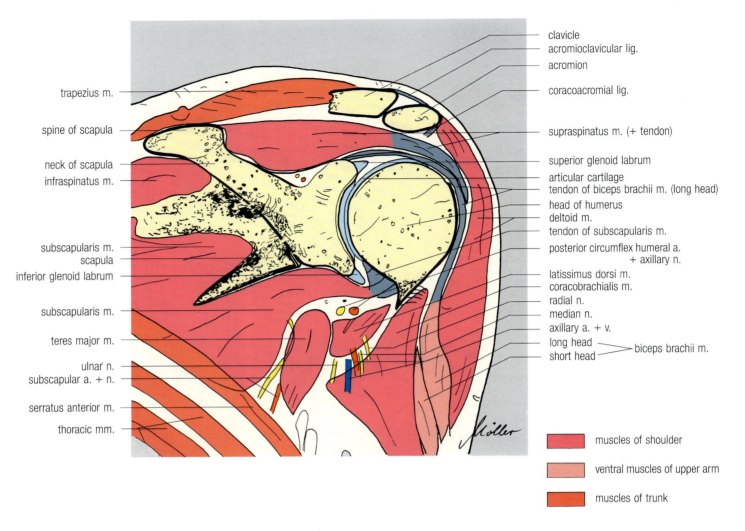

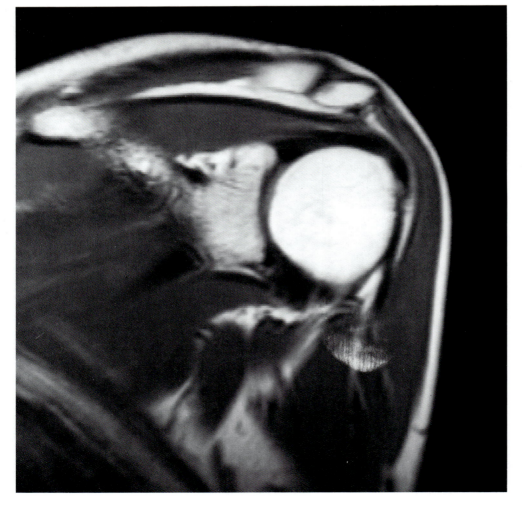

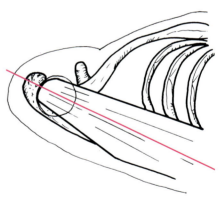

- muscles of shoulder
- ventral muscles of upper arm
- muscles of trunk

cranial / medial – lateral / caudal

Shoulder – Coronal

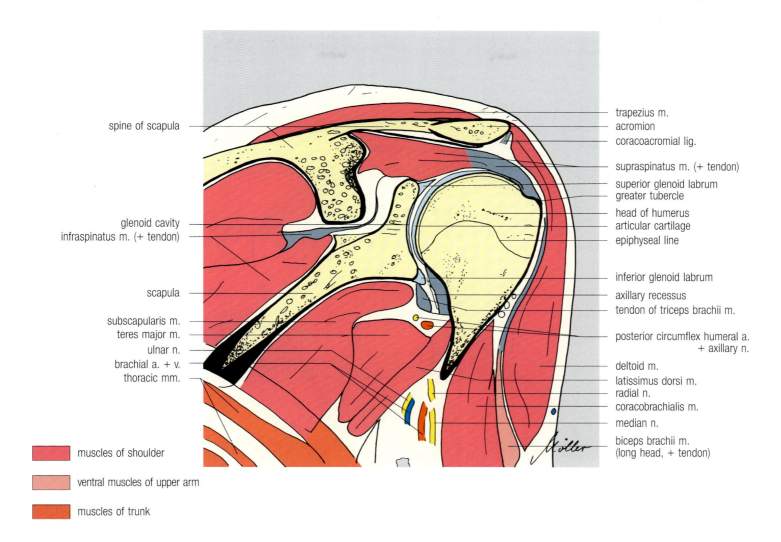

- spine of scapula
- glenoid cavity
- infraspinatus m. (+ tendon)
- scapula
- subscapularis m.
- teres major m.
- ulnar n.
- brachial a. + v.
- thoracic mm.

- trapezius m.
- acromion
- coracoacromial lig.
- supraspinatus m. (+ tendon)
- superior glenoid labrum
- greater tubercle
- head of humerus
- articular cartilage
- epiphyseal line
- inferior glenoid labrum
- axillary recessus
- tendon of triceps brachii m.
- posterior circumflex humeral a. + axillary n.
- deltoid m.
- latissimus dorsi m.
- radial n.
- coracobrachialis m.
- median n.
- biceps brachii m. (long head, + tendon)

- muscles of shoulder
- ventral muscles of upper arm
- muscles of trunk

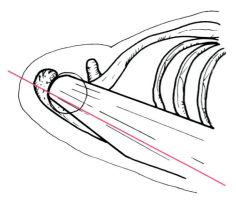

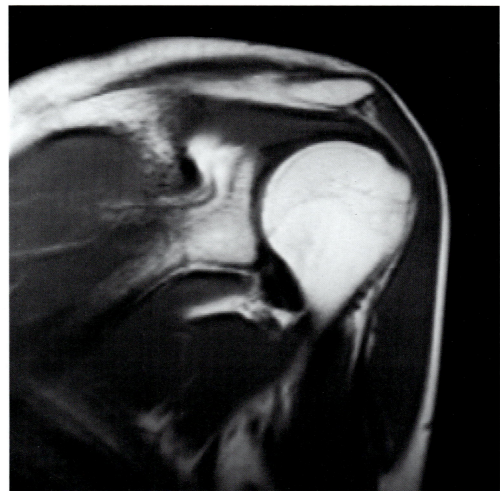

cranial / medial – lateral / caudal

Shoulder – Coronal

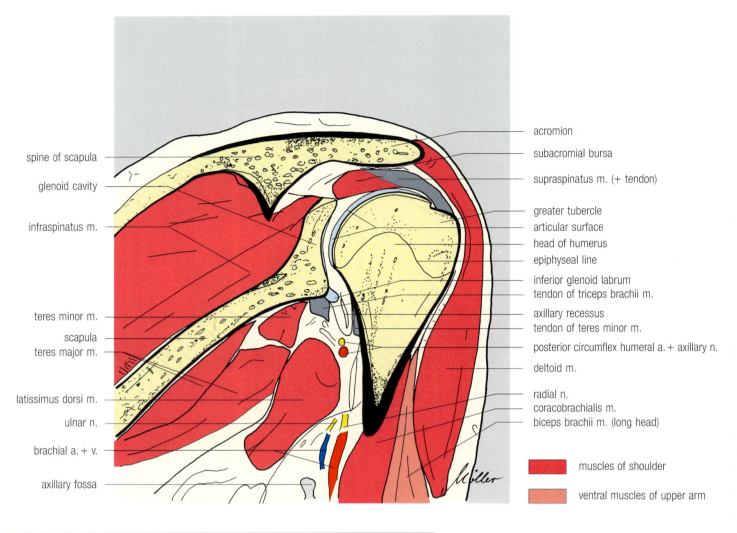

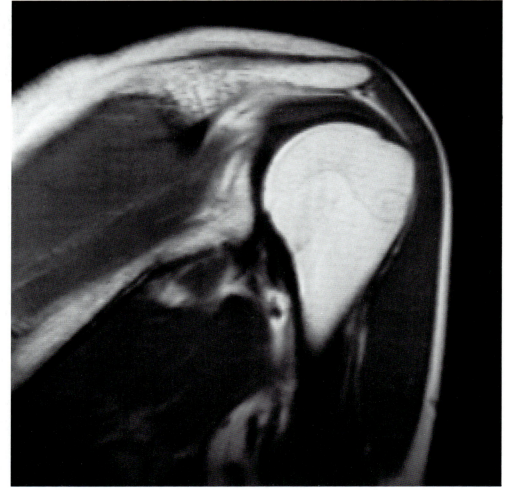

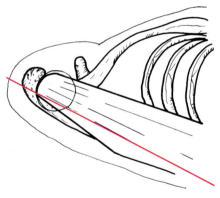

cranial — medial — lateral — caudal

Shoulder – Coronal

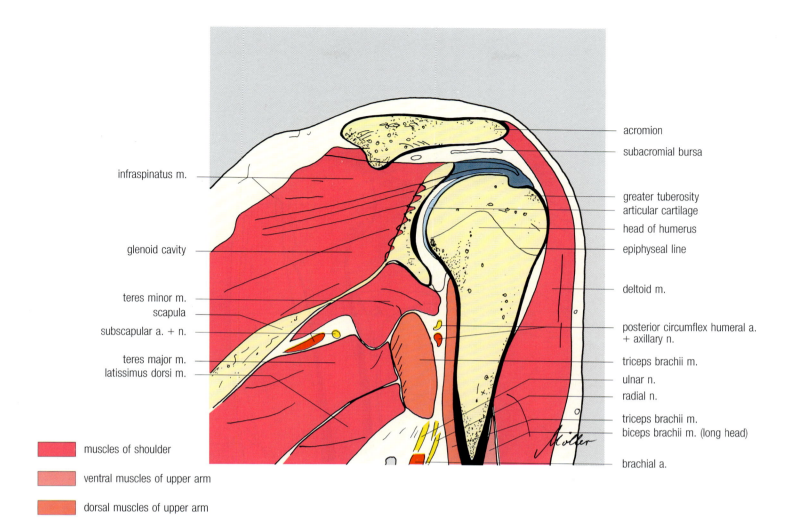

- muscles of shoulder
- ventral muscles of upper arm
- dorsal muscles of upper arm

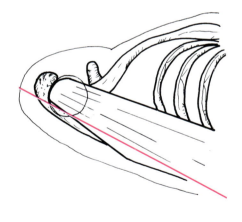

cranial
medial — lateral
caudal

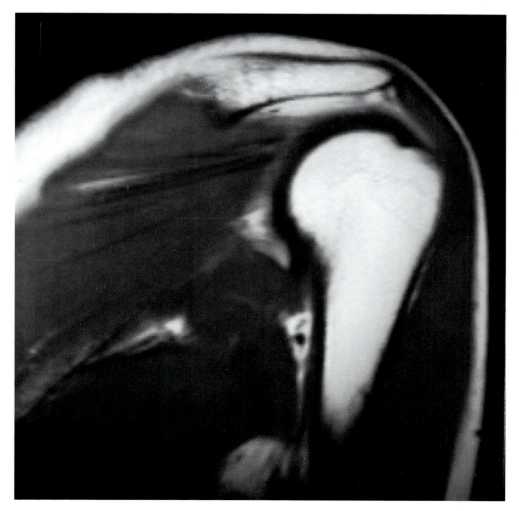

54 Shoulder – Coronal

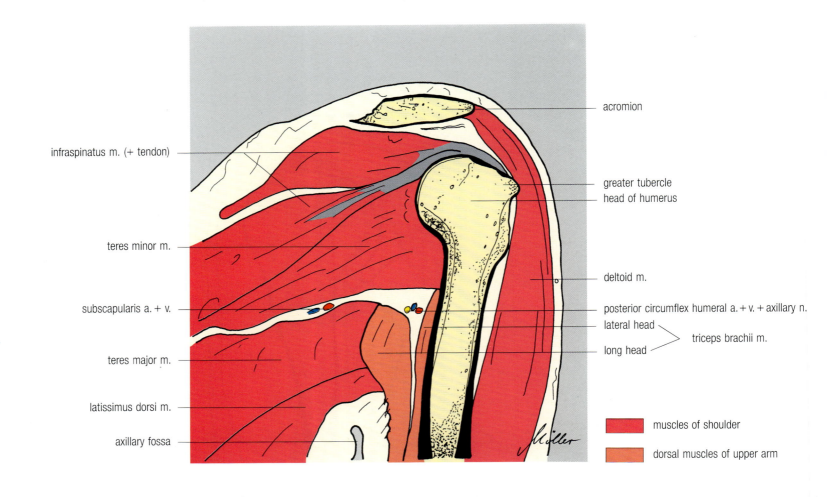

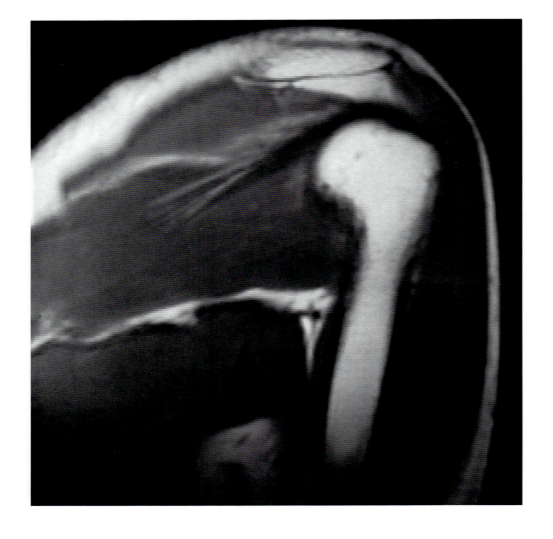

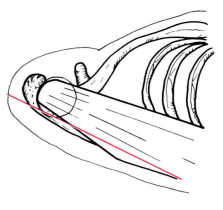

Shoulder – Coronal

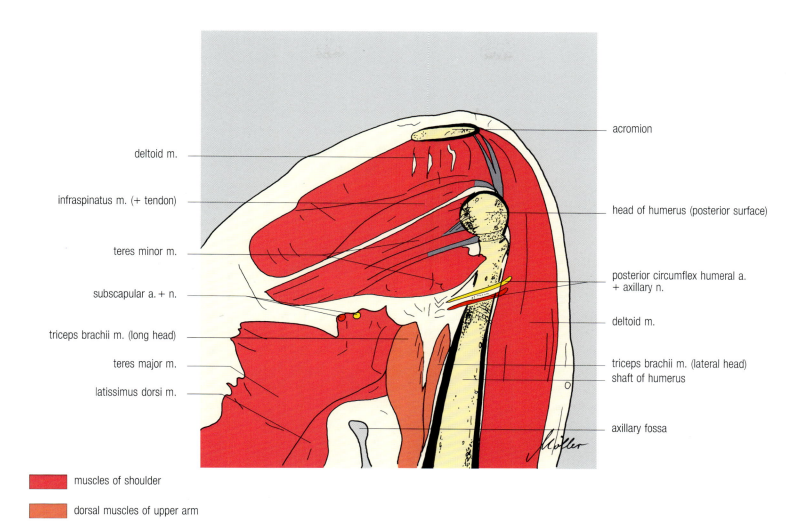

- muscles of shoulder
- dorsal muscles of upper arm

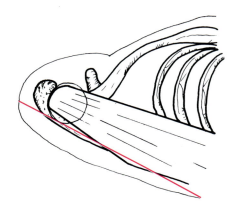

medial — cranial / caudal — lateral

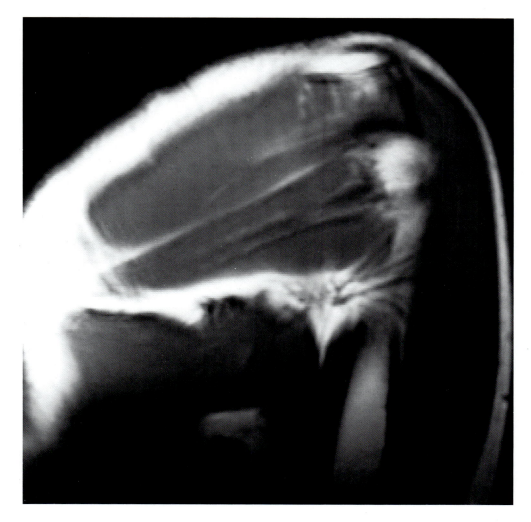

Shoulder – Sagittal

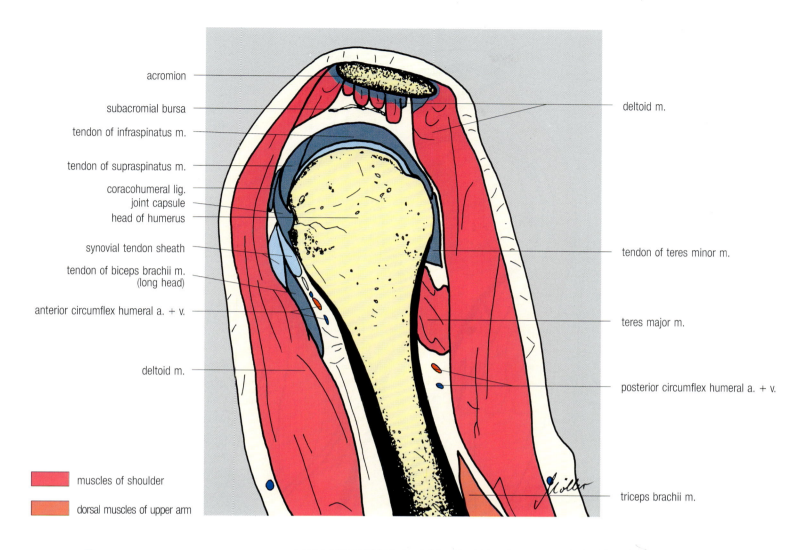

- acromion
- subacromial bursa
- tendon of infraspinatus m.
- tendon of supraspinatus m.
- coracohumeral lig.
- joint capsule
- head of humerus
- synovial tendon sheath
- tendon of biceps brachii m. (long head)
- anterior circumflex humeral a. + v.
- deltoid m.
- deltoid m.
- tendon of teres minor m.
- teres major m.
- posterior circumflex humeral a. + v.
- triceps brachii m.

■ muscles of shoulder
■ dorsal muscles of upper arm

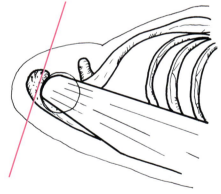

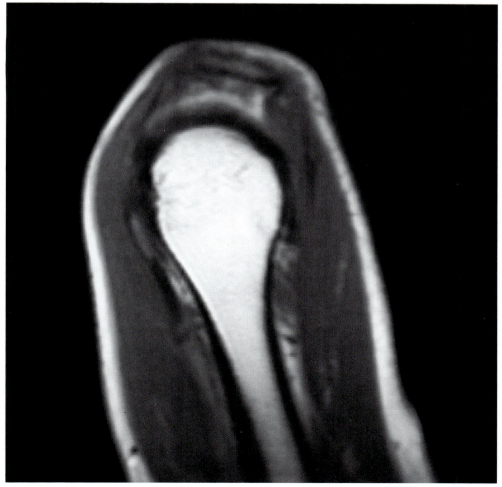

cranial
ventral — dorsal
caudal

57

58 Shoulder – Sagittal

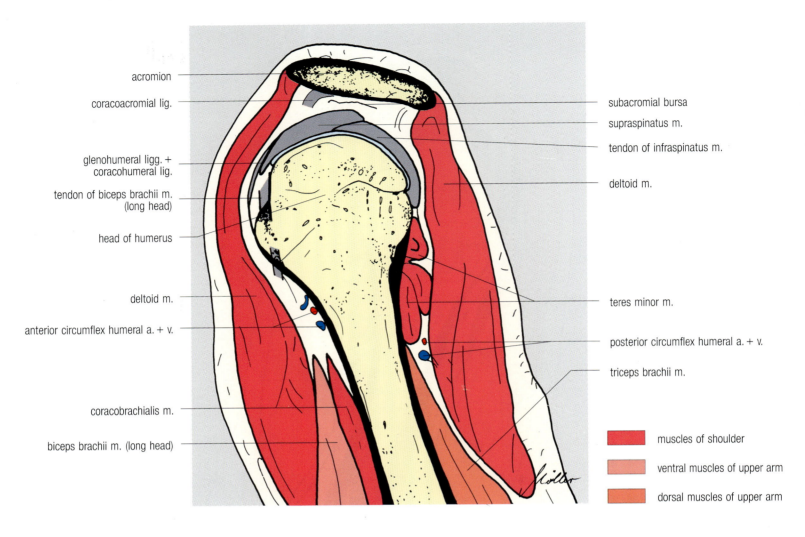

- acromion
- coracoacromial lig.
- glenohumeral ligg. + coracohumeral lig.
- tendon of biceps brachii m. (long head)
- head of humerus
- deltoid m.
- anterior circumflex humeral a. + v.
- coracobrachialis m.
- biceps brachii m. (long head)
- subacromial bursa
- supraspinatus m.
- tendon of infraspinatus m.
- deltoid m.
- teres minor m.
- posterior circumflex humeral a. + v.
- triceps brachii m.

■ muscles of shoulder
■ ventral muscles of upper arm
■ dorsal muscles of upper arm

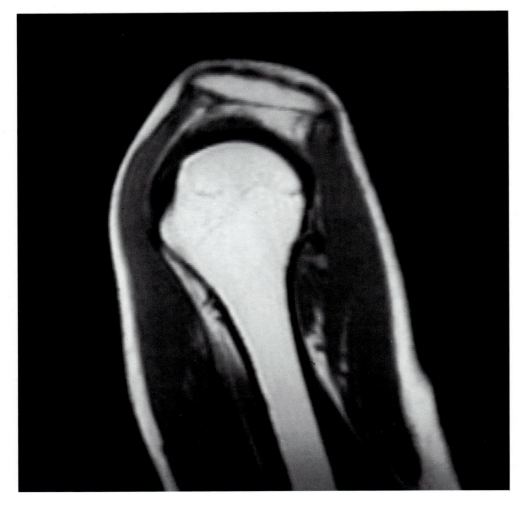

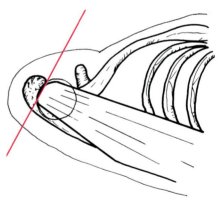

cranial
ventral   dorsal
caudal

Shoulder – Sagittal

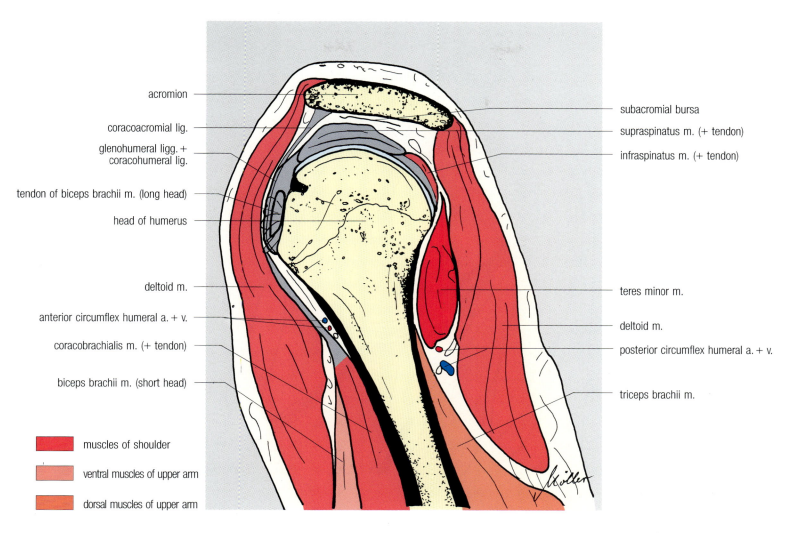

- acromion
- coracoacromial lig.
- glenohumeral ligg. + coracohumeral lig.
- tendon of biceps brachii m. (long head)
- head of humerus
- deltoid m.
- anterior circumflex humeral a. + v.
- coracobrachialis m. (+ tendon)
- biceps brachii m. (short head)
- subacromial bursa
- supraspinatus m. (+ tendon)
- infraspinatus m. (+ tendon)
- teres minor m.
- deltoid m.
- posterior circumflex humeral a. + v.
- triceps brachii m.

■ muscles of shoulder
■ ventral muscles of upper arm
■ dorsal muscles of upper arm

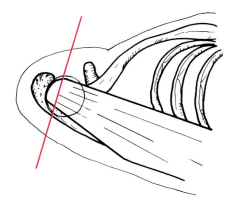

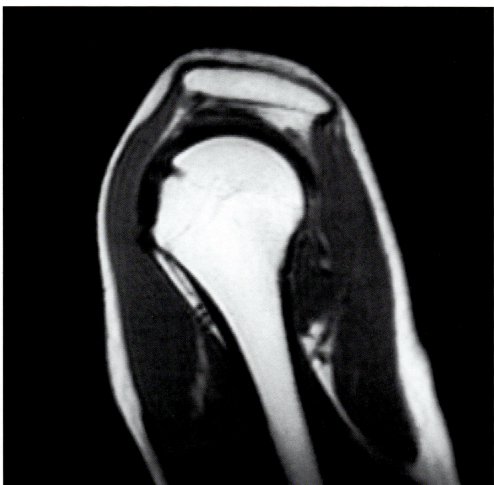

cranial
ventral — dorsal
caudal

Shoulder – Sagittal

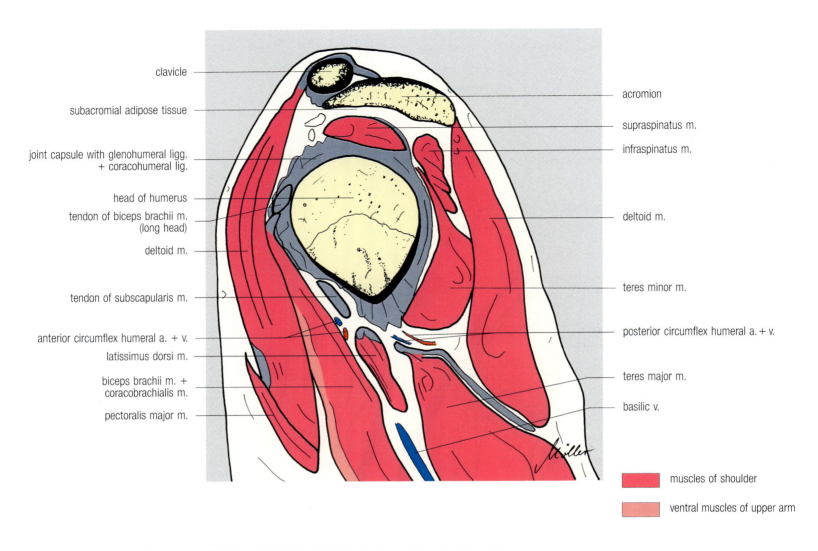

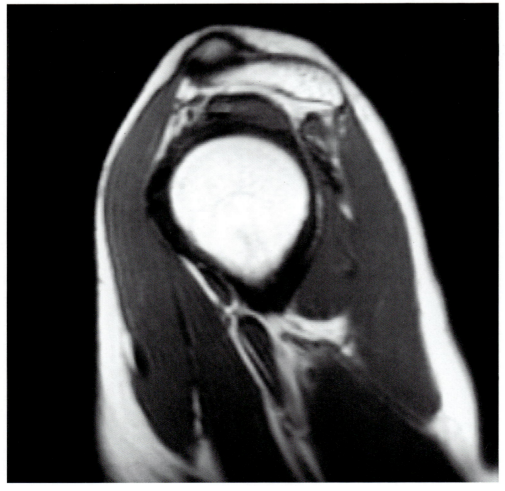

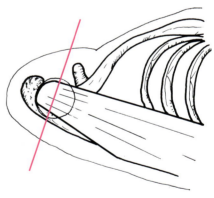

Shoulder – Sagittal

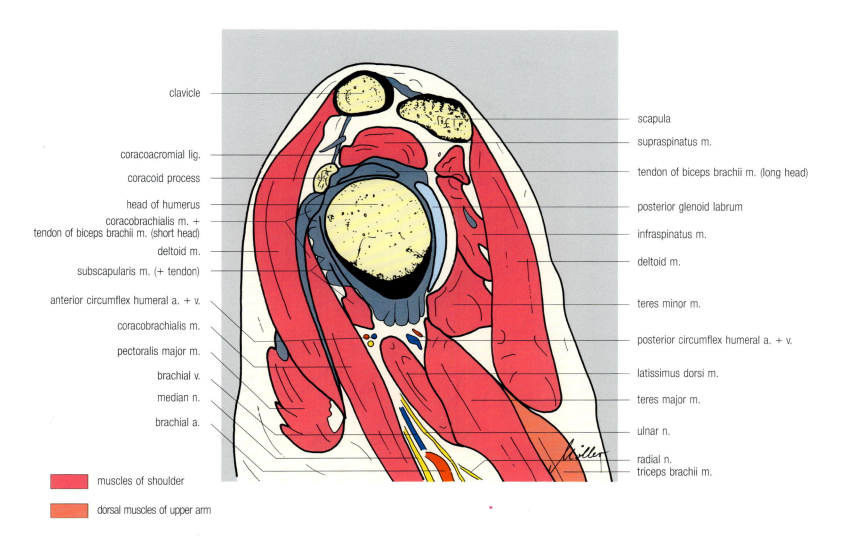

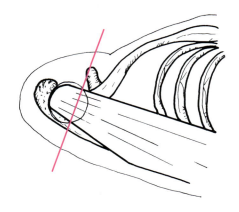

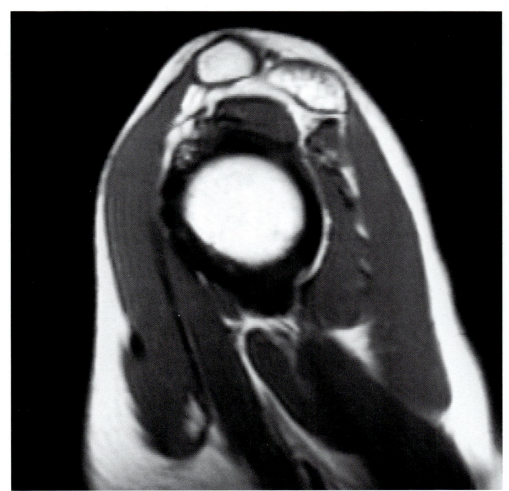

Shoulder – Sagittal

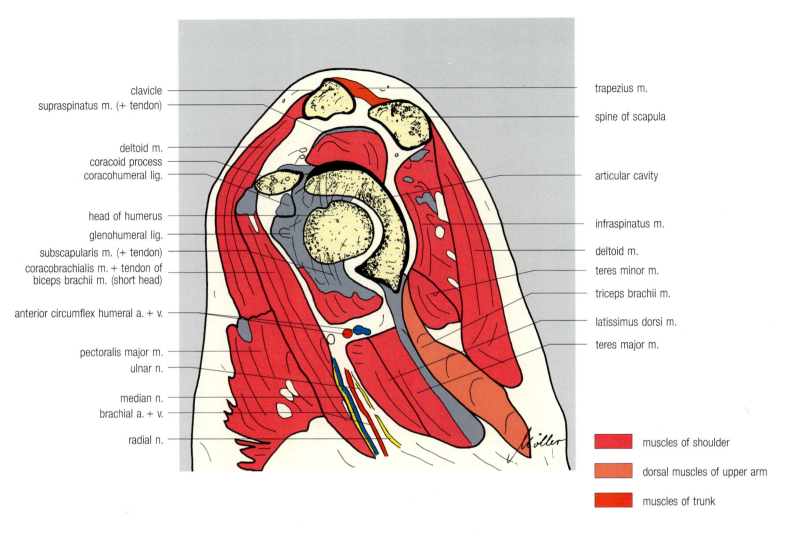

- clavicle
- supraspinatus m. (+ tendon)
- deltoid m.
- coracoid process
- coracohumeral lig.
- head of humerus
- glenohumeral lig.
- subscapularis m. (+ tendon)
- coracobrachialis m. + tendon of biceps brachii m. (short head)
- anterior circumflex humeral a. + v.
- pectoralis major m.
- ulnar n.
- median n.
- brachial a. + v.
- radial n.

- trapezius m.
- spine of scapula
- articular cavity
- infraspinatus m.
- deltoid m.
- teres minor m.
- triceps brachii m.
- latissimus dorsi m.
- teres major m.

■ muscles of shoulder
■ dorsal muscles of upper arm
■ muscles of trunk

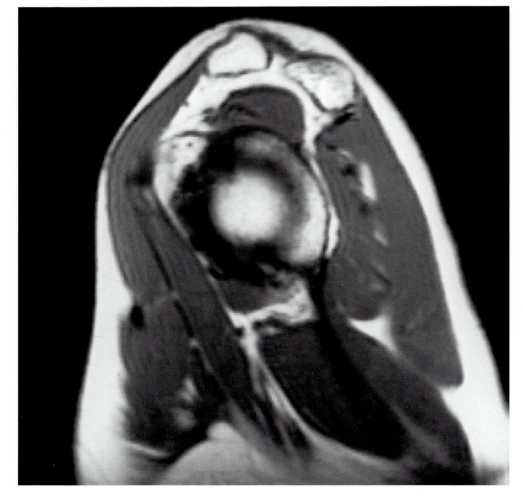

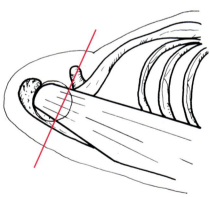

cranial
ventral — dorsal
caudal

Shoulder – Sagittal 63

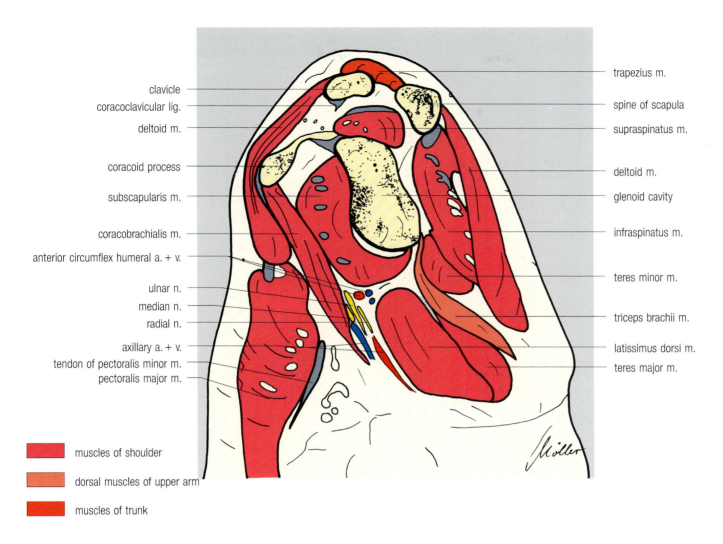

- clavicle
- coracoclavicular lig.
- deltoid m.
- coracoid process
- subscapularis m.
- coracobrachialis m.
- anterior circumflex humeral a. + v.
- ulnar n.
- median n.
- radial n.
- axillary a. + v.
- tendon of pectoralis minor m.
- pectoralis major m.

- trapezius m.
- spine of scapula
- supraspinatus m.
- deltoid m.
- glenoid cavity
- infraspinatus m.
- teres minor m.
- triceps brachii m.
- latissimus dorsi m.
- teres major m.

- muscles of shoulder
- dorsal muscles of upper arm
- muscles of trunk

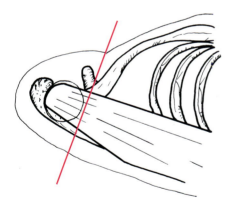

cranial
ventral — dorsal
caudal

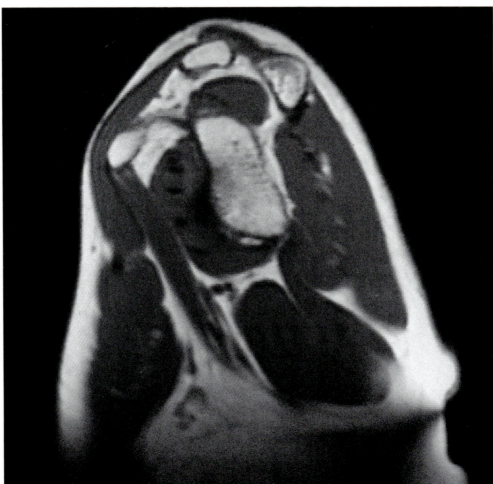

Upper Arm

Coronal
Sagittal

Upper Arm – Coronal

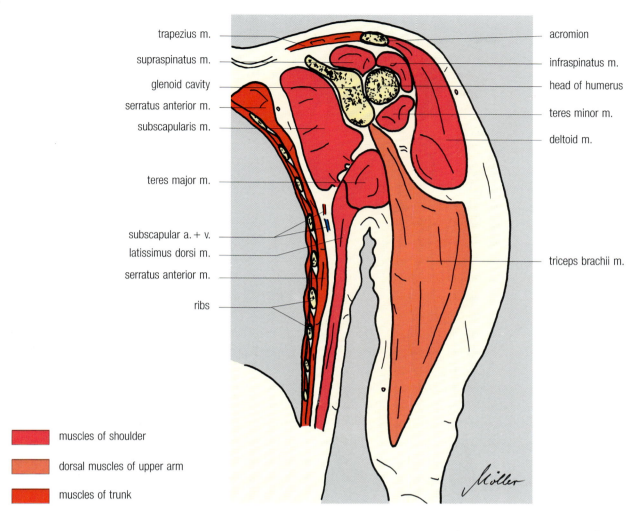

- muscles of shoulder
- dorsal muscles of upper arm
- muscles of trunk

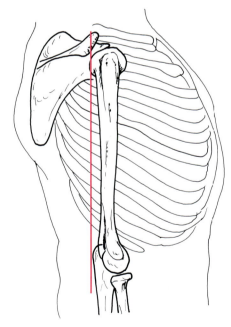

cranial
medial — lateral
caudal

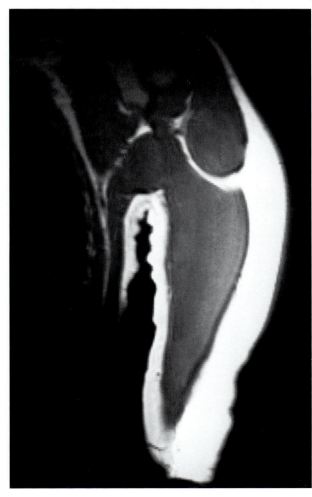

68 Upper Arm – Coronal

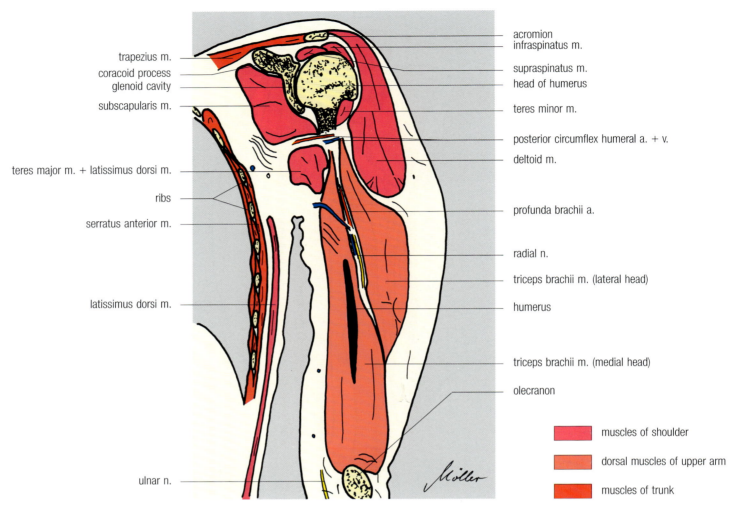

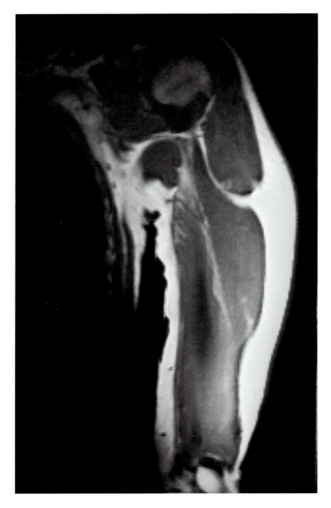

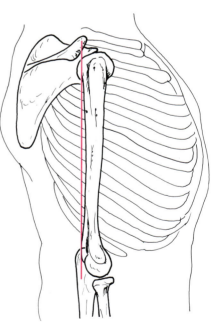

cranial
medial lateral
caudal

Upper Arm – Coronal

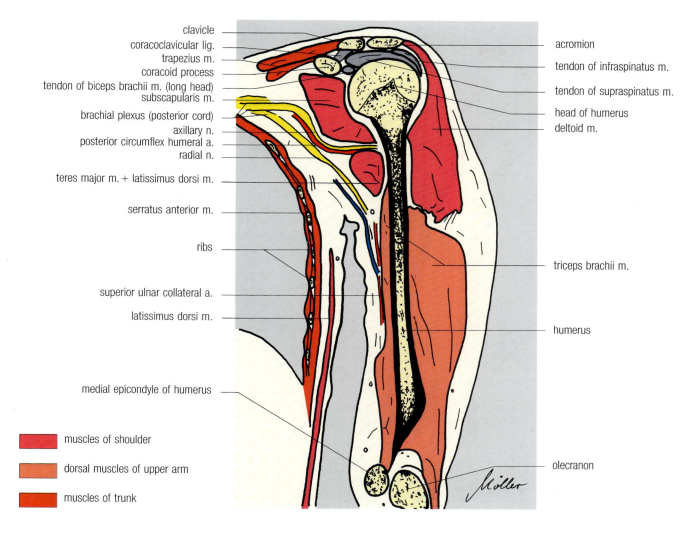

- clavicle
- coracoclavicular lig.
- trapezius m.
- coracoid process
- tendon of biceps brachii m. (long head)
- subscapularis m.
- brachial plexus (posterior cord)
- axillary n.
- posterior circumflex humeral a.
- radial n.
- teres major m. + latissimus dorsi m.
- serratus anterior m.
- ribs
- superior ulnar collateral a.
- latissimus dorsi m.
- medial epicondyle of humerus

- acromion
- tendon of infraspinatus m.
- tendon of supraspinatus m.
- head of humerus
- deltoid m.
- triceps brachii m.
- humerus
- olecranon

- ■ muscles of shoulder
- ■ dorsal muscles of upper arm
- ■ muscles of trunk

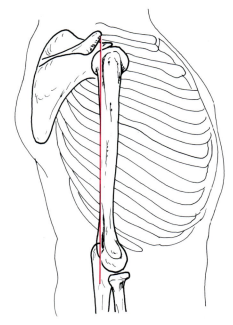

cranial
medial — lateral
caudal

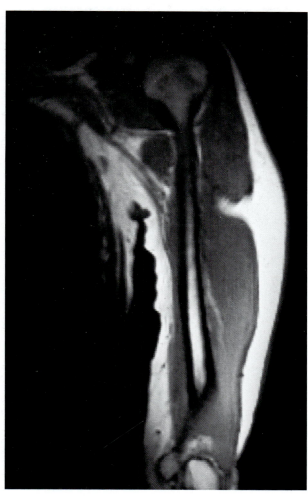

Upper Arm – Coronal

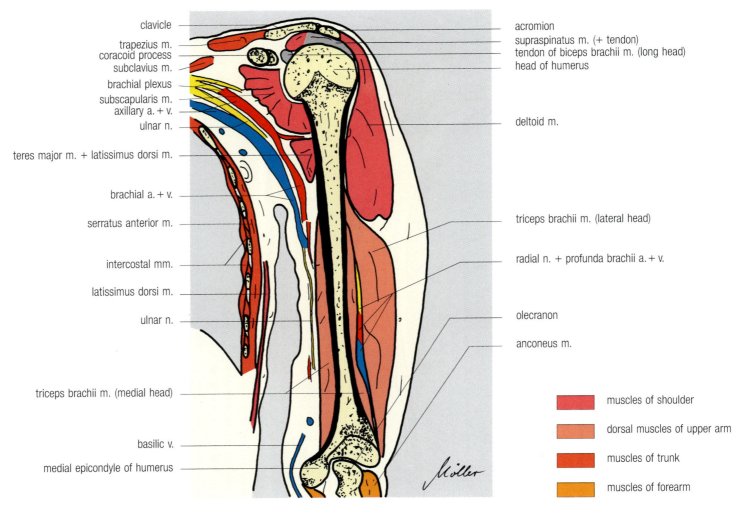

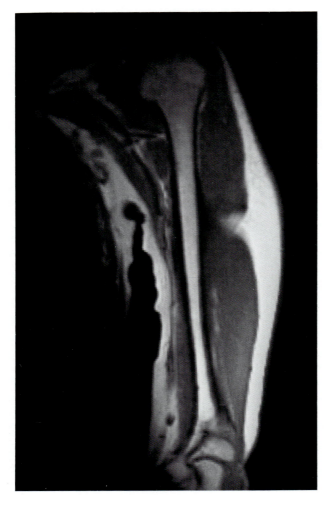

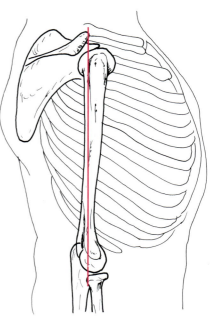

Upper Arm – Coronal

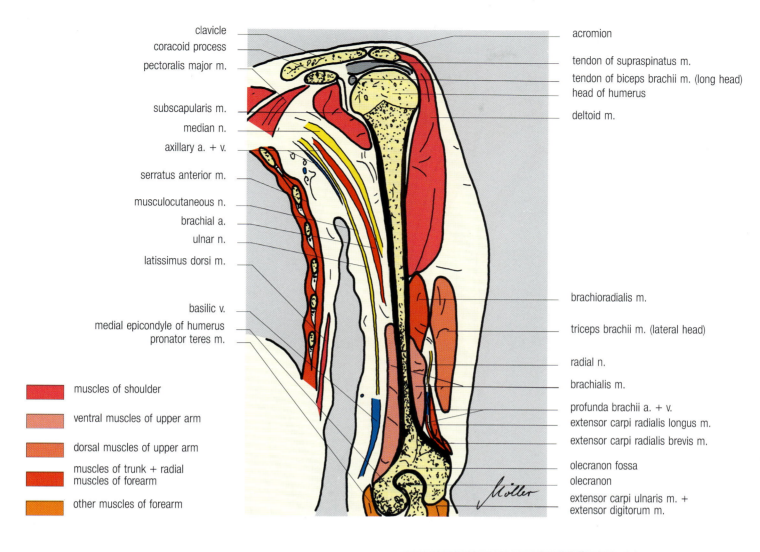

- clavicle
- coracoid process
- pectoralis major m.
- subscapularis m.
- median n.
- axillary a. + v.
- serratus anterior m.
- musculocutaneous n.
- brachial a.
- ulnar n.
- latissimus dorsi m.
- basilic v.
- medial epicondyle of humerus
- pronator teres m.

- acromion
- tendon of supraspinatus m.
- tendon of biceps brachii m. (long head)
- head of humerus
- deltoid m.
- brachioradialis m.
- triceps brachii m. (lateral head)
- radial n.
- brachialis m.
- profunda brachii a. + v.
- extensor carpi radialis longus m.
- extensor carpi radialis brevis m.
- olecranon fossa
- olecranon
- extensor carpi ulnaris m. + extensor digitorum m.

- ■ muscles of shoulder
- ■ ventral muscles of upper arm
- ■ dorsal muscles of upper arm
- ■ muscles of trunk + radial muscles of forearm
- ■ other muscles of forearm

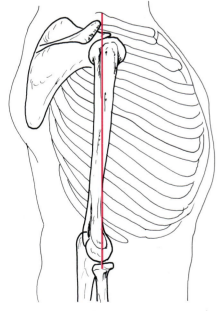

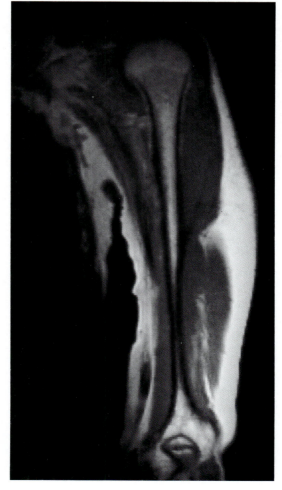

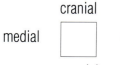

cranial / medial – lateral / caudal

Upper Arm – Coronal

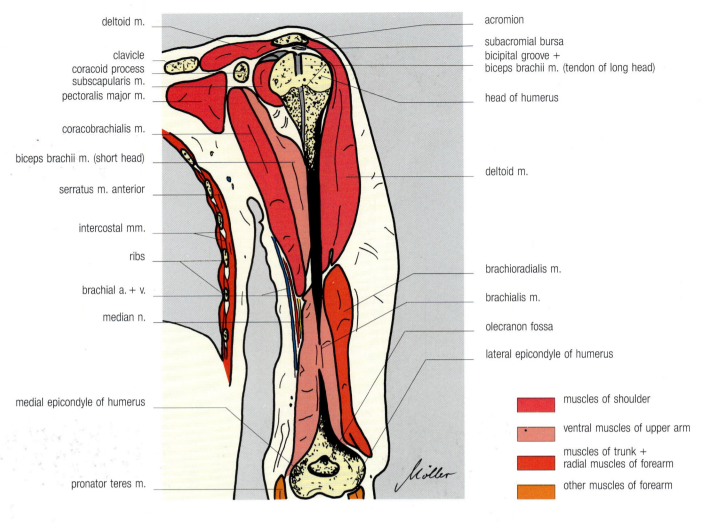

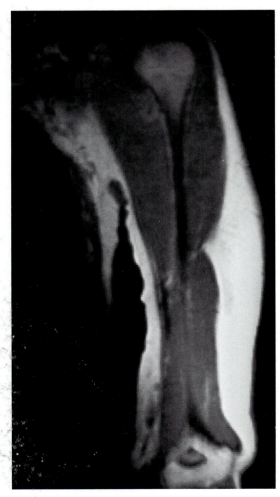

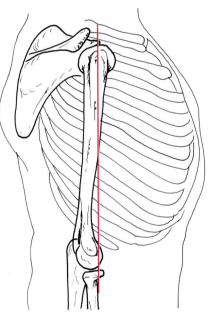

Upper Arm – Coronal

73

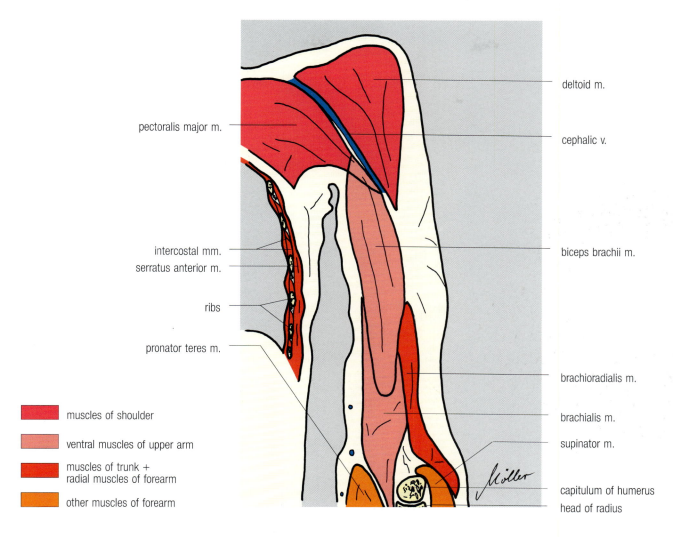

- deltoid m.
- pectoralis major m.
- cephalic v.
- intercostal mm.
- serratus anterior m.
- biceps brachii m.
- ribs
- pronator teres m.
- brachioradialis m.
- brachialis m.
- supinator m.
- capitulum of humerus
- head of radius

■ muscles of shoulder
■ ventral muscles of upper arm
■ muscles of trunk + radial muscles of forearm
■ other muscles of forearm

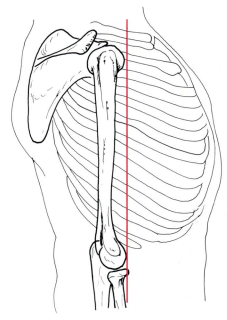

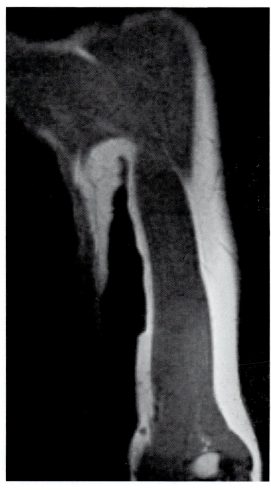

```
          cranial
medial  □  lateral
         caudal
```

Upper Arm – Sagittal

75

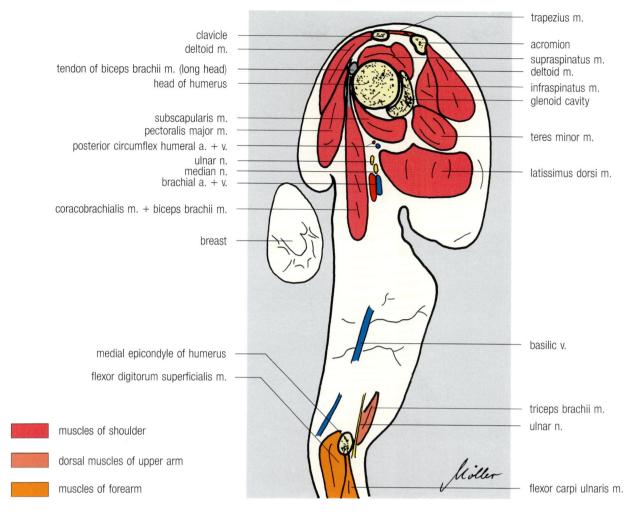

- muscles of shoulder
- dorsal muscles of upper arm
- muscles of forearm

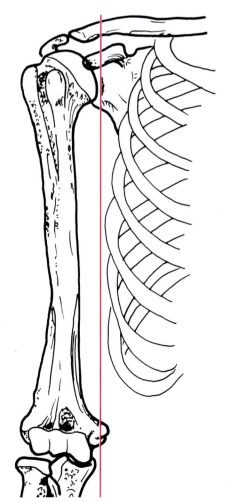
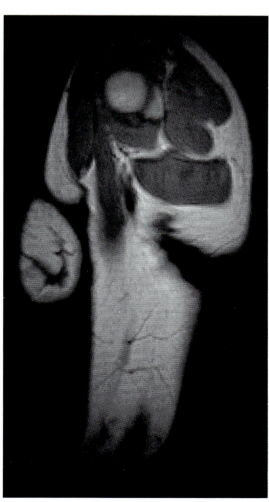

cranial
ventral — dorsal
caudal

Upper Arm – Sagittal

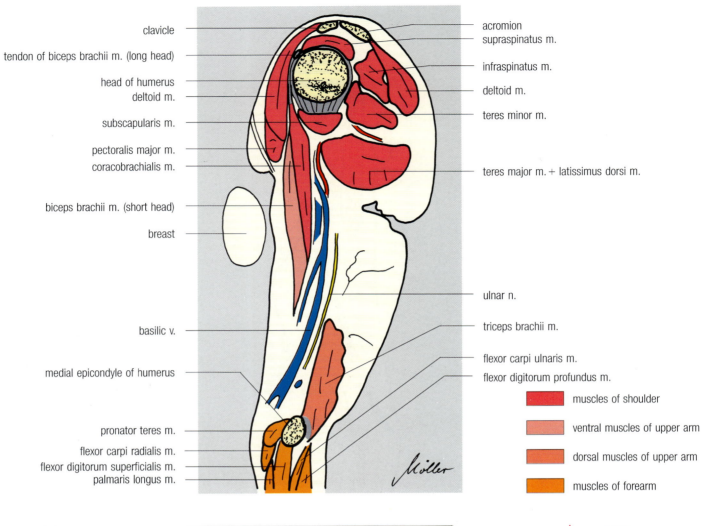

- clavicle
- tendon of biceps brachii m. (long head)
- head of humerus
- deltoid m.
- subscapularis m.
- pectoralis major m.
- coracobrachialis m.
- biceps brachii m. (short head)
- breast
- basilic v.
- medial epicondyle of humerus
- pronator teres m.
- flexor carpi radialis m.
- flexor digitorum superficialis m.
- palmaris longus m.
- acromion
- supraspinatus m.
- infraspinatus m.
- deltoid m.
- teres minor m.
- teres major m. + latissimus dorsi m.
- ulnar n.
- triceps brachii m.
- flexor carpi ulnaris m.
- flexor digitorum profundus m.

- muscles of shoulder
- ventral muscles of upper arm
- dorsal muscles of upper arm
- muscles of forearm

cranial / ventral / dorsal / caudal

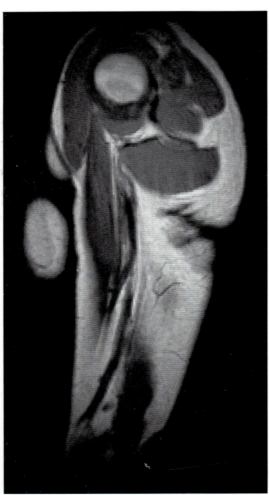
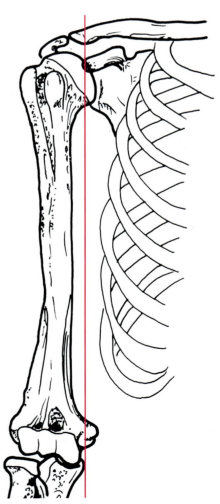

Upper Arm – Sagittal

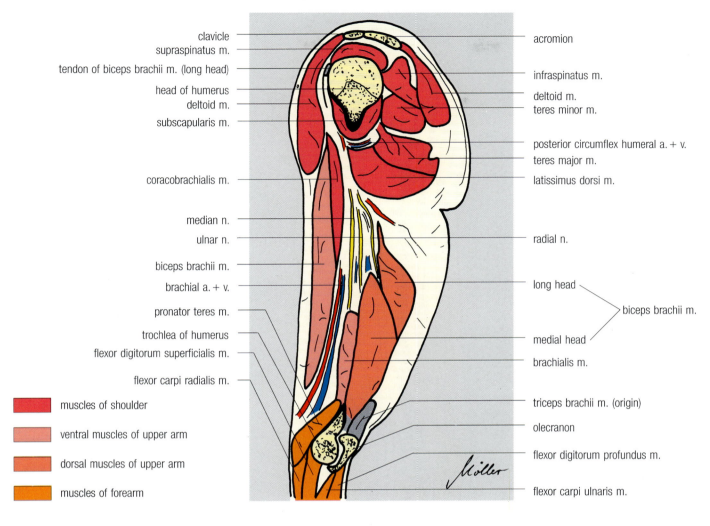

- clavicle
- supraspinatus m.
- tendon of biceps brachii m. (long head)
- head of humerus
- deltoid m.
- subscapularis m.
- coracobrachialis m.
- median n.
- ulnar n.
- biceps brachii m.
- brachial a. + v.
- pronator teres m.
- trochlea of humerus
- flexor digitorum superficialis m.
- flexor carpi radialis m.

- acromion
- infraspinatus m.
- deltoid m.
- teres minor m.
- posterior circumflex humeral a. + v.
- teres major m.
- latissimus dorsi m.
- radial n.
- long head ⎫ biceps brachii m.
- medial head ⎭
- brachialis m.
- triceps brachii m. (origin)
- olecranon
- flexor digitorum profundus m.
- flexor carpi ulnaris m.

- ■ muscles of shoulder
- ■ ventral muscles of upper arm
- ■ dorsal muscles of upper arm
- ■ muscles of forearm

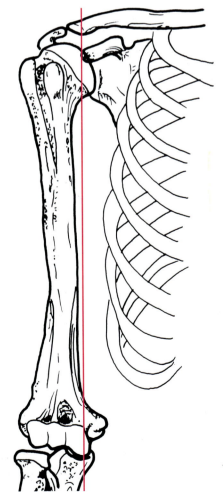

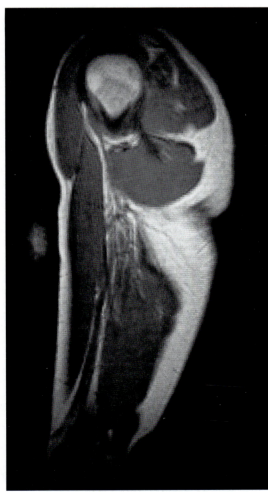

cranial
ventral — dorsal
caudal

Upper Arm – Sagittal

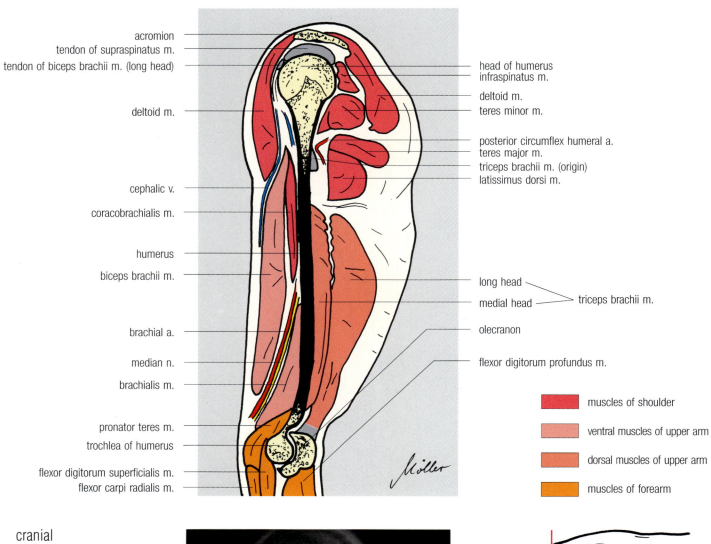

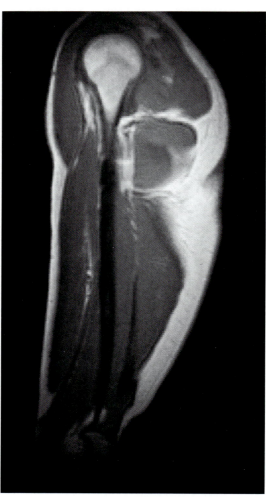

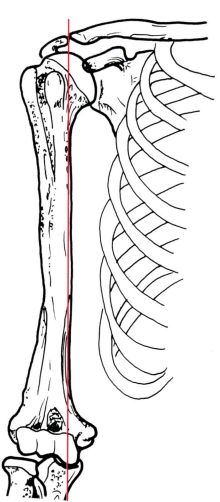

Upper Arm – Sagittal

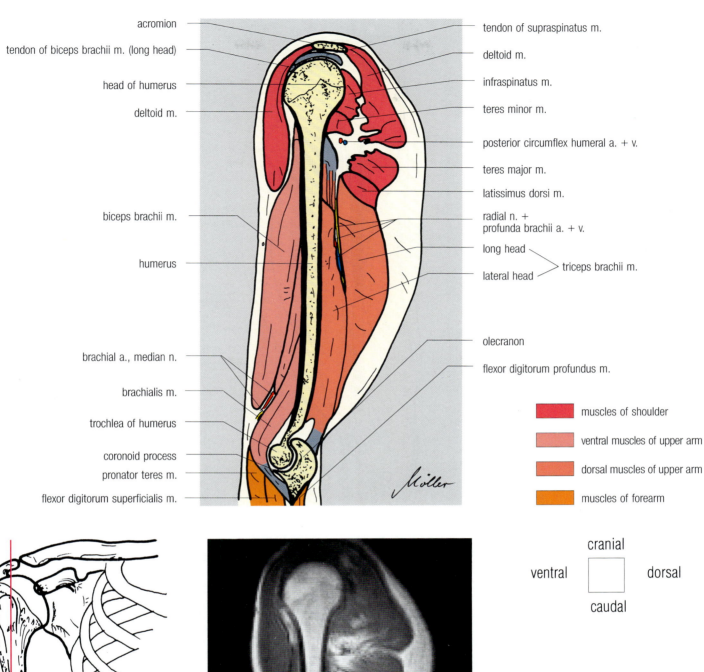
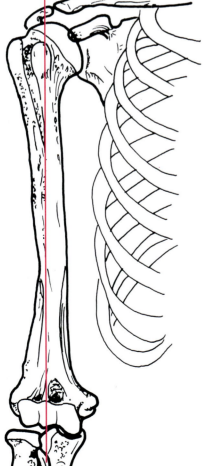
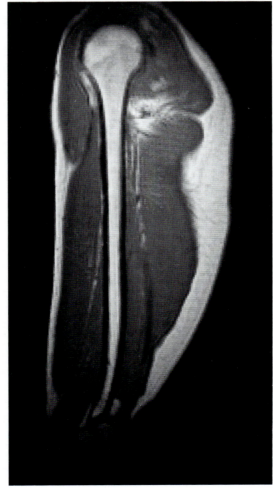

Upper Arm – Sagittal

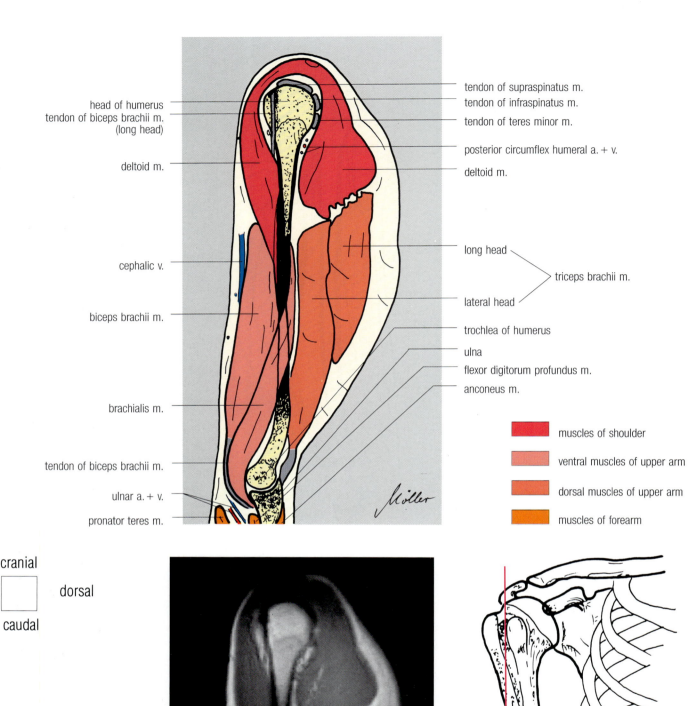

Upper Arm – Sagittal

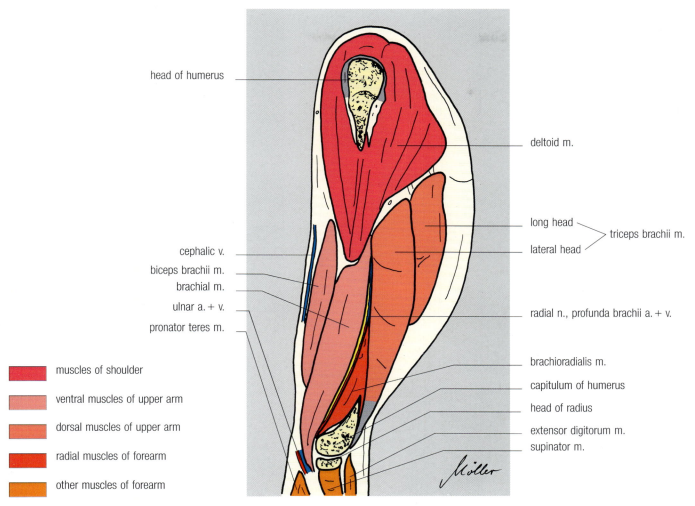

- muscles of shoulder
- ventral muscles of upper arm
- dorsal muscles of upper arm
- radial muscles of forearm
- other muscles of forearm

head of humerus
deltoid m.
long head — triceps brachii m.
lateral head
cephalic v.
biceps brachii m.
brachial m.
ulnar a. + v.
pronator teres m.
radial n., profunda brachii a. + v.
brachioradialis m.
capitulum of humerus
head of radius
extensor digitorum m.
supinator m.

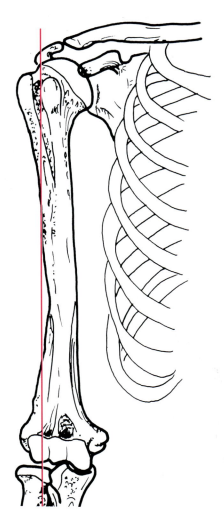

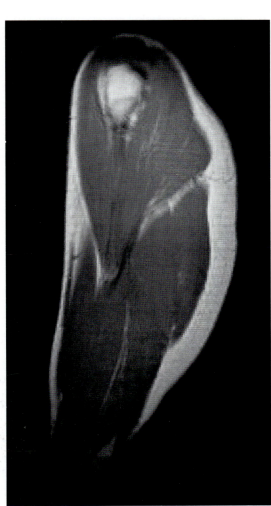

cranial
ventral — dorsal
caudal

Elbow

Coronal
Sagittal

Elbow – Coronal

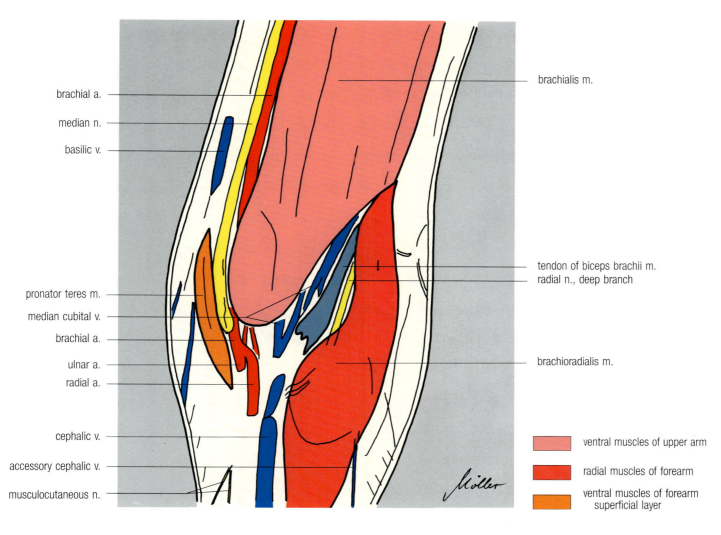

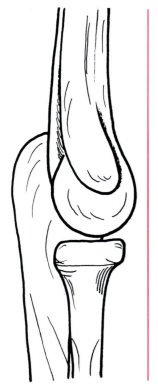

Elbow – Coronal

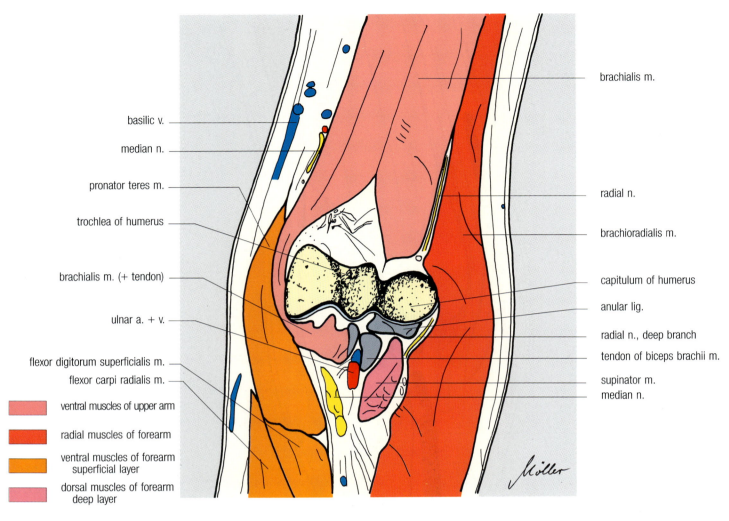

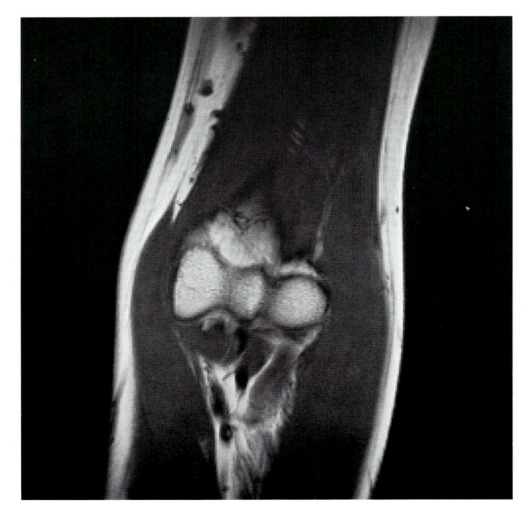 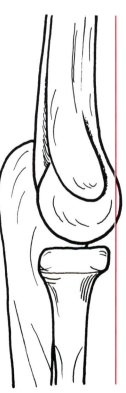

Elbow – Coronal

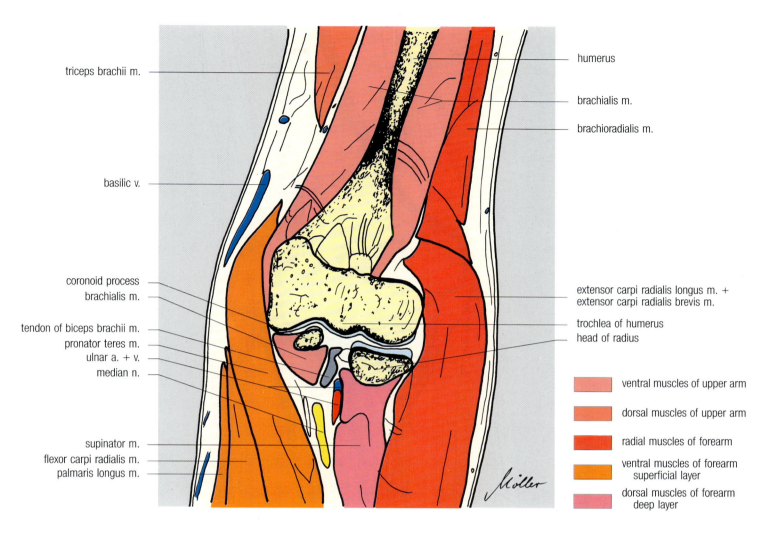

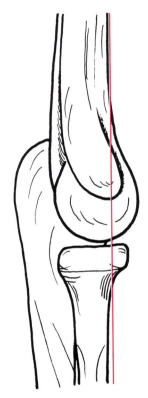

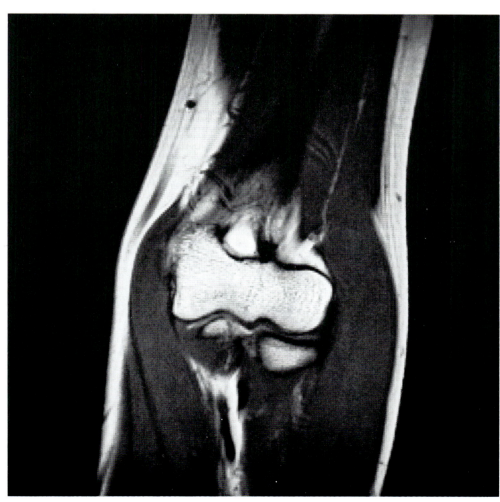

Elbow – Coronal

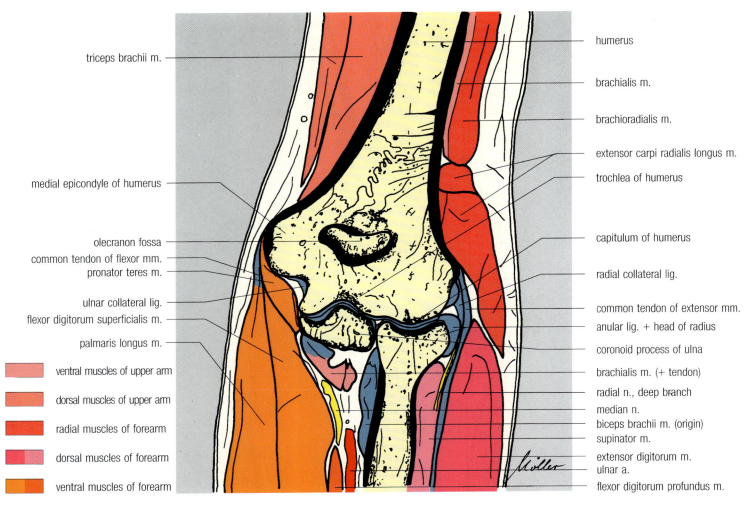

- triceps brachii m.
- medial epicondyle of humerus
- olecranon fossa
- common tendon of flexor mm.
- pronator teres m.
- ulnar collateral lig.
- flexor digitorum superficialis m.
- palmaris longus m.
- ventral muscles of upper arm
- dorsal muscles of upper arm
- radial muscles of forearm
- dorsal muscles of forearm
- ventral muscles of forearm
- humerus
- brachialis m.
- brachioradialis m.
- extensor carpi radialis longus m.
- trochlea of humerus
- capitulum of humerus
- radial collateral lig.
- common tendon of extensor mm.
- anular lig. + head of radius
- coronoid process of ulna
- brachialis m. (+ tendon)
- radial n., deep branch
- median n.
- biceps brachii m. (origin)
- supinator m.
- extensor digitorum m.
- ulnar a.
- flexor digitorum profundus m.

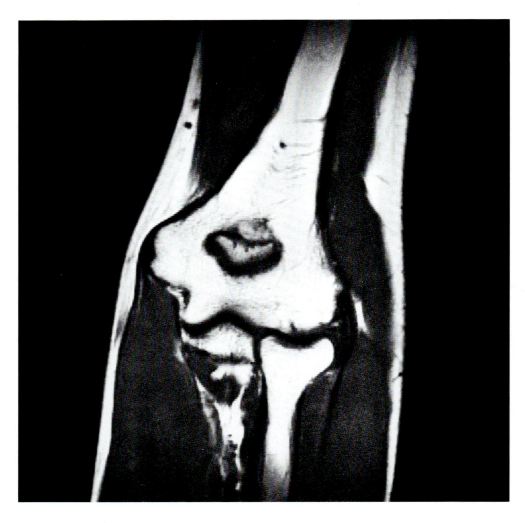

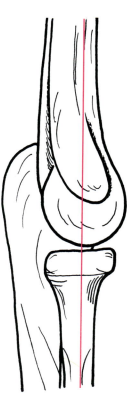

proximal
ulnar — radial
medial — lateral
distal

Elbow – Coronal

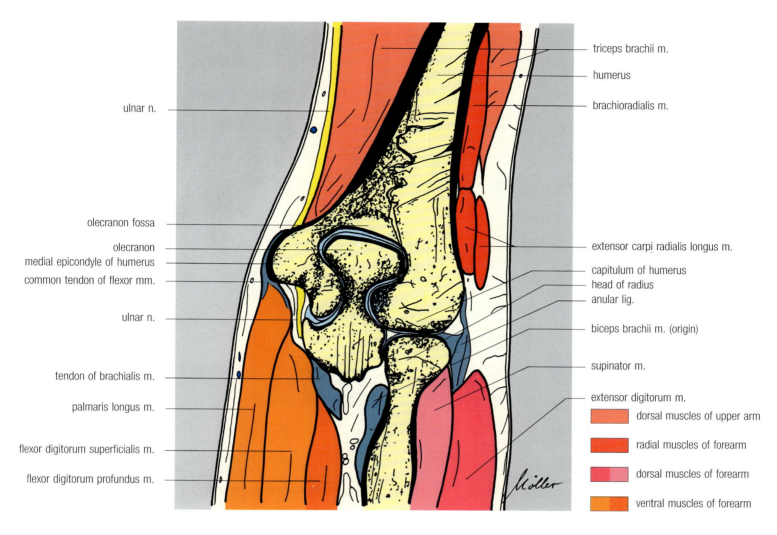

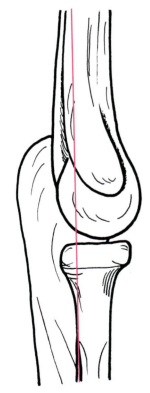
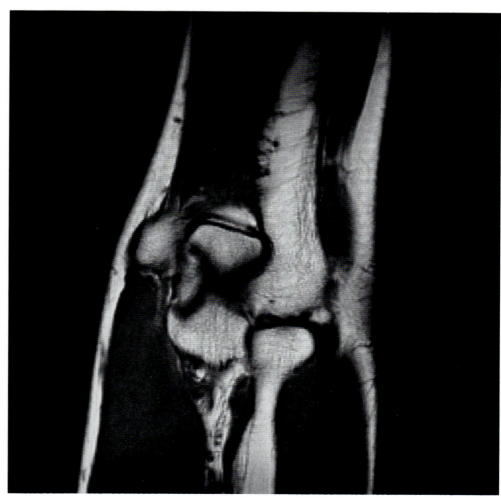

Elbow – Coronal

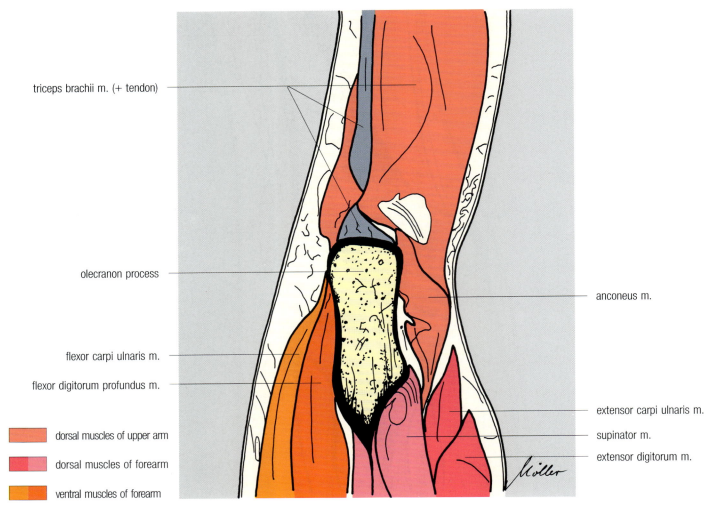

- triceps brachii m. (+ tendon)
- olecranon process
- flexor carpi ulnaris m.
- flexor digitorum profundus m.
- anconeus m.
- extensor carpi ulnaris m.
- supinator m.
- extensor digitorum m.

■ dorsal muscles of upper arm
■ dorsal muscles of forearm
■ ventral muscles of forearm

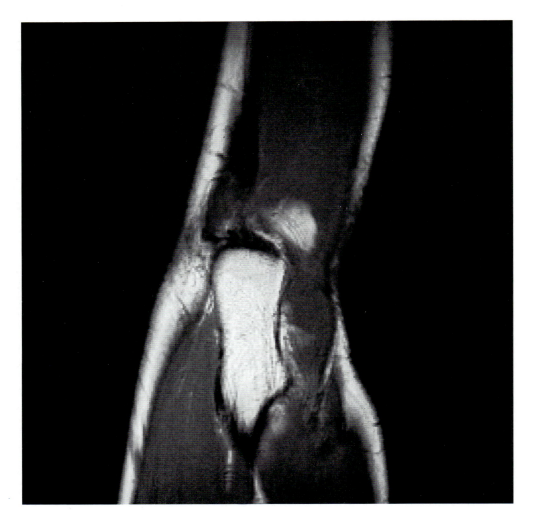

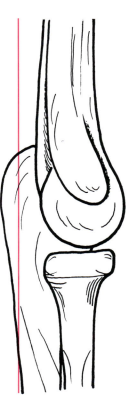

proximal
ulnar — radial
medial — lateral
distal

Elbow – Sagittal

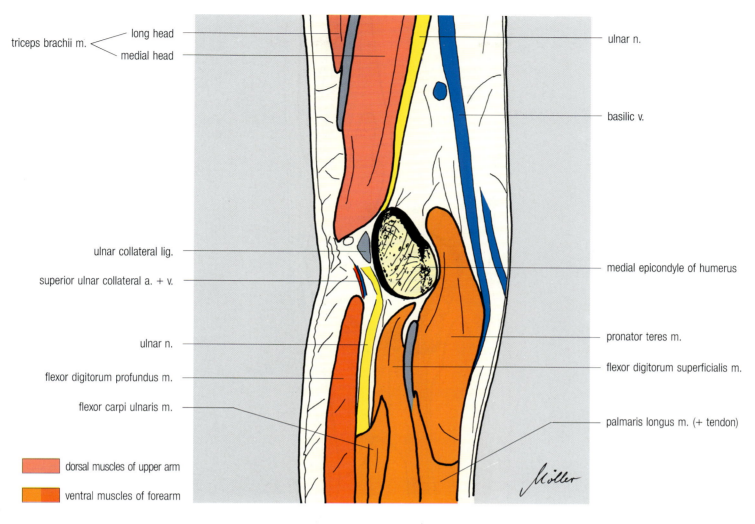

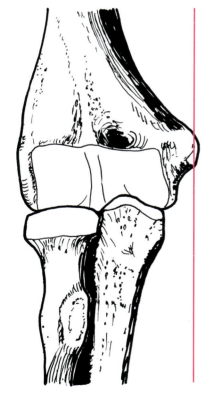

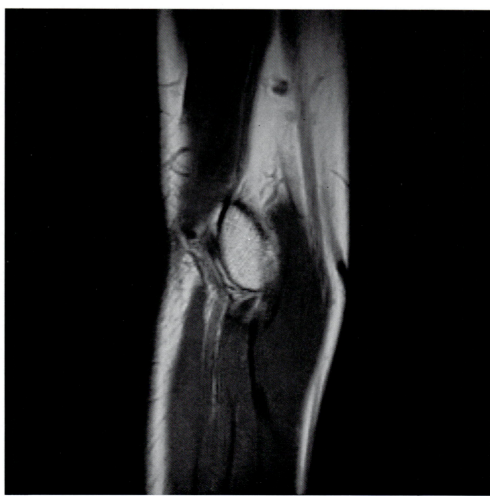

Elbow – Sagittal

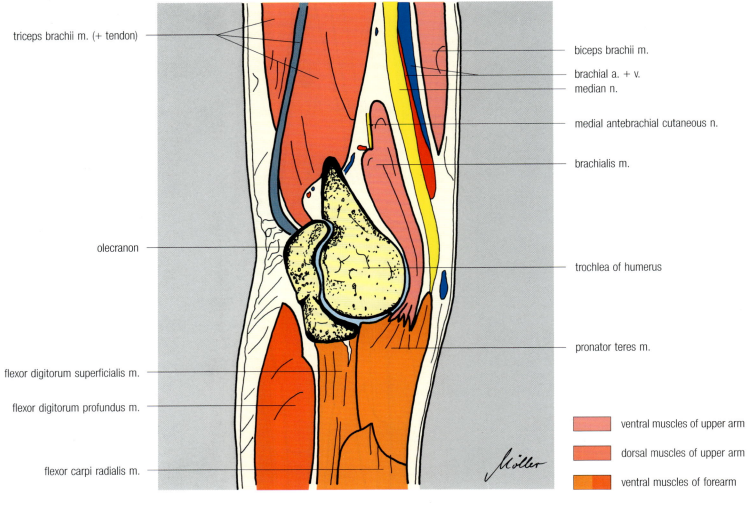

- triceps brachii m. (+ tendon)
- olecranon
- flexor digitorum superficialis m.
- flexor digitorum profundus m.
- flexor carpi radialis m.
- biceps brachii m.
- brachial a. + v.
- median n.
- medial antebrachial cutaneous n.
- brachialis m.
- trochlea of humerus
- pronator teres m.

■ ventral muscles of upper arm
■ dorsal muscles of upper arm
■ ventral muscles of forearm

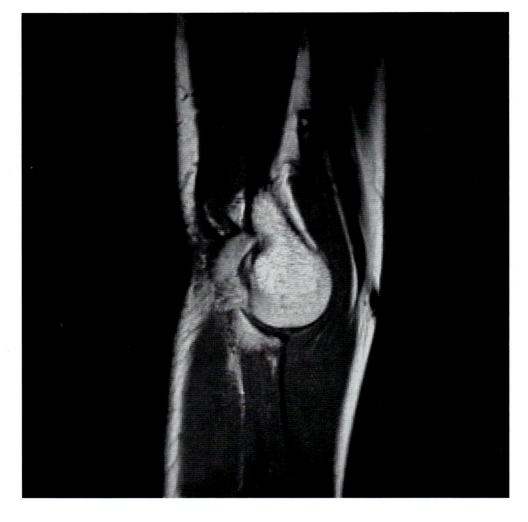

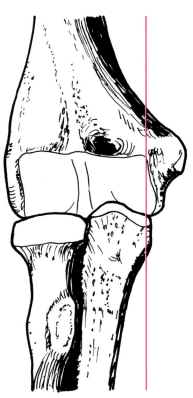

proximal
dorsal — ventral
distal

Elbow – Sagittal

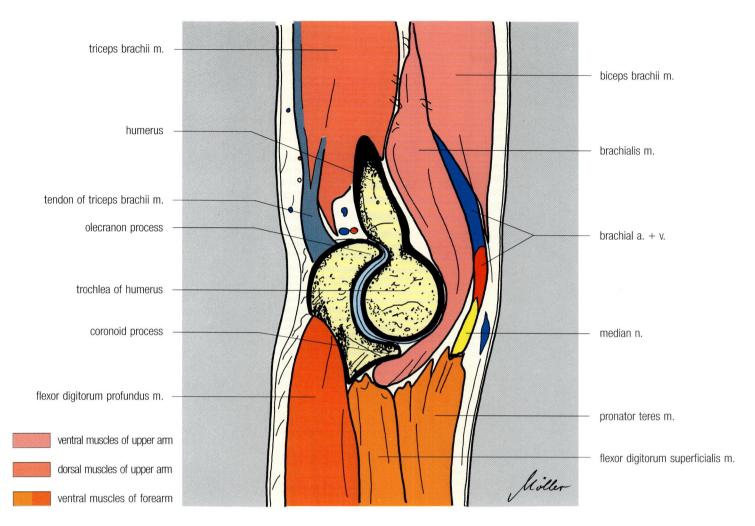

- triceps brachii m.
- humerus
- tendon of triceps brachii m.
- olecranon process
- trochlea of humerus
- coronoid process
- flexor digitorum profundus m.
- biceps brachii m.
- brachialis m.
- brachial a. + v.
- median n.
- pronator teres m.
- flexor digitorum superficialis m.

■ ventral muscles of upper arm
■ dorsal muscles of upper arm
■ ventral muscles of forearm

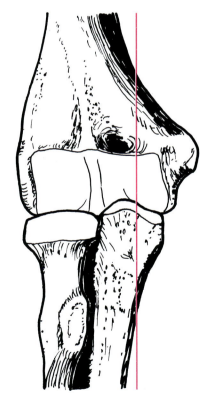

proximal
dorsal — ventral
distal

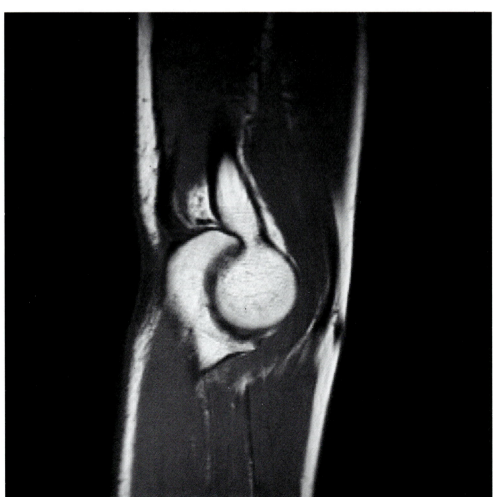

Elbow – Sagittal

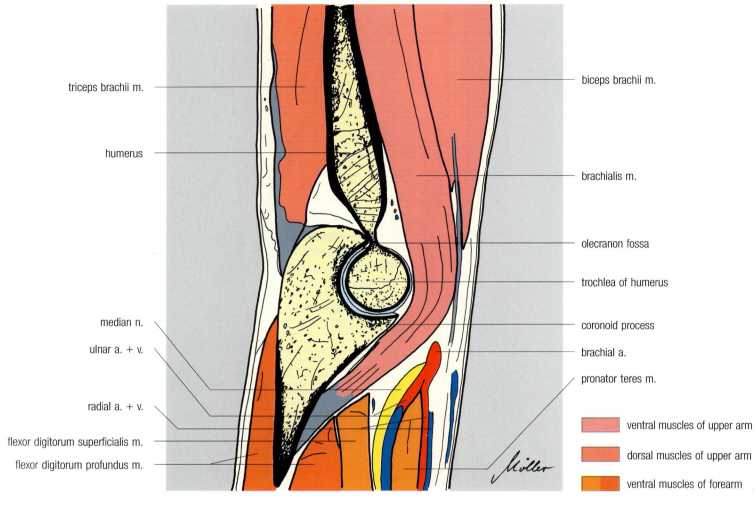
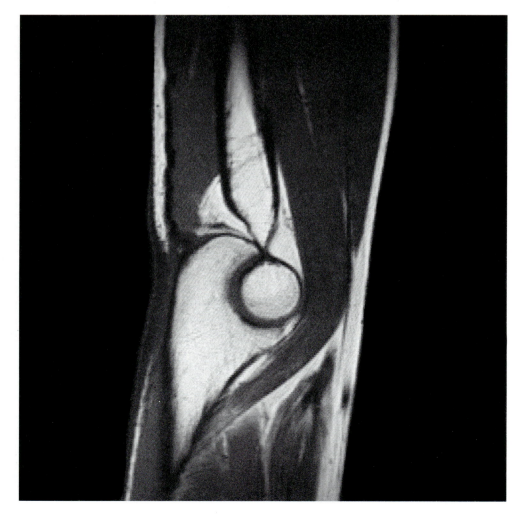
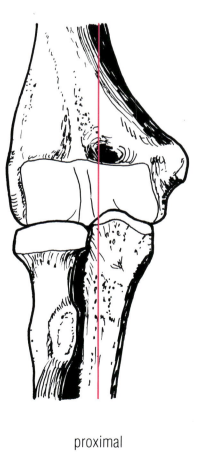

Elbow – Sagittal 95

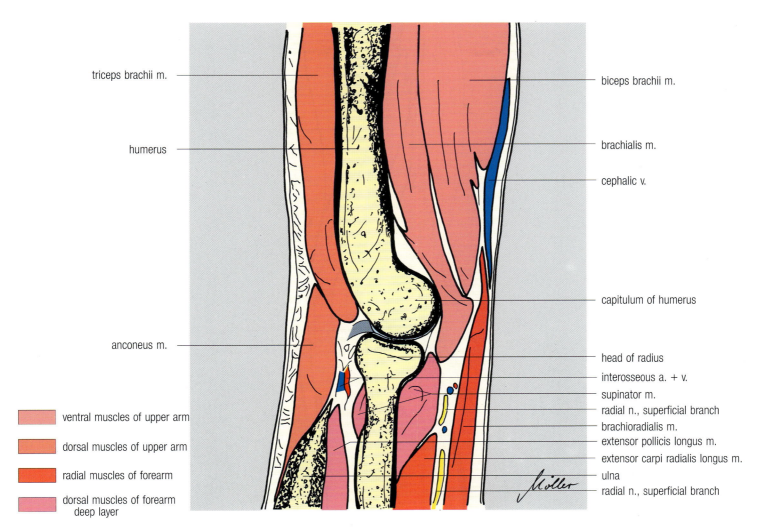

- triceps brachii m.
- humerus
- anconeus m.

- ventral muscles of upper arm
- dorsal muscles of upper arm
- radial muscles of forearm
- dorsal muscles of forearm deep layer

- biceps brachii m.
- brachialis m.
- cephalic v.
- capitulum of humerus
- head of radius
- interosseous a. + v.
- supinator m.
- radial n., superficial branch
- brachioradialis m.
- extensor pollicis longus m.
- extensor carpi radialis longus m.
- ulna
- radial n., superficial branch

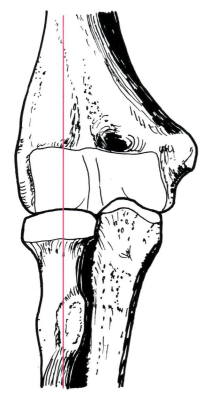

proximal
dorsal ventral
distal

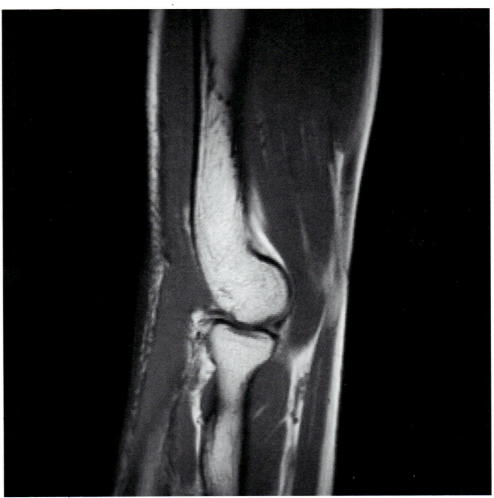

Elbow – Sagittal

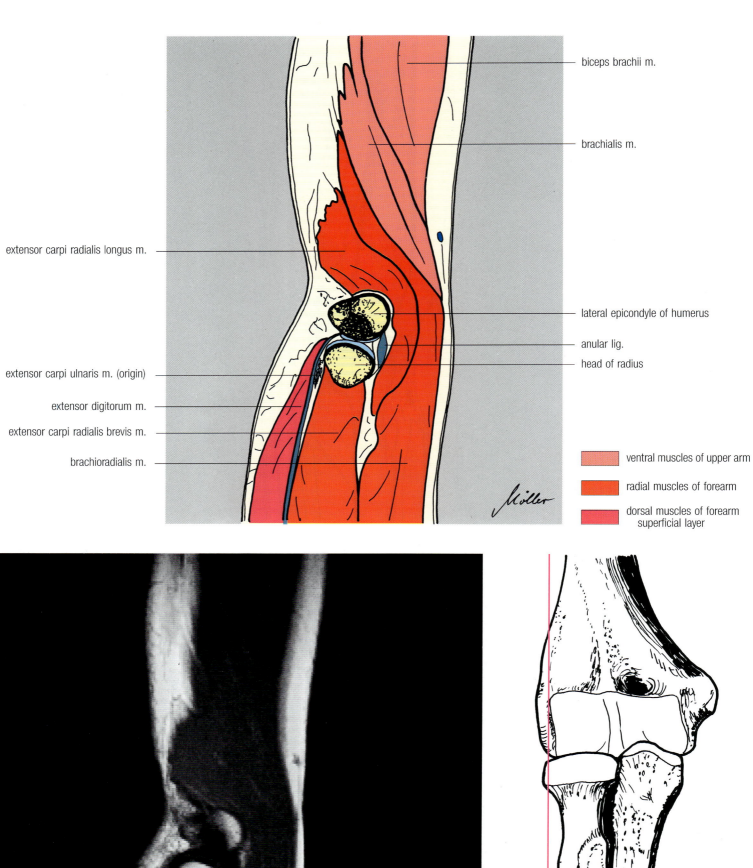

- biceps brachii m.
- brachialis m.
- extensor carpi radialis longus m.
- lateral epicondyle of humerus
- anular lig.
- head of radius
- extensor carpi ulnaris m. (origin)
- extensor digitorum m.
- extensor carpi radialis brevis m.
- brachioradialis m.

- ventral muscles of upper arm
- radial muscles of forearm
- dorsal muscles of forearm superficial layer

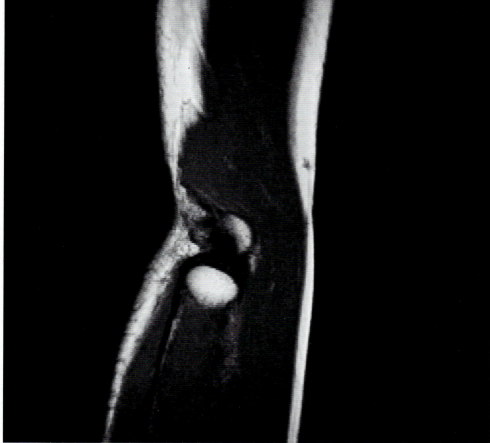

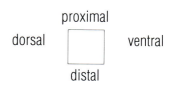

proximal
dorsal — ventral
distal

Forearm

Coronal
Sagittal

Forearm – Coronal

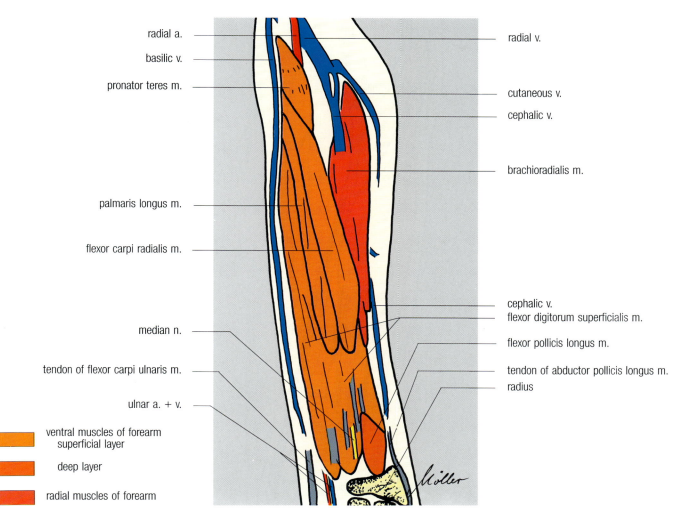

- radial a.
- basilic v.
- pronator teres m.
- palmaris longus m.
- flexor carpi radialis m.
- median n.
- tendon of flexor carpi ulnaris m.
- ulnar a. + v.
- radial v.
- cutaneous v.
- cephalic v.
- brachioradialis m.
- cephalic v.
- flexor digitorum superficialis m.
- flexor pollicis longus m.
- tendon of abductor pollicis longus m.
- radius

■ ventral muscles of forearm superficial layer
■ deep layer
■ radial muscles of forearm

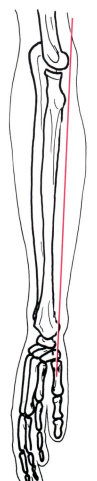

proximal
ulnar / medial   radial / lateral
distal

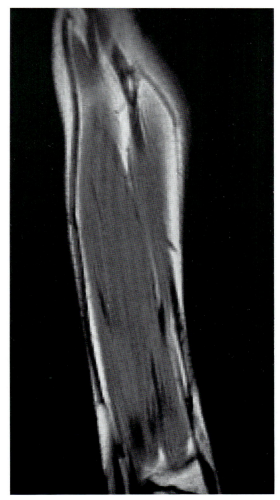

100 Forearm – Coronal

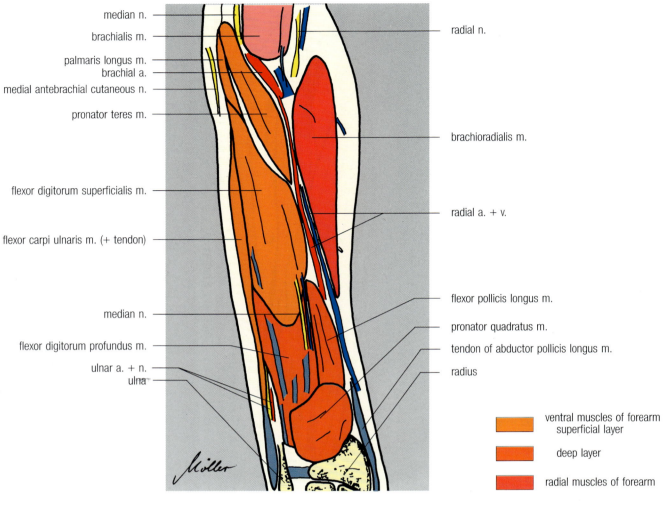

- median n.
- brachialis m.
- palmaris longus m.
- brachial a.
- medial antebrachial cutaneous n.
- pronator teres m.
- flexor digitorum superficialis m.
- flexor carpi ulnaris m. (+ tendon)
- median n.
- flexor digitorum profundus m.
- ulnar a. + n.
- ulna
- radial n.
- brachioradialis m.
- radial a. + v.
- flexor pollicis longus m.
- pronator quadratus m.
- tendon of abductor pollicis longus m.
- radius

■ ventral muscles of forearm superficial layer
■ deep layer
■ radial muscles of forearm

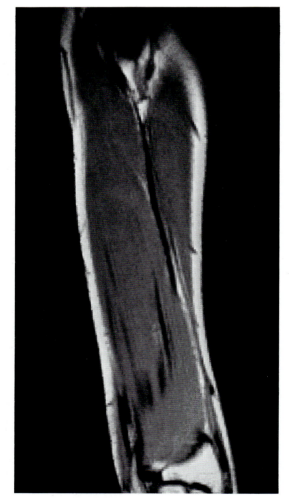

proximal
ulnar — radial
medial — lateral
distal

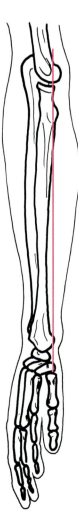

Forearm – Coronal

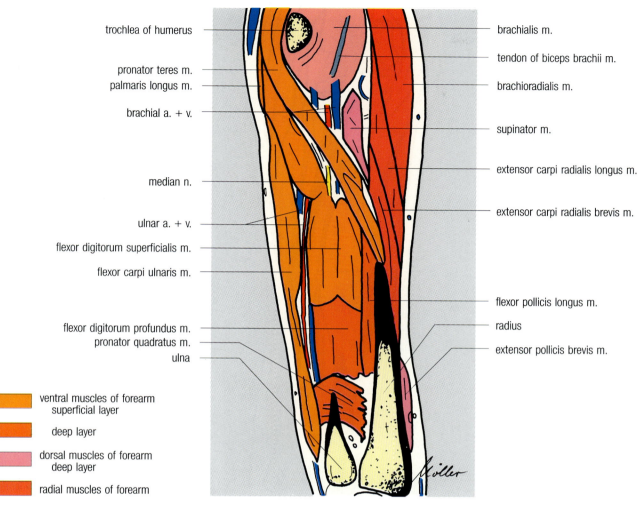

- trochlea of humerus
- pronator teres m.
- palmaris longus m.
- brachial a. + v.
- median n.
- ulnar a. + v.
- flexor digitorum superficialis m.
- flexor carpi ulnaris m.
- flexor digitorum profundus m.
- pronator quadratus m.
- ulna
- brachialis m.
- tendon of biceps brachii m.
- brachioradialis m.
- supinator m.
- extensor carpi radialis longus m.
- extensor carpi radialis brevis m.
- flexor pollicis longus m.
- radius
- extensor pollicis brevis m.

- ventral muscles of forearm superficial layer
- deep layer
- dorsal muscles of forearm deep layer
- radial muscles of forearm

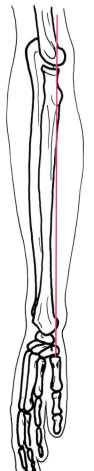

proximal
ulnar — radial
medial — lateral
distal

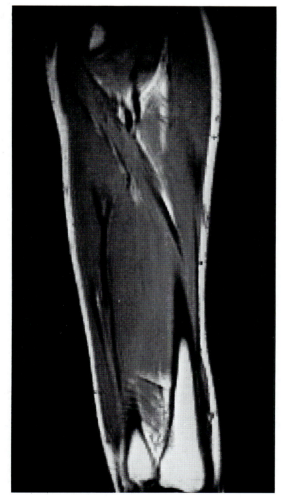

Forearm – Coronal

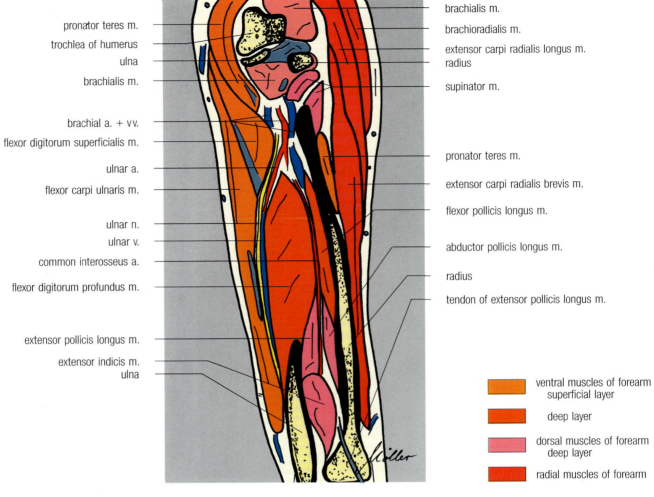

- pronator teres m.
- trochlea of humerus
- ulna
- brachialis m.
- brachial a. + vv.
- flexor digitorum superficialis m.
- ulnar a.
- flexor carpi ulnaris m.
- ulnar n.
- ulnar v.
- common interosseus a.
- flexor digitorum profundus m.
- extensor pollicis longus m.
- extensor indicis m.
- ulna

- brachialis m.
- brachioradialis m.
- extensor carpi radialis longus m.
- radius
- supinator m.
- pronator teres m.
- extensor carpi radialis brevis m.
- flexor pollicis longus m.
- abductor pollicis longus m.
- radius
- tendon of extensor pollicis longus m.

- ventral muscles of forearm superficial layer
- deep layer
- dorsal muscles of forearm deep layer
- radial muscles of forearm

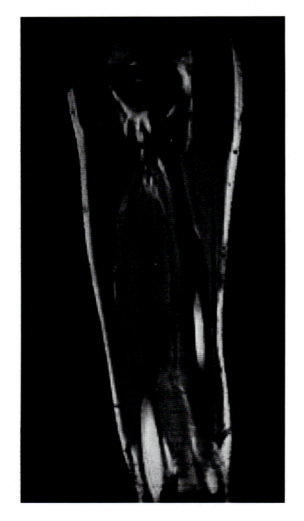

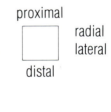

proximal
ulnar — radial
medial — lateral
distal

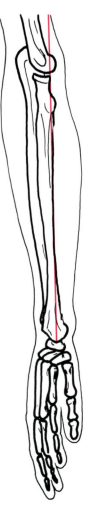

Forearm – Coronal

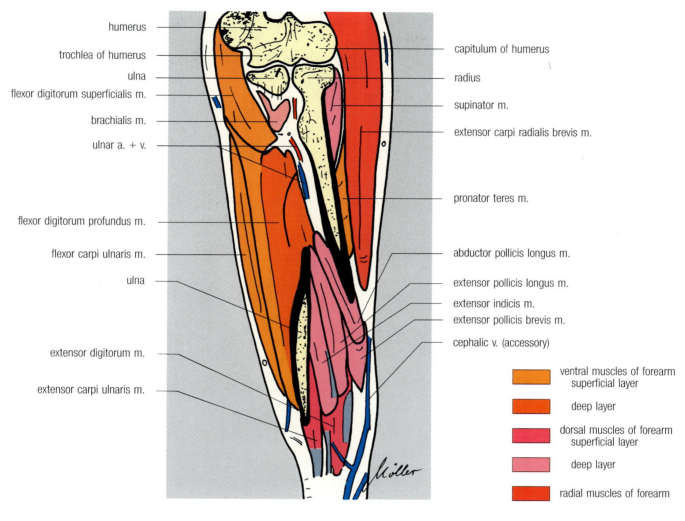
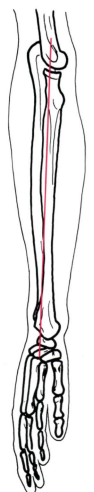
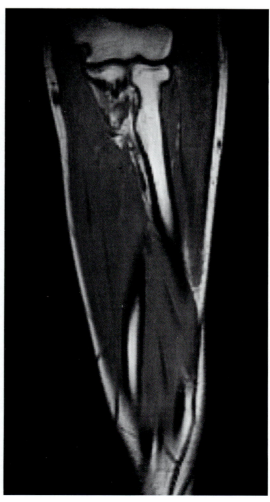

Forearm – Coronal

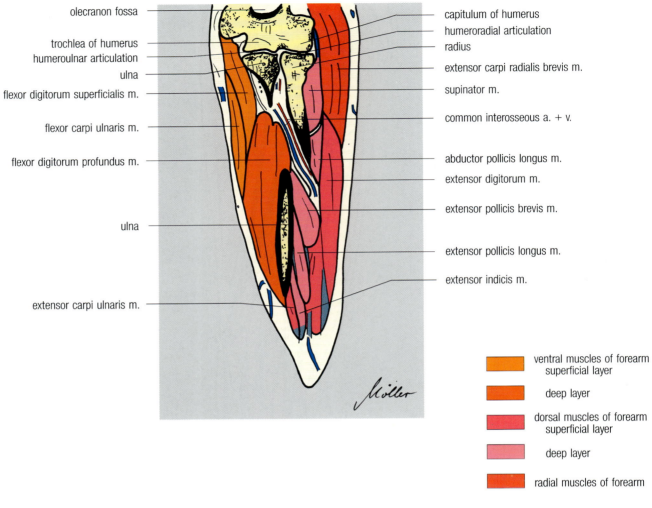

- olecranon fossa
- trochlea of humerus
- humeroulnar articulation
- ulna
- flexor digitorum superficialis m.
- flexor carpi ulnaris m.
- flexor digitorum profundus m.
- ulna
- extensor carpi ulnaris m.
- capitulum of humerus
- humeroradial articulation
- radius
- extensor carpi radialis brevis m.
- supinator m.
- common interosseous a. + v.
- abductor pollicis longus m.
- extensor digitorum m.
- extensor pollicis brevis m.
- extensor pollicis longus m.
- extensor indicis m.

■ ventral muscles of forearm superficial layer
■ deep layer
■ dorsal muscles of forearm superficial layer
■ deep layer
■ radial muscles of forearm

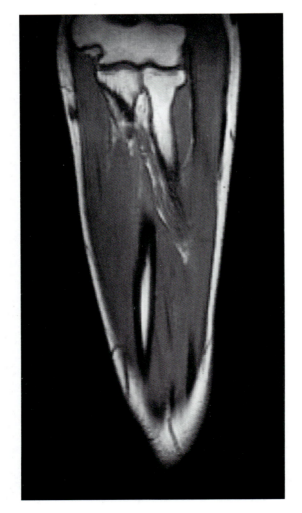

proximal / distal / ulnar medial / radial lateral

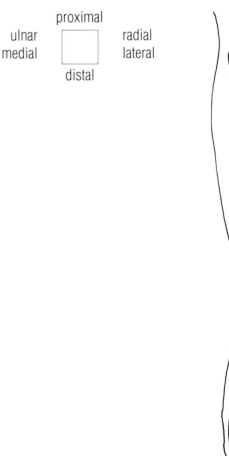

Forearm – Coronal

105

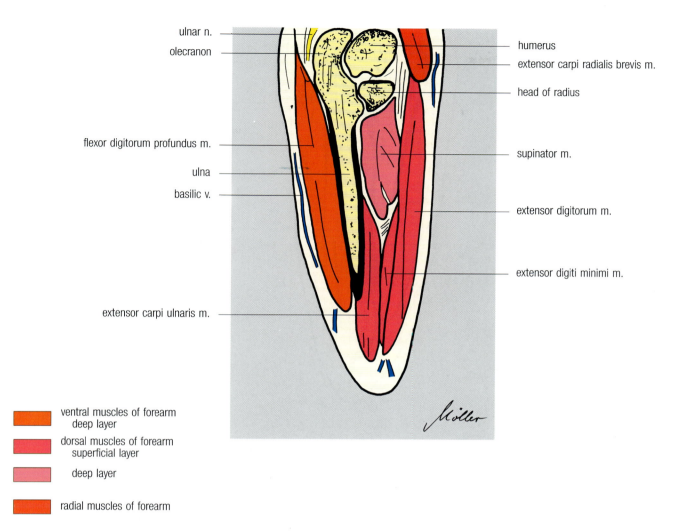

- ulnar n.
- olecranon
- flexor digitorum profundus m.
- ulna
- basilic v.
- extensor carpi ulnaris m.
- humerus
- extensor carpi radialis brevis m.
- head of radius
- supinator m.
- extensor digitorum m.
- extensor digiti minimi m.

■ ventral muscles of forearm deep layer
■ dorsal muscles of forearm superficial layer
■ deep layer
■ radial muscles of forearm

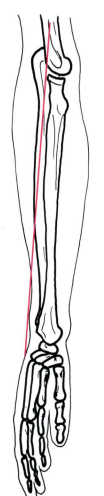

proximal — distal
ulnar medial — radial lateral

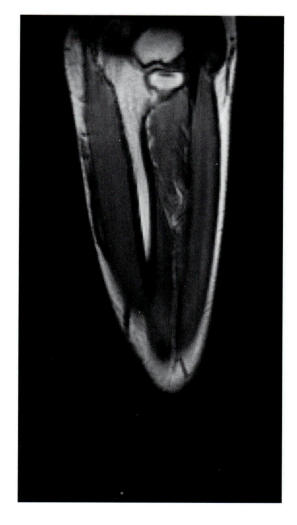

106 Forearm – Coronal

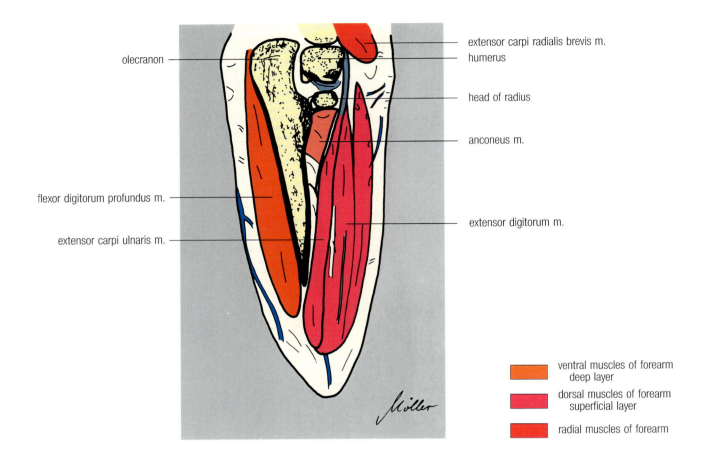

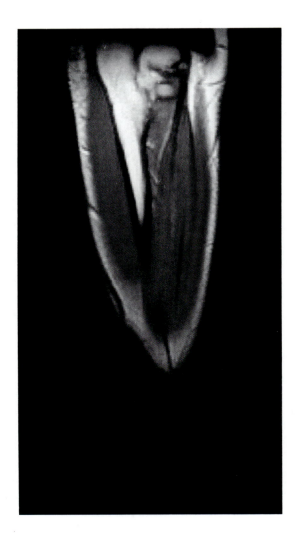
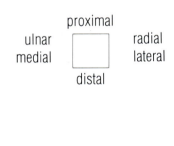
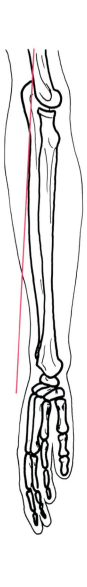

Forearm – Sagittal

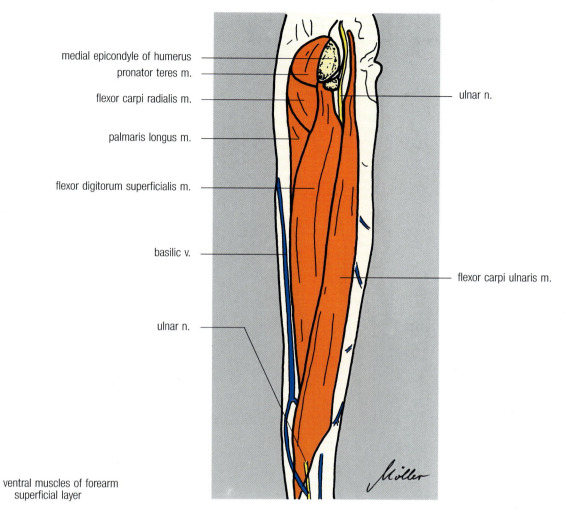

- medial epicondyle of humerus
- pronator teres m.
- flexor carpi radialis m.
- palmaris longus m.
- flexor digitorum superficialis m.
- basilic v.
- ulnar n.
- ulnar n.
- flexor carpi ulnaris m.

■ ventral muscles of forearm superficial layer

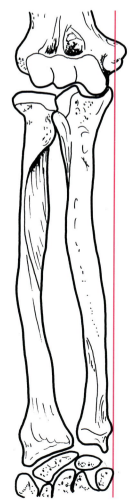

proximal

ventral — dorsal

distal

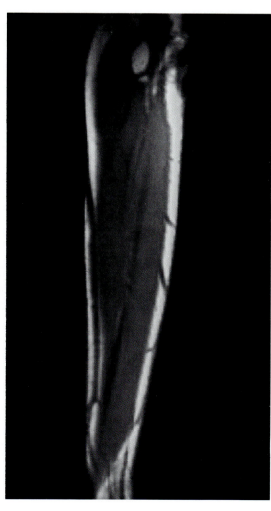

108 Forearm – Sagittal

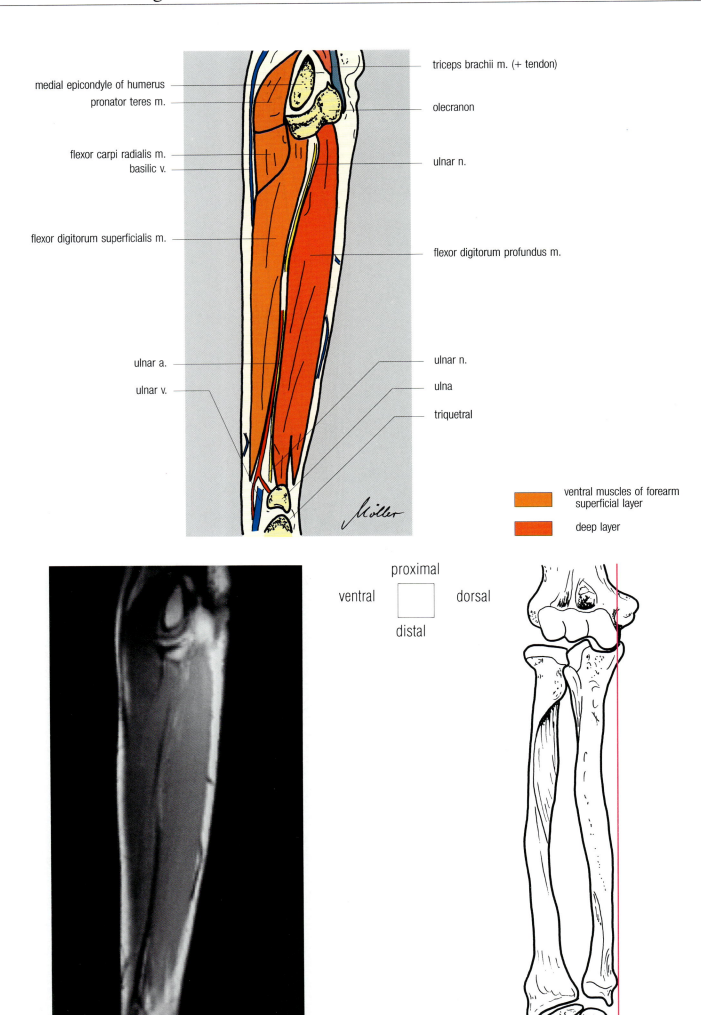

Forearm – Sagittal

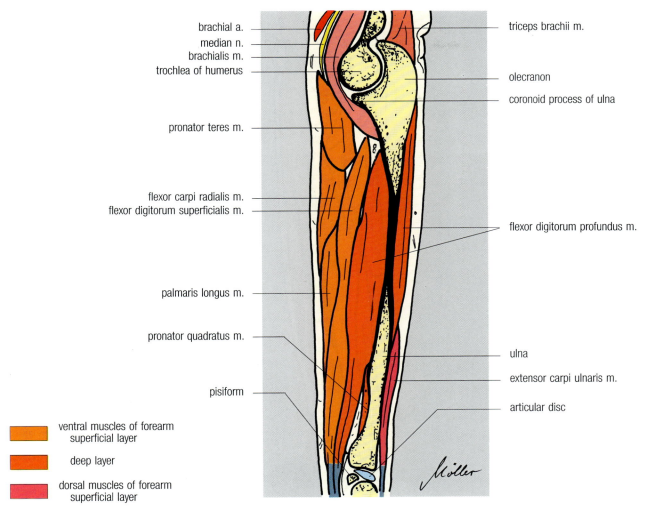

- brachial a.
- median n.
- brachialis m.
- trochlea of humerus
- pronator teres m.
- flexor carpi radialis m.
- flexor digitorum superficialis m.
- palmaris longus m.
- pronator quadratus m.
- pisiform
- triceps brachii m.
- olecranon
- coronoid process of ulna
- flexor digitorum profundus m.
- ulna
- extensor carpi ulnaris m.
- articular disc

■ ventral muscles of forearm superficial layer
■ deep layer
■ dorsal muscles of forearm superficial layer

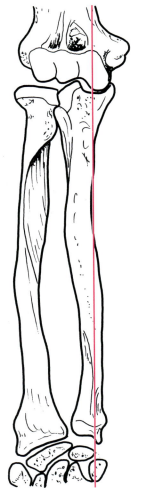

proximal
ventral ☐ dorsal
distal

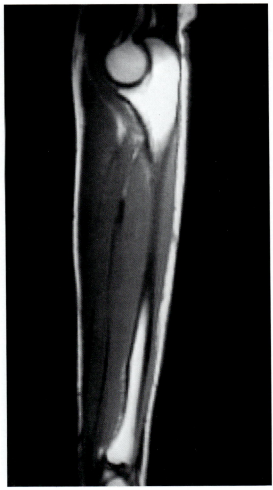

Forearm – Sagittal

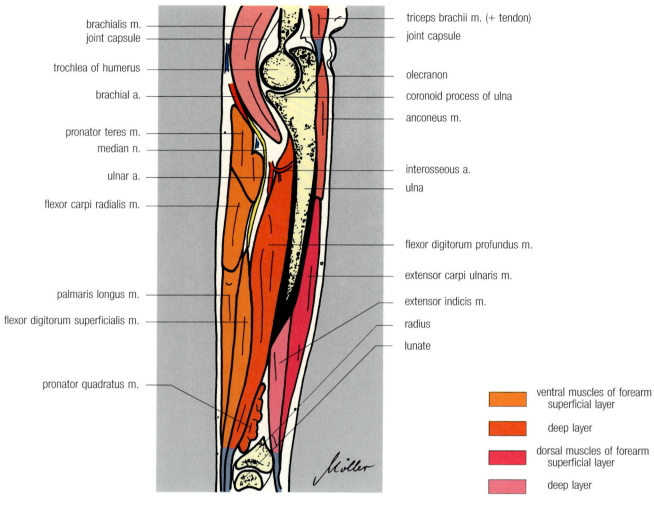

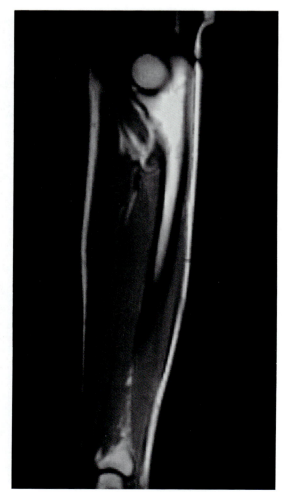

Forearm – Sagittal

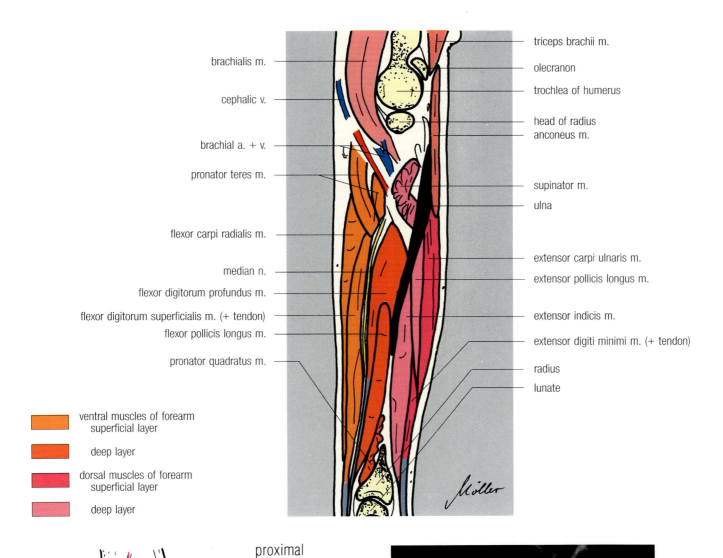
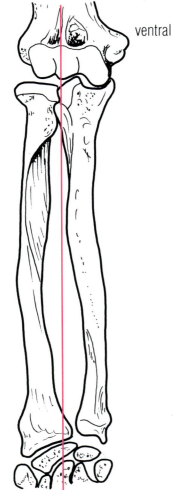
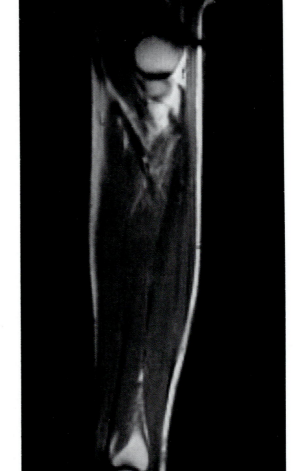

112 Forearm – Sagittal

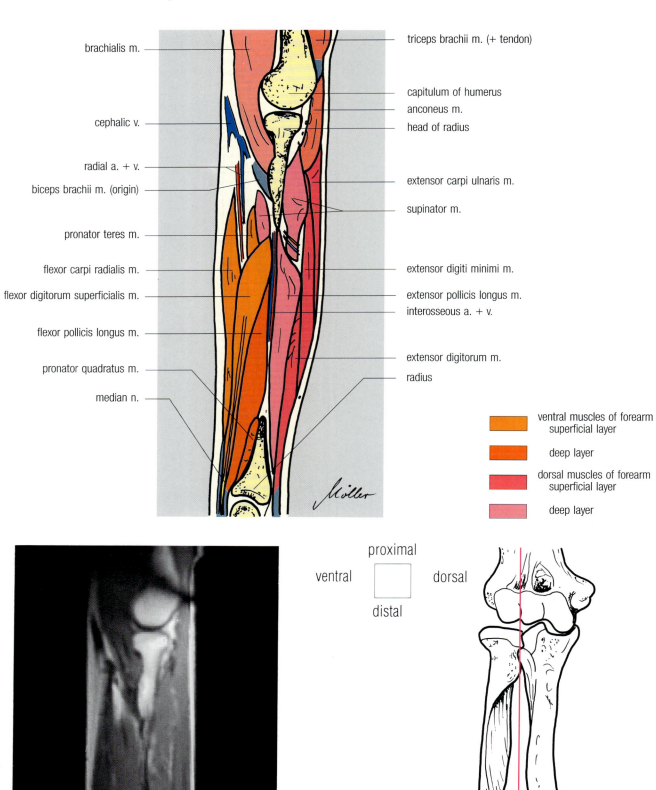

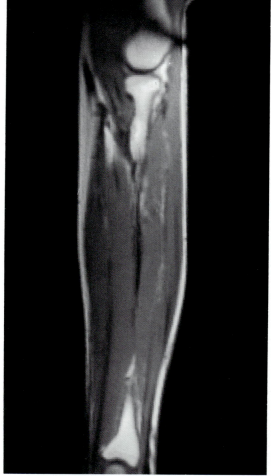
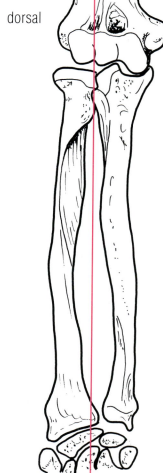

Forearm – Sagittal

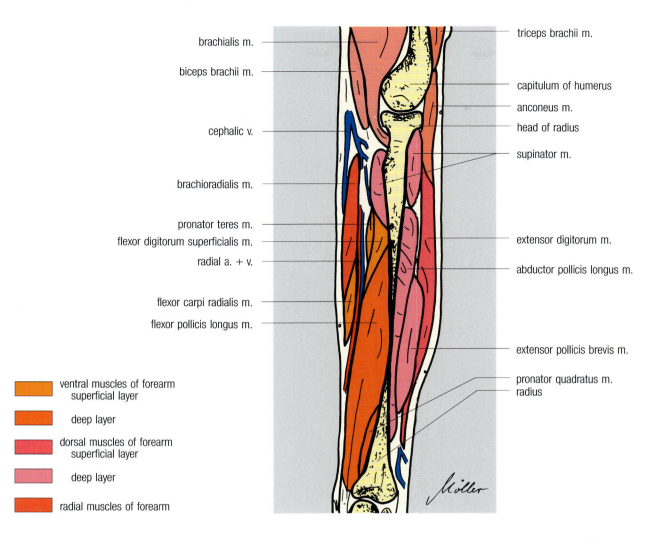

- brachialis m.
- biceps brachii m.
- cephalic v.
- brachioradialis m.
- pronator teres m.
- flexor digitorum superficialis m.
- radial a. + v.
- flexor carpi radialis m.
- flexor pollicis longus m.

- triceps brachii m.
- capitulum of humerus
- anconeus m.
- head of radius
- supinator m.
- extensor digitorum m.
- abductor pollicis longus m.
- extensor pollicis brevis m.
- pronator quadratus m.
- radius

- ventral muscles of forearm superficial layer
- deep layer
- dorsal muscles of forearm superficial layer
- deep layer
- radial muscles of forearm

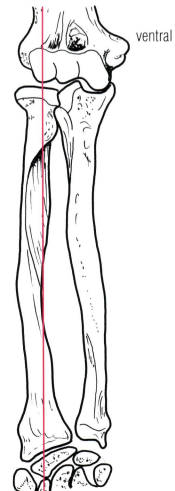

proximal
ventral dorsal
distal

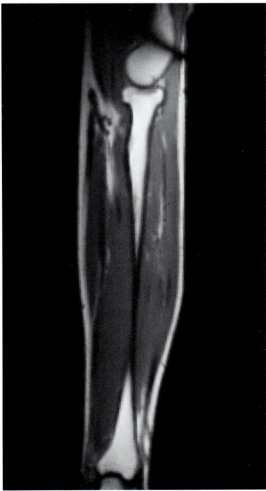

Forearm – Sagittal

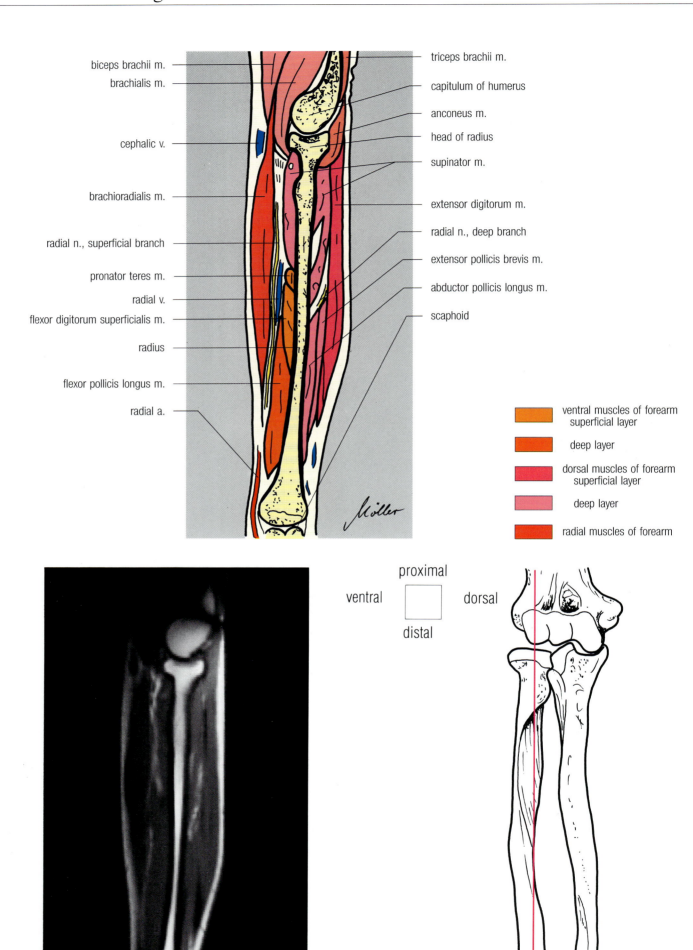

Forearm – Sagittal

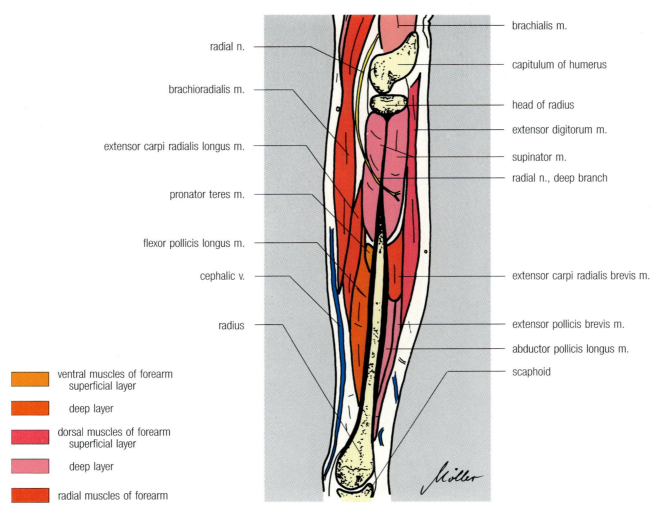

- radial n.
- brachioradialis m.
- extensor carpi radialis longus m.
- pronator teres m.
- flexor pollicis longus m.
- cephalic v.
- radius

- brachialis m.
- capitulum of humerus
- head of radius
- extensor digitorum m.
- supinator m.
- radial n., deep branch
- extensor carpi radialis brevis m.
- extensor pollicis brevis m.
- abductor pollicis longus m.
- scaphoid

- ventral muscles of forearm superficial layer
- deep layer
- dorsal muscles of forearm superficial layer
- deep layer
- radial muscles of forearm

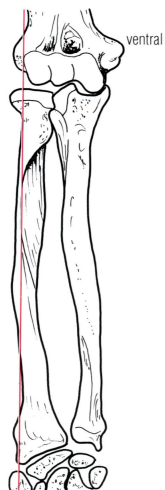

proximal
ventral — dorsal
distal

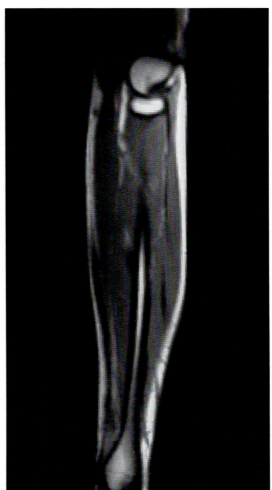

Forearm – Sagittal

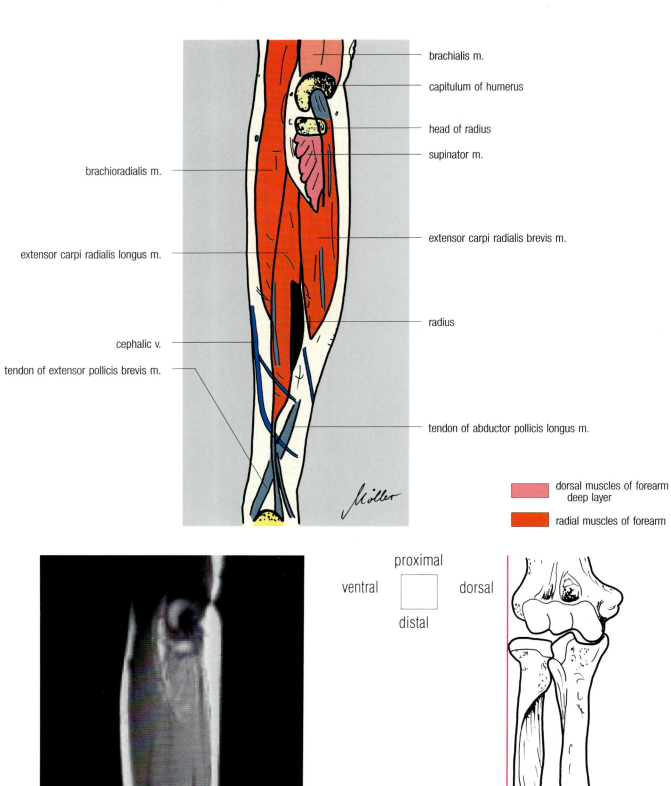

- brachialis m.
- capitulum of humerus
- head of radius
- supinator m.
- brachioradialis m.
- extensor carpi radialis brevis m.
- extensor carpi radialis longus m.
- radius
- cephalic v.
- tendon of extensor pollicis brevis m.
- tendon of abductor pollicis longus m.

dorsal muscles of forearm deep layer

radial muscles of forearm

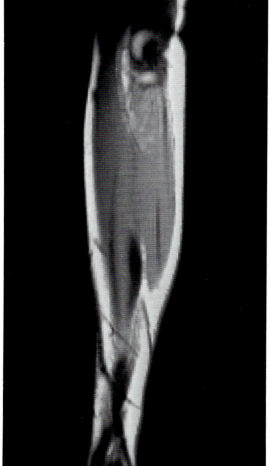

proximal
ventral — dorsal
distal

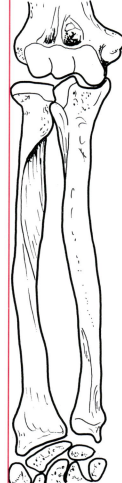

Wrist and Hand
Coronal
Sagittal

Wrist and Hand – Coronal

119

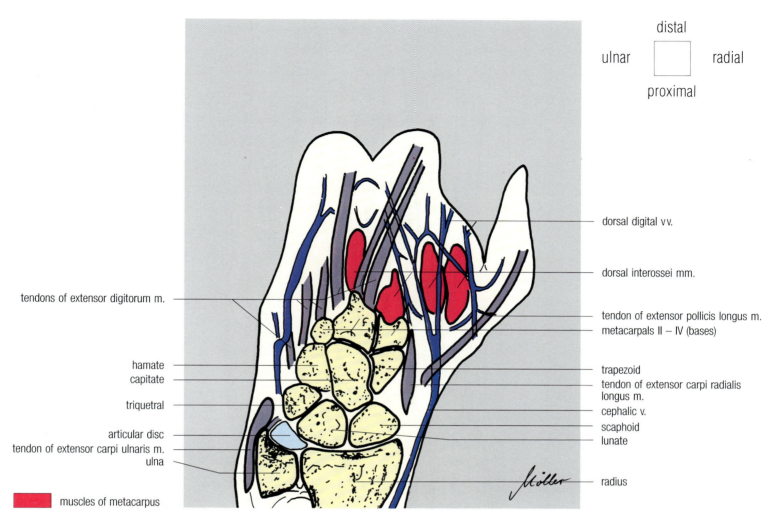

distal
ulnar   radial
proximal

- dorsal digital vv.
- dorsal interossei mm.
- tendons of extensor digitorum m.
- tendon of extensor pollicis longus m.
- metacarpals II – IV (bases)
- hamate
- capitate
- trapezoid
- tendon of extensor carpi radialis longus m.
- triquetral
- cephalic v.
- articular disc
- scaphoid
- tendon of extensor carpi ulnaris m.
- lunate
- ulna
- radius

■ muscles of metacarpus

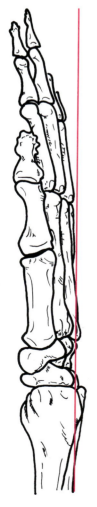

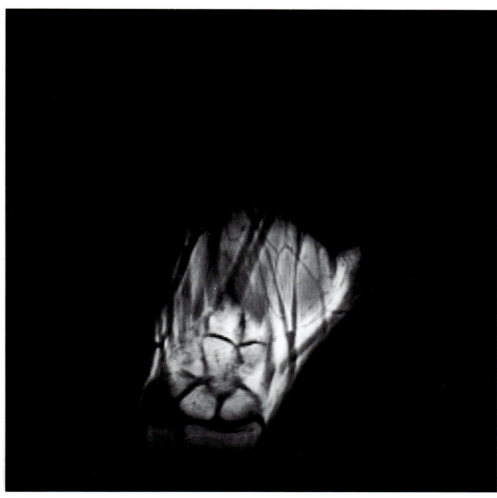

Wrist and Hand – Coronal

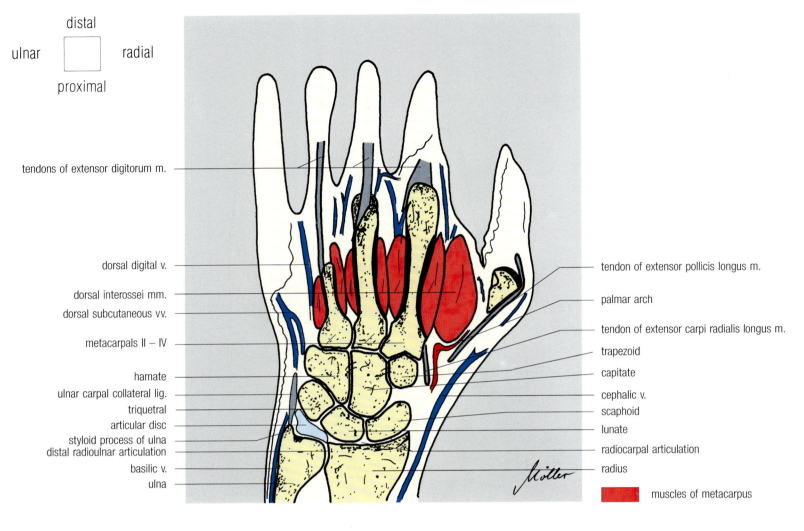

distal
ulnar □ radial
proximal

- tendons of extensor digitorum m.
- dorsal digital v.
- dorsal interossei mm.
- dorsal subcutaneous vv.
- metacarpals II – IV
- hamate
- ulnar carpal collateral lig.
- triquetral
- articular disc
- styloid process of ulna
- distal radioulnar articulation
- basilic v.
- ulna

- tendon of extensor pollicis longus m.
- palmar arch
- tendon of extensor carpi radialis longus m.
- trapezoid
- capitate
- cephalic v.
- scaphoid
- lunate
- radiocarpal articulation
- radius

■ muscles of metacarpus

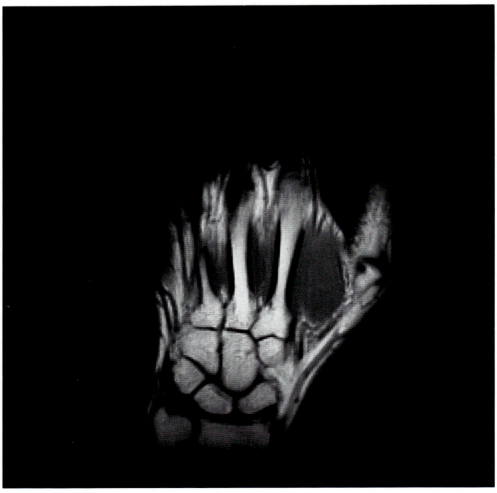
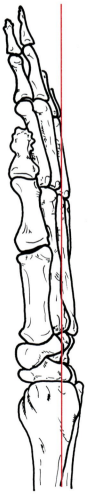

Wrist and Hand – Coronal

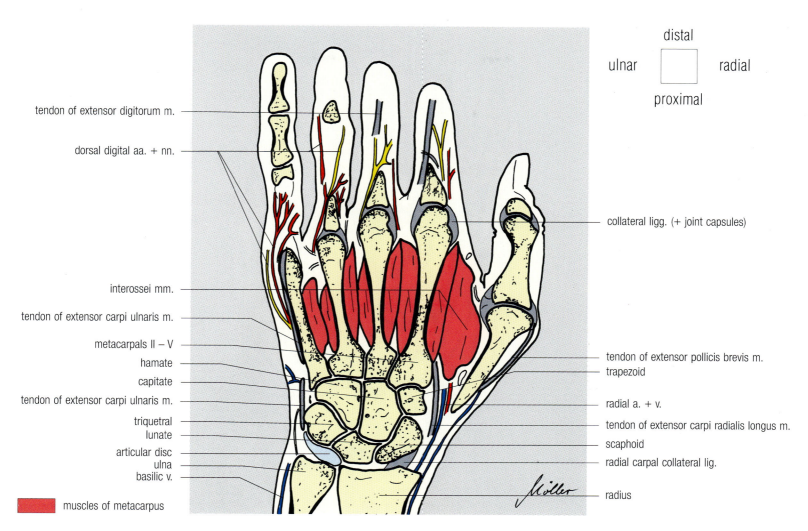

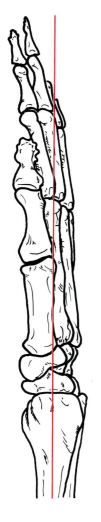
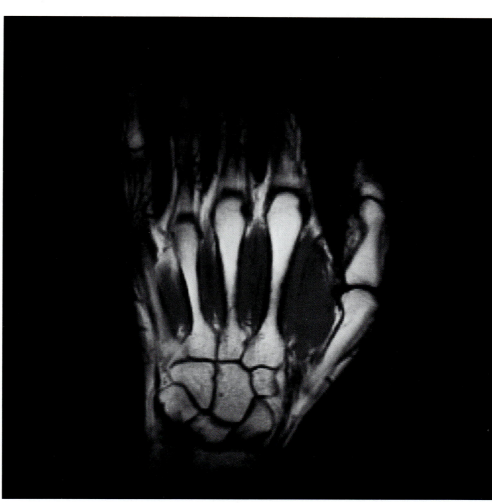

Wrist and Hand – Coronal

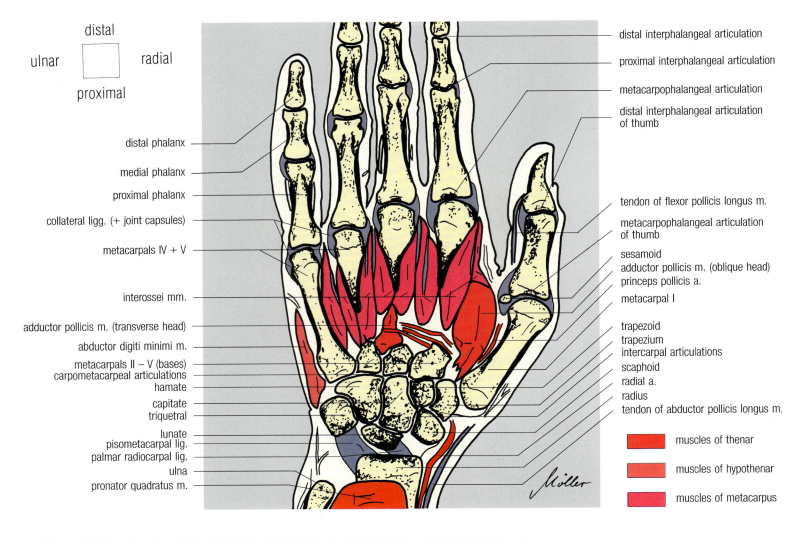
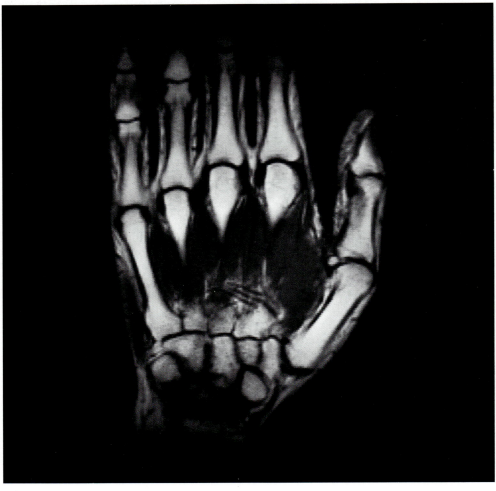
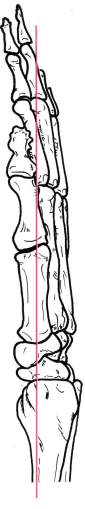

Wrist and Hand – Coronal

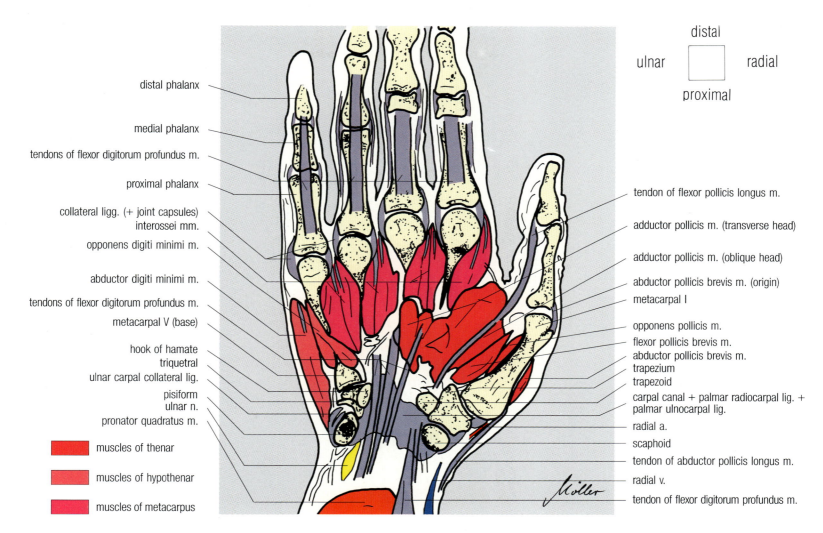

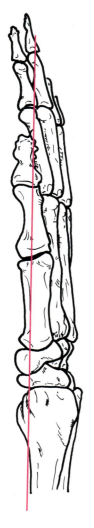
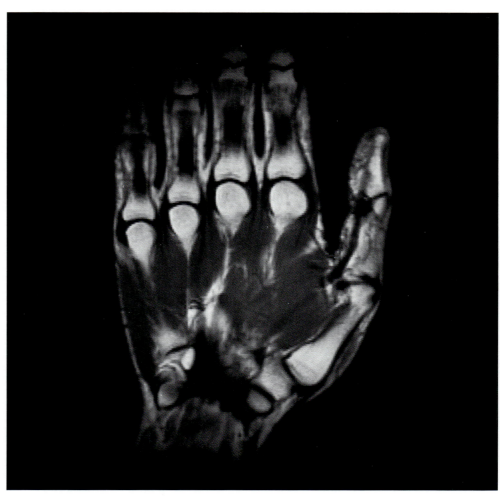

124 Wrist and Hand – Coronal

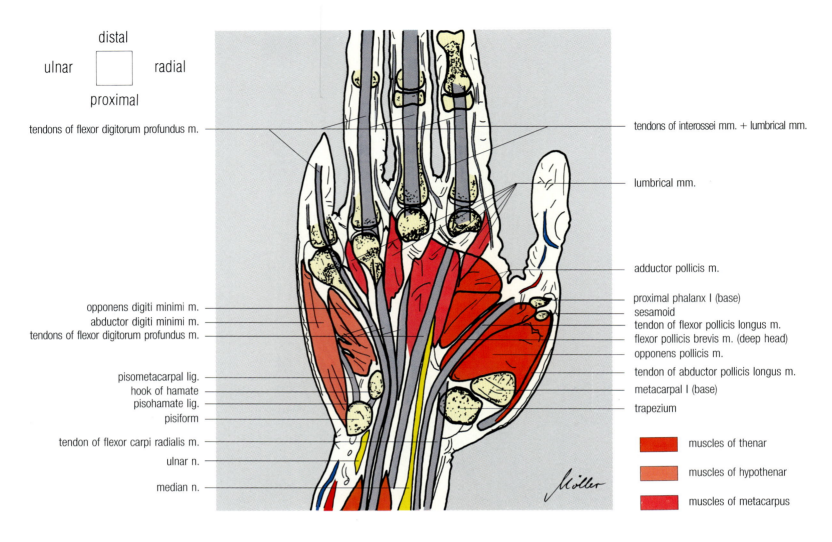

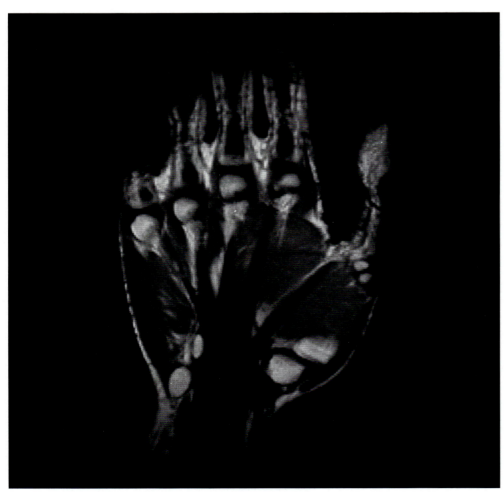
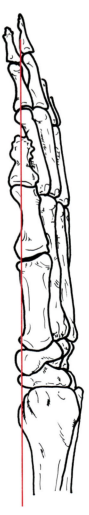

Wrist and Hand – Coronal

125

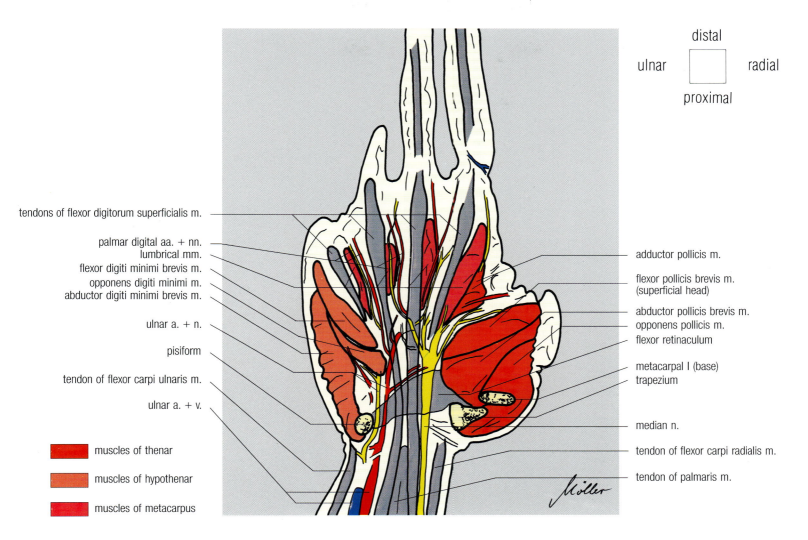

distal
ulnar   radial
proximal

- tendons of flexor digitorum superficialis m.
- palmar digital aa. + nn.
- lumbrical mm.
- flexor digiti minimi brevis m.
- opponens digiti minimi m.
- abductor digiti minimi brevis m.
- ulnar a. + n.
- pisiform
- tendon of flexor carpi ulnaris m.
- ulnar a. + v.

- adductor pollicis m.
- flexor pollicis brevis m. (superficial head)
- abductor pollicis brevis m.
- opponens pollicis m.
- flexor retinaculum
- metacarpal I (base)
- trapezium
- median n.
- tendon of flexor carpi radialis m.
- tendon of palmaris m.

- muscles of thenar
- muscles of hypothenar
- muscles of metacarpus

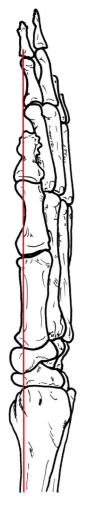

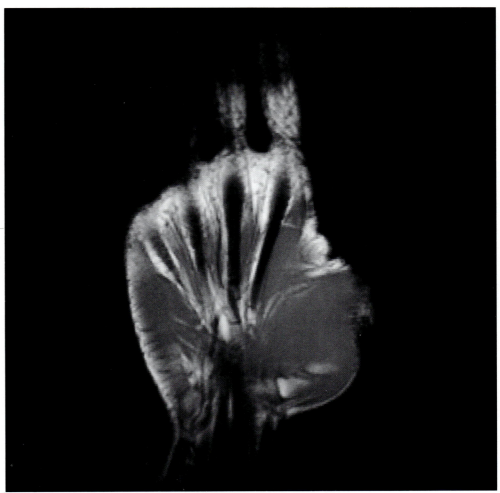

Wrist and Hand – Sagittal

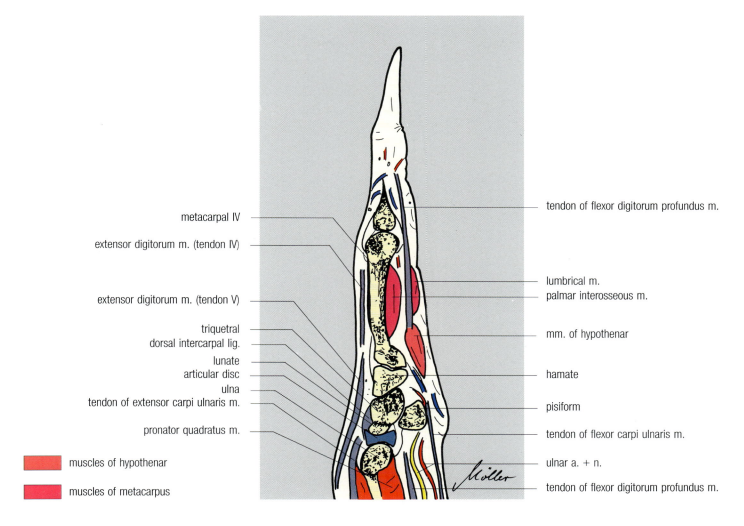

- metacarpal IV
- extensor digitorum m. (tendon IV)
- extensor digitorum m. (tendon V)
- triquetral
- dorsal intercarpal lig.
- lunate
- articular disc
- ulna
- tendon of extensor carpi ulnaris m.
- pronator quadratus m.

- tendon of flexor digitorum profundus m.
- lumbrical m.
- palmar interosseous m.
- mm. of hypothenar
- hamate
- pisiform
- tendon of flexor carpi ulnaris m.
- ulnar a. + n.
- tendon of flexor digitorum profundus m.

■ muscles of hypothenar
■ muscles of metacarpus

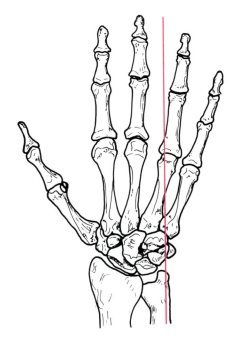

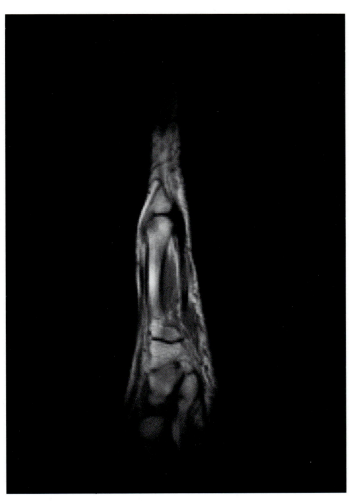

distal
dorsal · palmar
proximal

Wrist and Hand – Sagittal

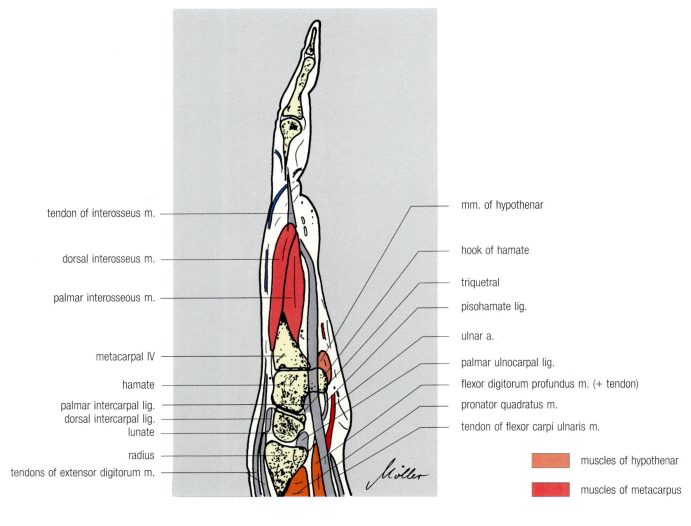

- tendon of interosseus m.
- dorsal interosseus m.
- palmar interosseous m.
- metacarpal IV
- hamate
- palmar intercarpal lig.
- dorsal intercarpal lig.
- lunate
- radius
- tendons of extensor digitorum m.

- mm. of hypothenar
- hook of hamate
- triquetral
- pisohamate lig.
- ulnar a.
- palmar ulnocarpal lig.
- flexor digitorum profundus m. (+ tendon)
- pronator quadratus m.
- tendon of flexor carpi ulnaris m.

■ muscles of hypothenar
■ muscles of metacarpus

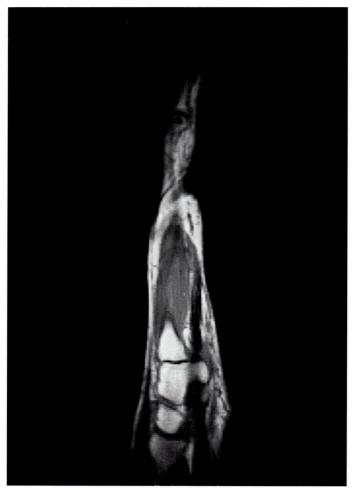

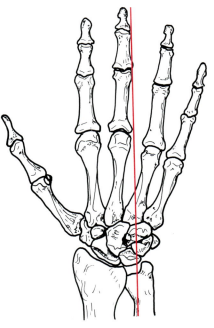

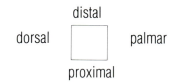

Wrist and Hand – Sagittal

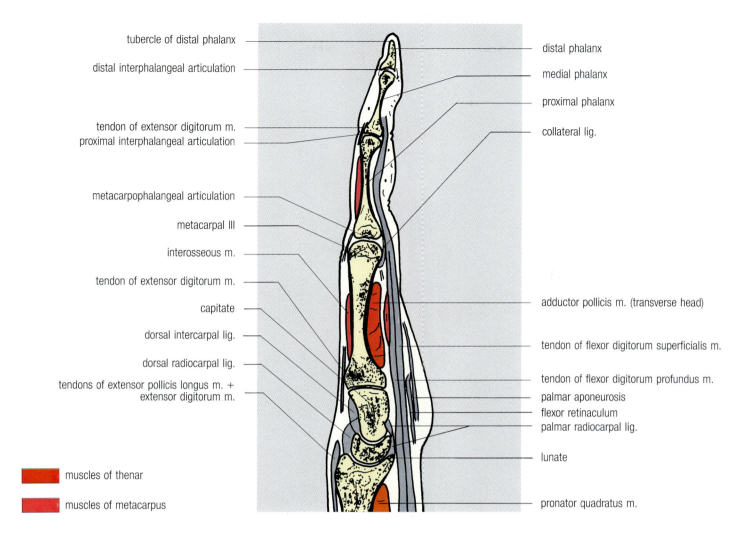

- tubercle of distal phalanx
- distal interphalangeal articulation
- tendon of extensor digitorum m.
- proximal interphalangeal articulation
- metacarpophalangeal articulation
- metacarpal III
- interosseous m.
- tendon of extensor digitorum m.
- capitate
- dorsal intercarpal lig.
- dorsal radiocarpal lig.
- tendons of extensor pollicis longus m. + extensor digitorum m.

- distal phalanx
- medial phalanx
- proximal phalanx
- collateral lig.
- adductor pollicis m. (transverse head)
- tendon of flexor digitorum superficialis m.
- tendon of flexor digitorum profundus m.
- palmar aponeurosis
- flexor retinaculum
- palmar radiocarpal lig.
- lunate
- pronator quadratus m.

■ muscles of thenar
■ muscles of metacarpus

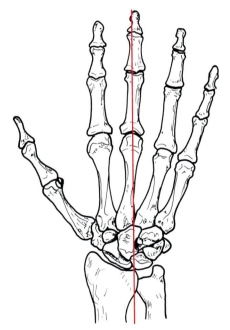

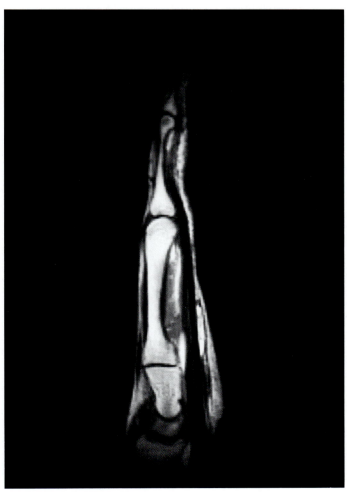

dorsal — distal / palmar / proximal

130 Wrist and Hand – Sagittal

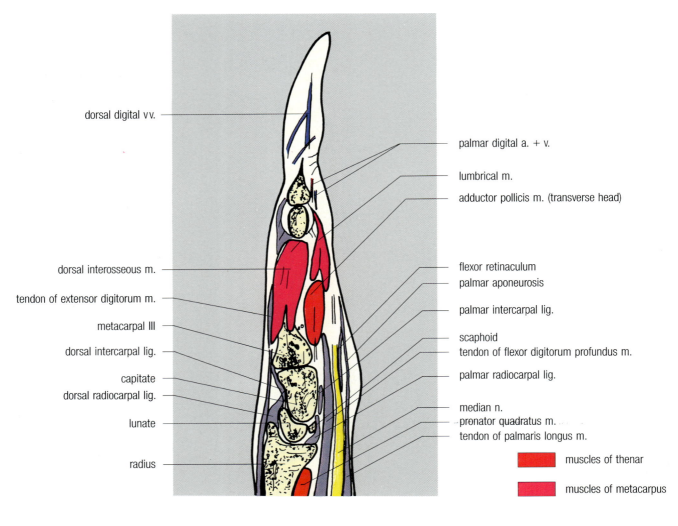

- dorsal digital v v.
- dorsal interosseous m.
- tendon of extensor digitorum m.
- metacarpal III
- dorsal intercarpal lig.
- capitate
- dorsal radiocarpal lig.
- lunate
- radius

- palmar digital a. + v.
- lumbrical m.
- adductor pollicis m. (transverse head)
- flexor retinaculum
- palmar aponeurosis
- palmar intercarpal lig.
- scaphoid
- tendon of flexor digitorum profundus m.
- palmar radiocarpal lig.
- median n.
- pronator quadratus m.
- tendon of palmaris longus m.

■ muscles of thenar
■ muscles of metacarpus

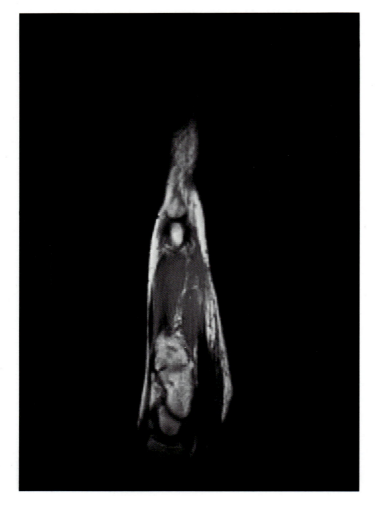

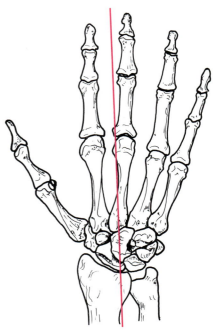

distal
dorsal ☐ palmar
proximal

Wrist and Hand – Sagittal

131

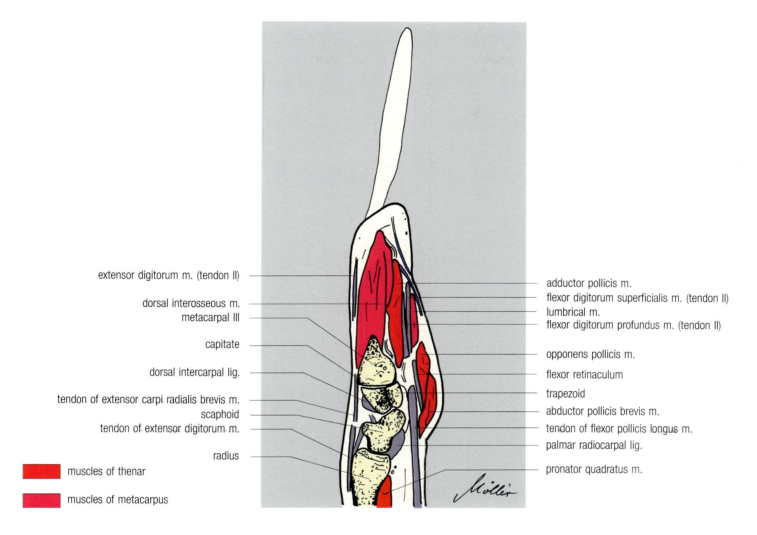

- extensor digitorum m. (tendon II)
- dorsal interosseous m.
- metacarpal III
- capitate
- dorsal intercarpal lig.
- tendon of extensor carpi radialis brevis m.
- scaphoid
- tendon of extensor digitorum m.
- radius

- adductor pollicis m.
- flexor digitorum superficialis m. (tendon II)
- lumbrical m.
- flexor digitorum profundus m. (tendon II)
- opponens pollicis m.
- flexor retinaculum
- trapezoid
- abductor pollicis brevis m.
- tendon of flexor pollicis longus m.
- palmar radiocarpal lig.
- pronator quadratus m.

■ muscles of thenar
■ muscles of metacarpus

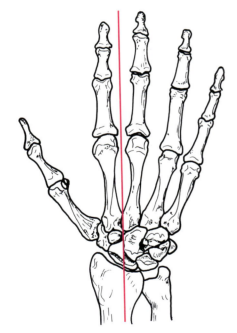

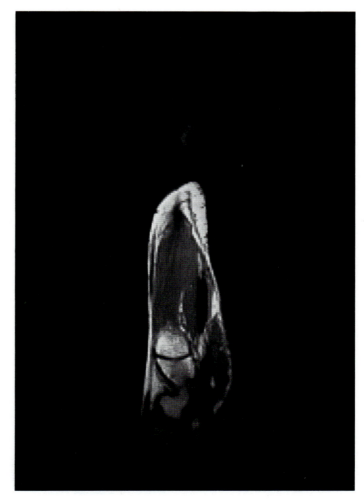

distal
dorsal — palmar
proximal

Wrist and Hand – Sagittal

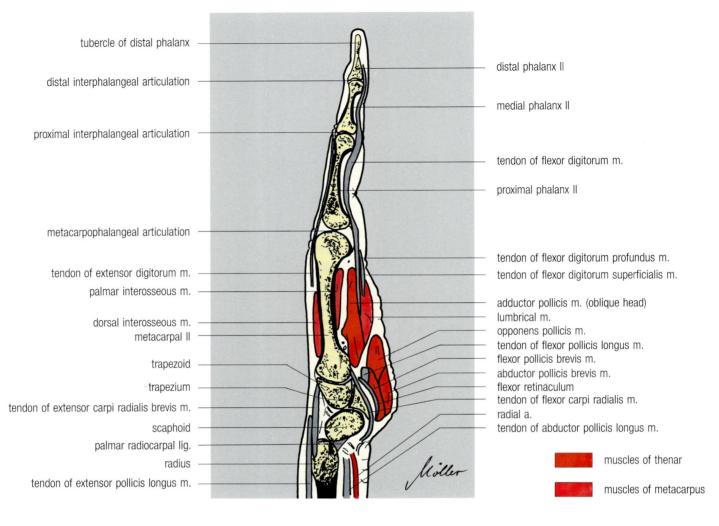

- tubercle of distal phalanx
- distal interphalangeal articulation
- proximal interphalangeal articulation
- metacarpophalangeal articulation
- tendon of extensor digitorum m.
- palmar interosseous m.
- dorsal interosseous m.
- metacarpal II
- trapezoid
- trapezium
- tendon of extensor carpi radialis brevis m.
- scaphoid
- palmar radiocarpal lig.
- radius
- tendon of extensor pollicis longus m.

- distal phalanx II
- medial phalanx II
- tendon of flexor digitorum m.
- proximal phalanx II
- tendon of flexor digitorum profundus m.
- tendon of flexor digitorum superficialis m.
- adductor pollicis m. (oblique head)
- lumbrical m.
- opponens pollicis m.
- tendon of flexor pollicis longus m.
- flexor pollicis brevis m.
- abductor pollicis brevis m.
- flexor retinaculum
- tendon of flexor carpi radialis m.
- radial a.
- tendon of abductor pollicis longus m.

■ muscles of thenar
■ muscles of metacarpus

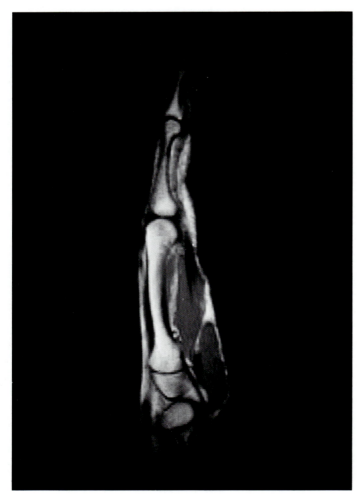

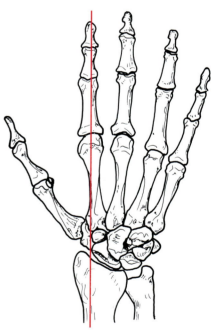

distal
dorsal palmar
proximal

Lower Limbs

Lower Limbs Axial

Hip

Thigh

Knee

Lower Leg

Ankle and Foot

Lower Limbs Axial – Hip

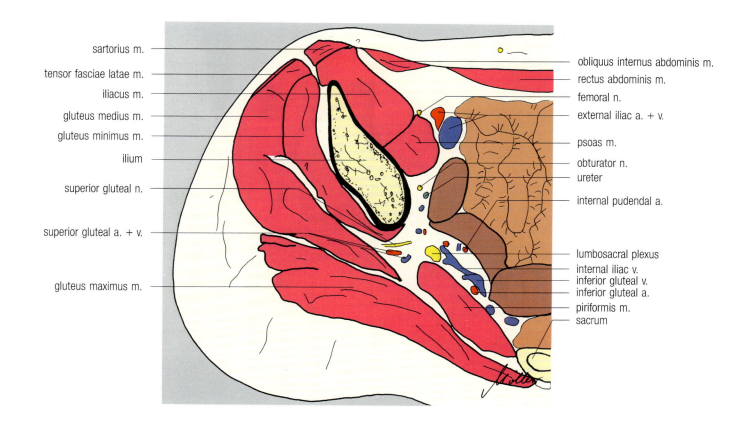

sartorius m.
tensor fasciae latae m.
iliacus m.
gluteus medius m.
gluteus minimus m.
ilium
superior gluteal n.
superior gluteal a. + v.
gluteus maximus m.

obliquus internus abdominis m.
rectus abdominis m.
femoral n.
external iliac a. + v.
psoas m.
obturator n.
ureter
internal pudendal a.
lumbosacral plexus
internal iliac v.
inferior gluteal v.
inferior gluteal a.
piriformis m.
sacrum

ventral
lateral | | medial
dorsal

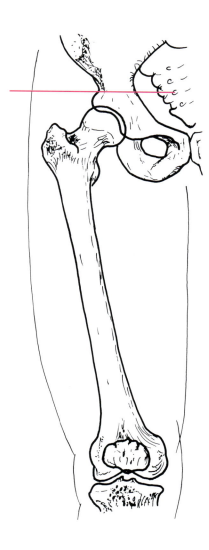

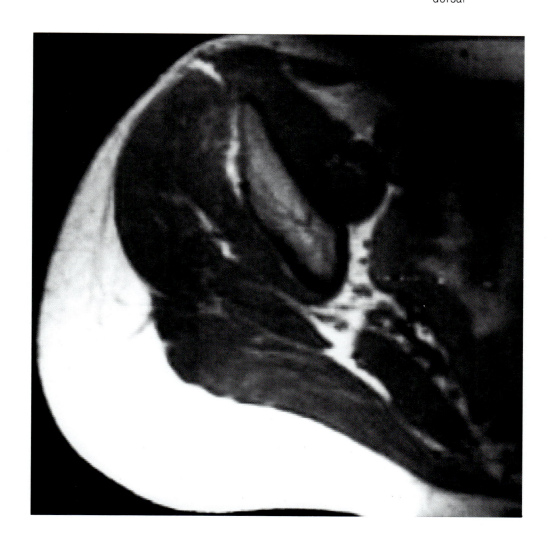

Lower Limbs Axial – Hip

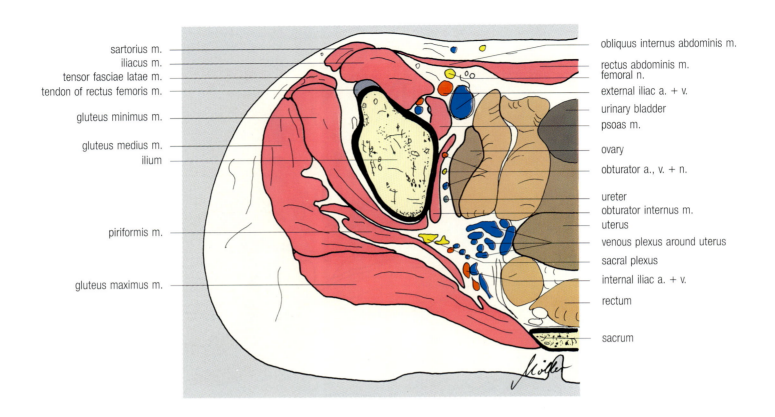

- sartorius m.
- iliacus m.
- tensor fasciae latae m.
- tendon of rectus femoris m.
- gluteus minimus m.
- gluteus medius m.
- ilium
- piriformis m.
- gluteus maximus m.
- obliquus internus abdominis m.
- rectus abdominis m.
- femoral n.
- external iliac a. + v.
- urinary bladder
- psoas m.
- ovary
- obturator a., v. + n.
- ureter
- obturator internus m.
- uterus
- venous plexus around uterus
- sacral plexus
- internal iliac a. + v.
- rectum
- sacrum

```
         ventral
lateral  ☐  medial
         dorsal
```

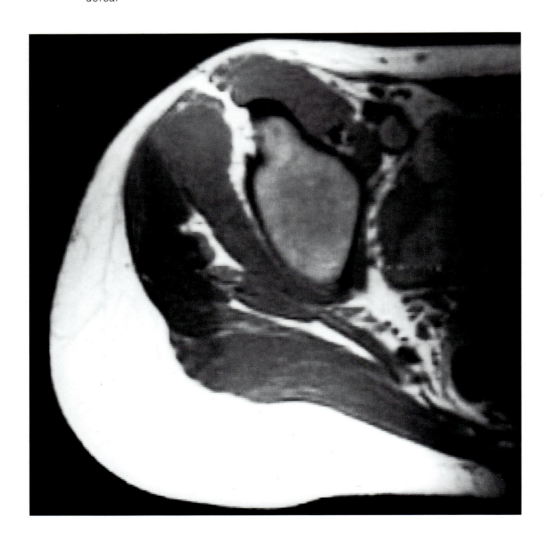
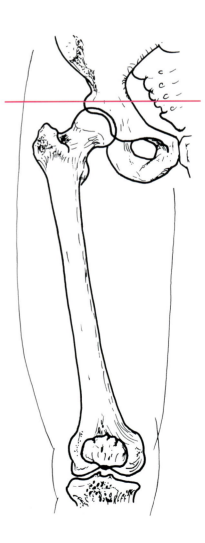

Lower Limbs Axial – Hip

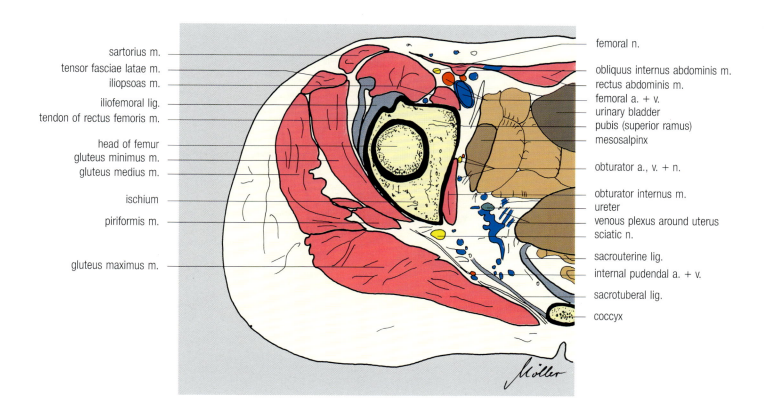

- sartorius m.
- tensor fasciae latae m.
- iliopsoas m.
- iliofemoral lig.
- tendon of rectus femoris m.
- head of femur
- gluteus minimus m.
- gluteus medius m.
- ischium
- piriformis m.
- gluteus maximus m.

- femoral n.
- obliquus internus abdominis m.
- rectus abdominis m.
- femoral a. + v.
- urinary bladder
- pubis (superior ramus)
- mesosalpinx
- obturator a., v. + n.
- obturator internus m.
- ureter
- venous plexus around uterus
- sciatic n.
- sacrouterine lig.
- internal pudendal a. + v.
- sacrotuberal lig.
- coccyx

```
        ventral
lateral  □  medial
        dorsal
```

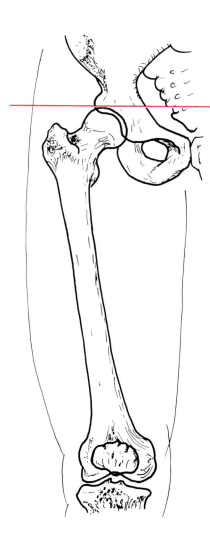

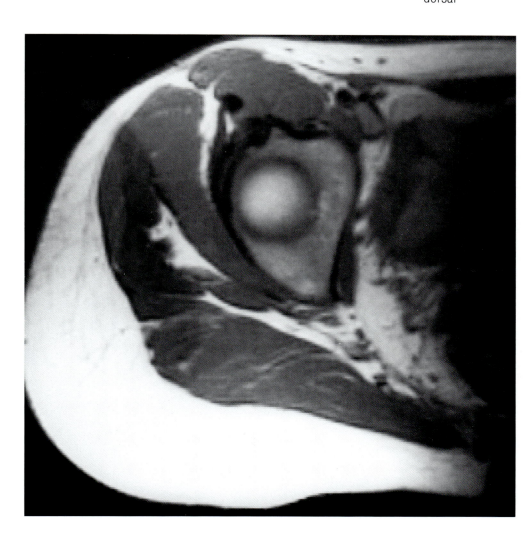

140 Lower Limbs Axial – Hip

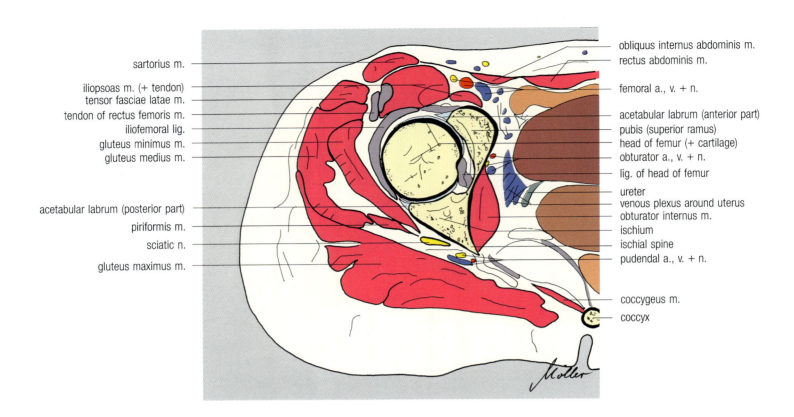

sartorius m.
iliopsoas m. (+ tendon)
tensor fasciae latae m.
tendon of rectus femoris m.
iliofemoral lig.
gluteus minimus m.
gluteus medius m.

acetabular labrum (posterior part)
piriformis m.
sciatic n.
gluteus maximus m.

obliquus internus abdominis m.
rectus abdominis m.
femoral a., v. + n.
acetabular labrum (anterior part)
pubis (superior ramus)
head of femur (+ cartilage)
obturator a., v. + n.
lig. of head of femur
ureter
venous plexus around uterus
obturator internus m.
ischium
ischial spine
pudendal a., v. + n.
coccygeus m.
coccyx

ventral
lateral | medial
dorsal

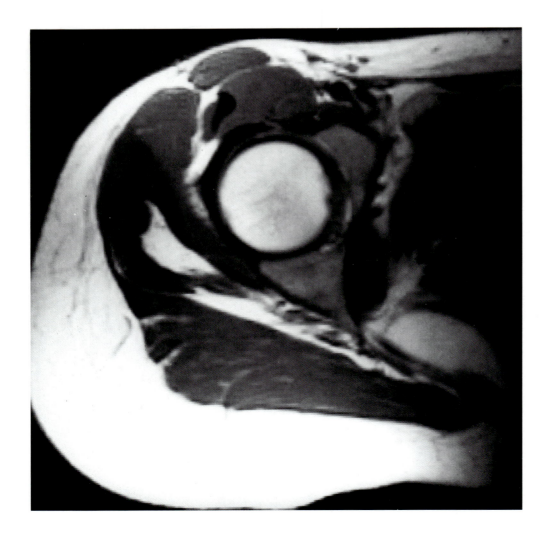
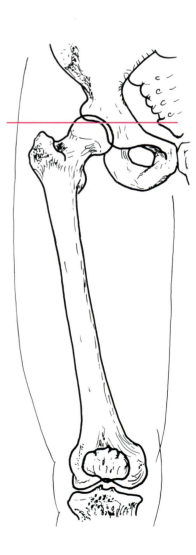

Lower Limbs Axial – Hip

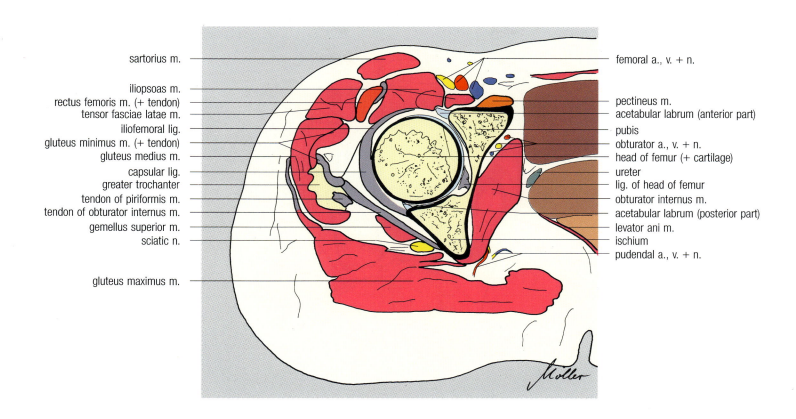

- sartorius m.
- iliopsoas m.
- rectus femoris m. (+ tendon)
- tensor fasciae latae m.
- iliofemoral lig.
- gluteus minimus m. (+ tendon)
- gluteus medius m.
- capsular lig.
- greater trochanter
- tendon of piriformis m.
- tendon of obturator internus m.
- gemellus superior m.
- sciatic n.
- gluteus maximus m.

- femoral a., v. + n.
- pectineus m.
- acetabular labrum (anterior part)
- pubis
- obturator a., v. + n.
- head of femur (+ cartilage)
- ureter
- lig. of head of femur
- obturator internus m.
- acetabular labrum (posterior part)
- levator ani m.
- ischium
- pudendal a., v. + n.

- adductor muscles
- quadriceps muscle group
- other muscles

ventral / lateral / medial / dorsal

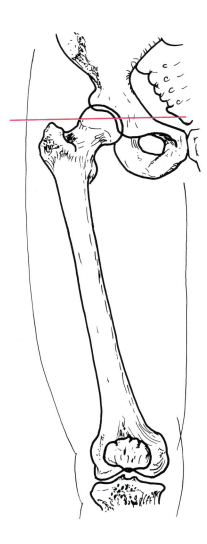

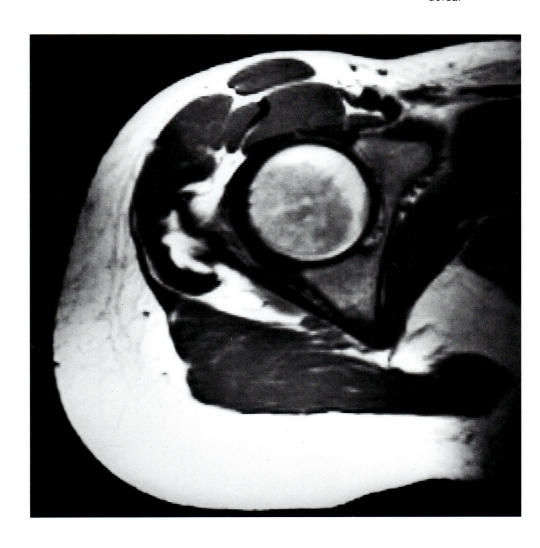

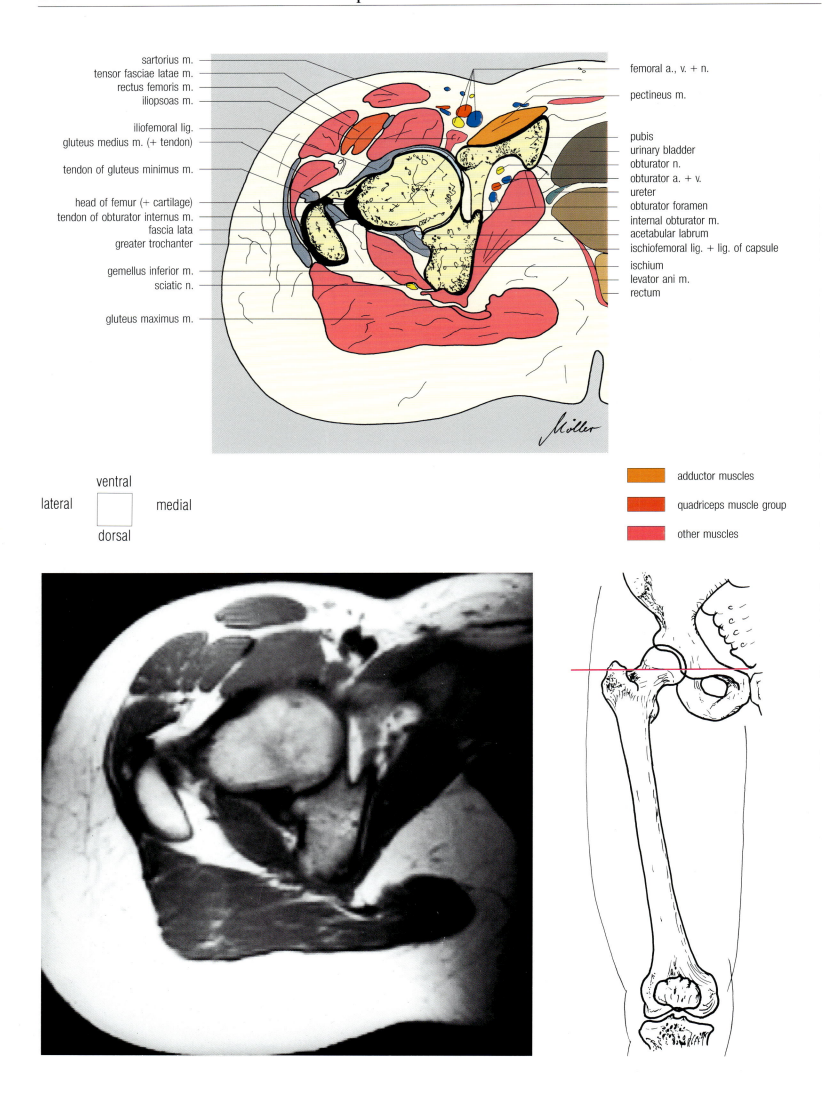

Lower Limbs Axial – Hip

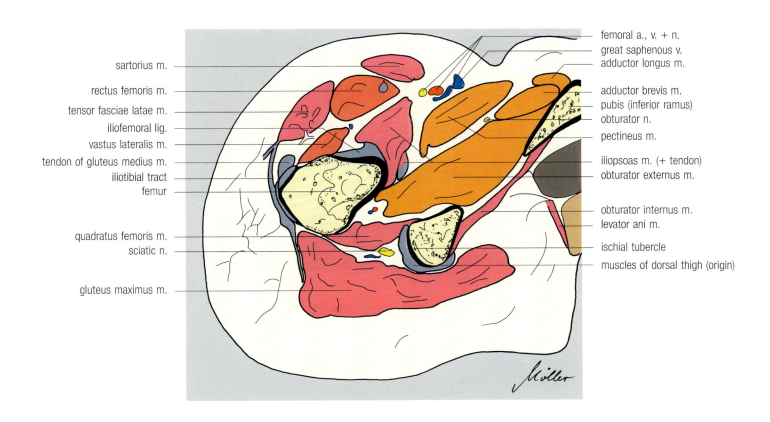

- sartorius m.
- rectus femoris m.
- tensor fasciae latae m.
- iliofemoral lig.
- vastus lateralis m.
- tendon of gluteus medius m.
- iliotibial tract
- femur
- quadratus femoris m.
- sciatic n.
- gluteus maximus m.

- femoral a., v. + n.
- great saphenous v.
- adductor longus m.
- adductor brevis m.
- pubis (inferior ramus)
- obturator n.
- pectineus m.
- iliopsoas m. (+ tendon)
- obturator externus m.
- obturator internus m.
- levator ani m.
- ischial tubercle
- muscles of dorsal thigh (origin)

- adductor muscles
- quadriceps muscle group
- other muscles

ventral / lateral / medial / dorsal

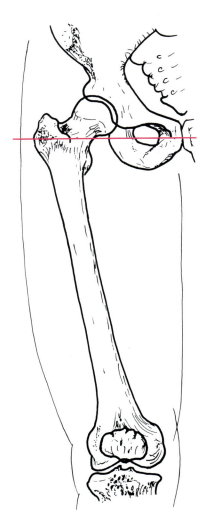

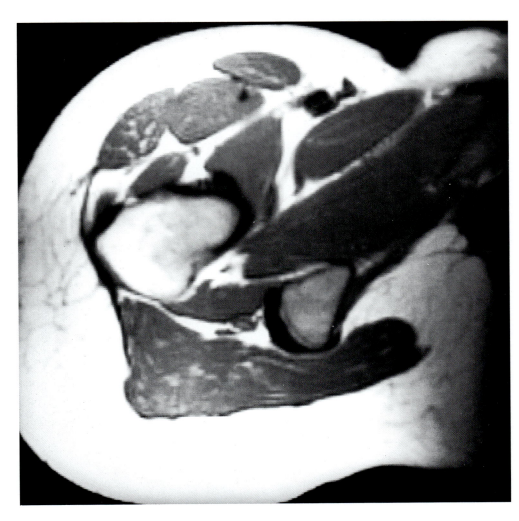

Lower Limbs Axial – Hip

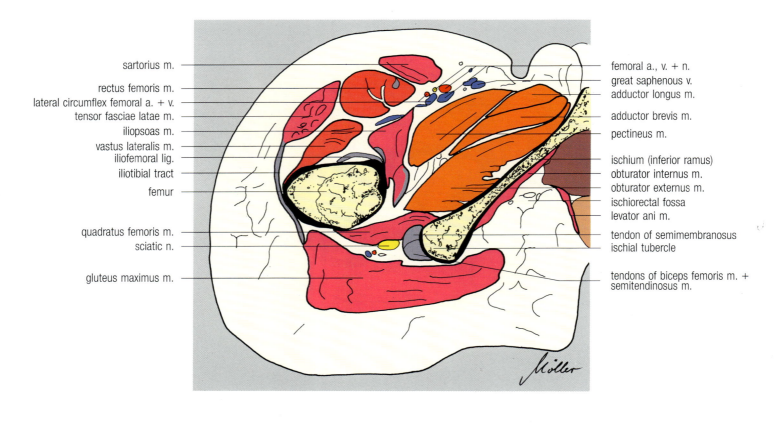

- sartorius m.
- rectus femoris m.
- lateral circumflex femoral a. + v.
- tensor fasciae latae m.
- iliopsoas m.
- vastus lateralis m.
- iliofemoral lig.
- iliotibial tract
- femur
- quadratus femoris m.
- sciatic n.
- gluteus maximus m.

- femoral a., v. + n.
- great saphenous v.
- adductor longus m.
- adductor brevis m.
- pectineus m.
- ischium (inferior ramus)
- obturator internus m.
- obturator externus m.
- ischiorectal fossa
- levator ani m.
- tendon of semimembranosus
- ischial tubercle
- tendons of biceps femoris m. + semitendinosus m.

lateral | ventral / dorsal | medial

- adductor muscles
- quadriceps muscle group
- other muscles

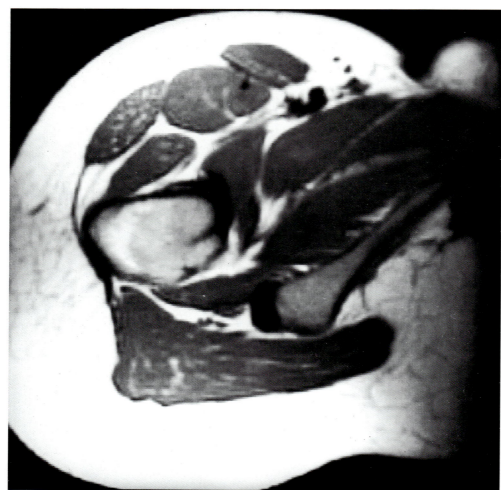

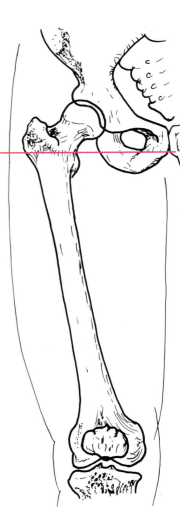

Lower Limbs Axial – Hip

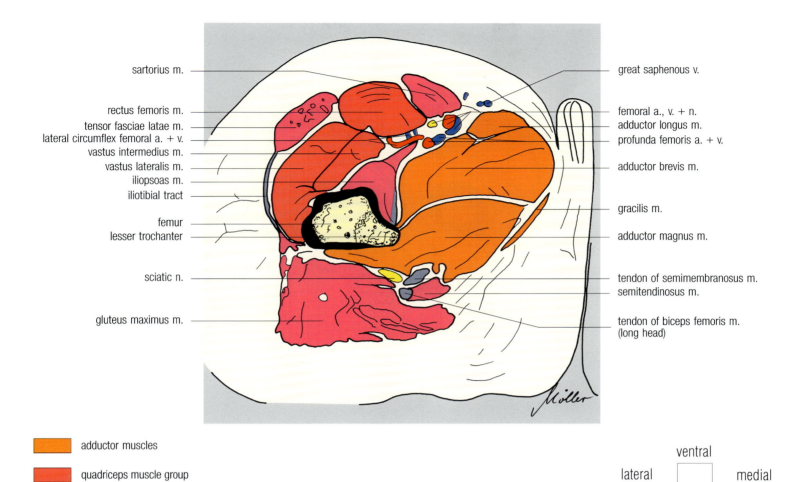

- sartorius m.
- rectus femoris m.
- tensor fasciae latae m.
- lateral circumflex femoral a. + v.
- vastus intermedius m.
- vastus lateralis m.
- iliopsoas m.
- iliotibial tract
- femur
- lesser trochanter
- sciatic n.
- gluteus maximus m.

- great saphenous v.
- femoral a., v. + n.
- adductor longus m.
- profunda femoris a. + v.
- adductor brevis m.
- gracilis m.
- adductor magnus m.
- tendon of semimembranosus m.
- semitendinosus m.
- tendon of biceps femoris m. (long head)

■ adductor muscles
■ quadriceps muscle group
■ other muscles

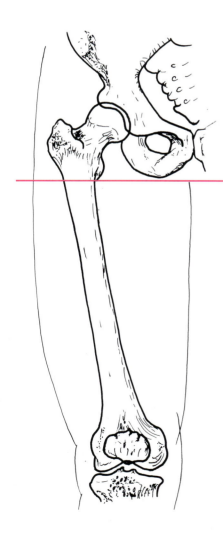

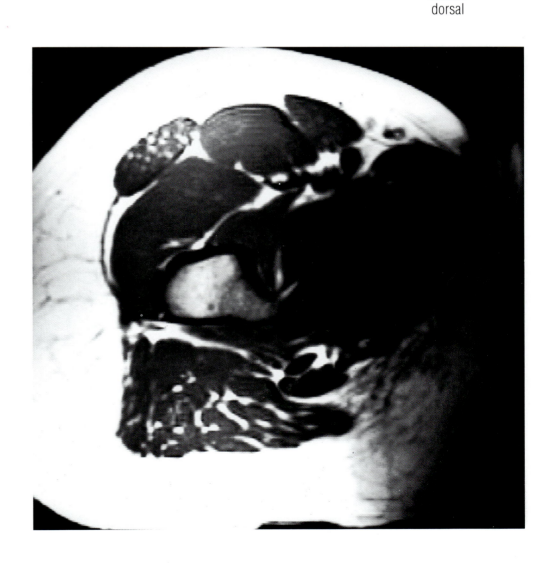

Lower Limbs Axial – Hip

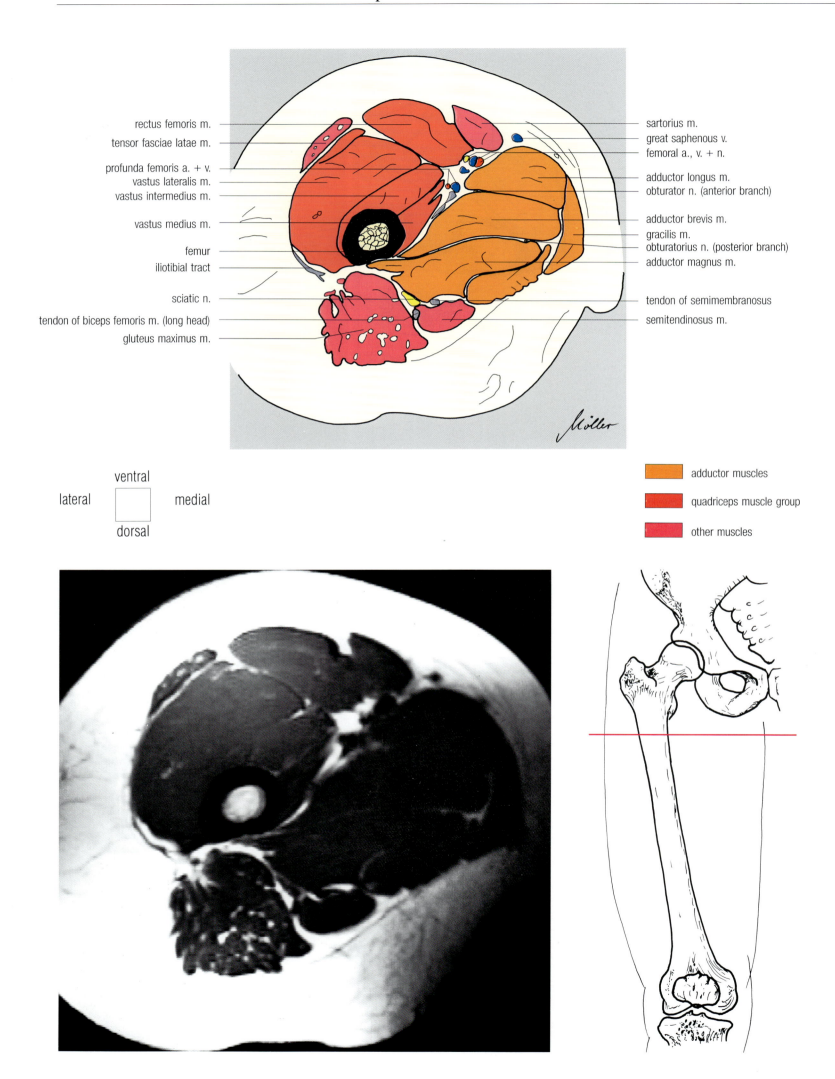

Lower Limbs Axial – Thigh 147

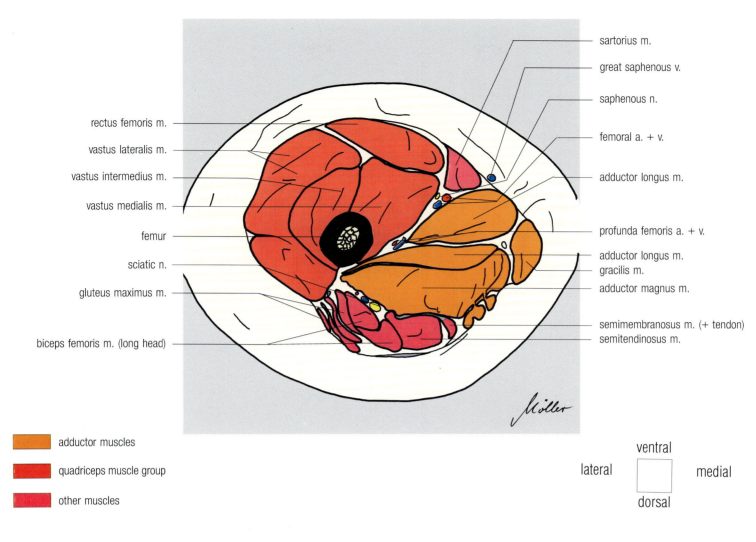

- adductor muscles
- quadriceps muscle group
- other muscles

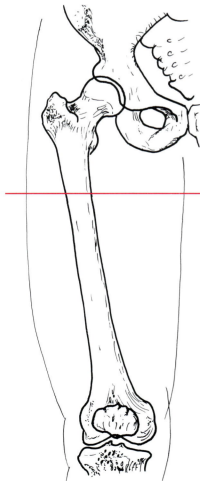

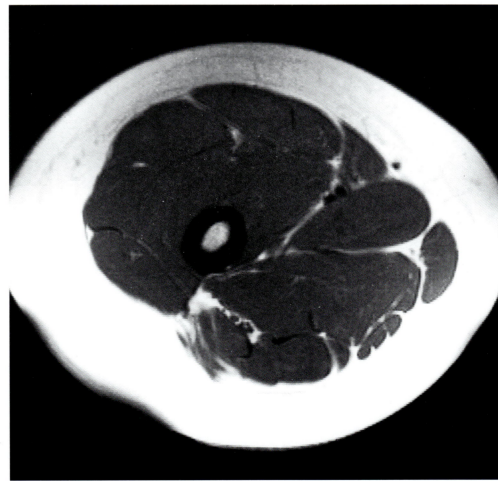

148 Lower Limbs Axial – Thigh

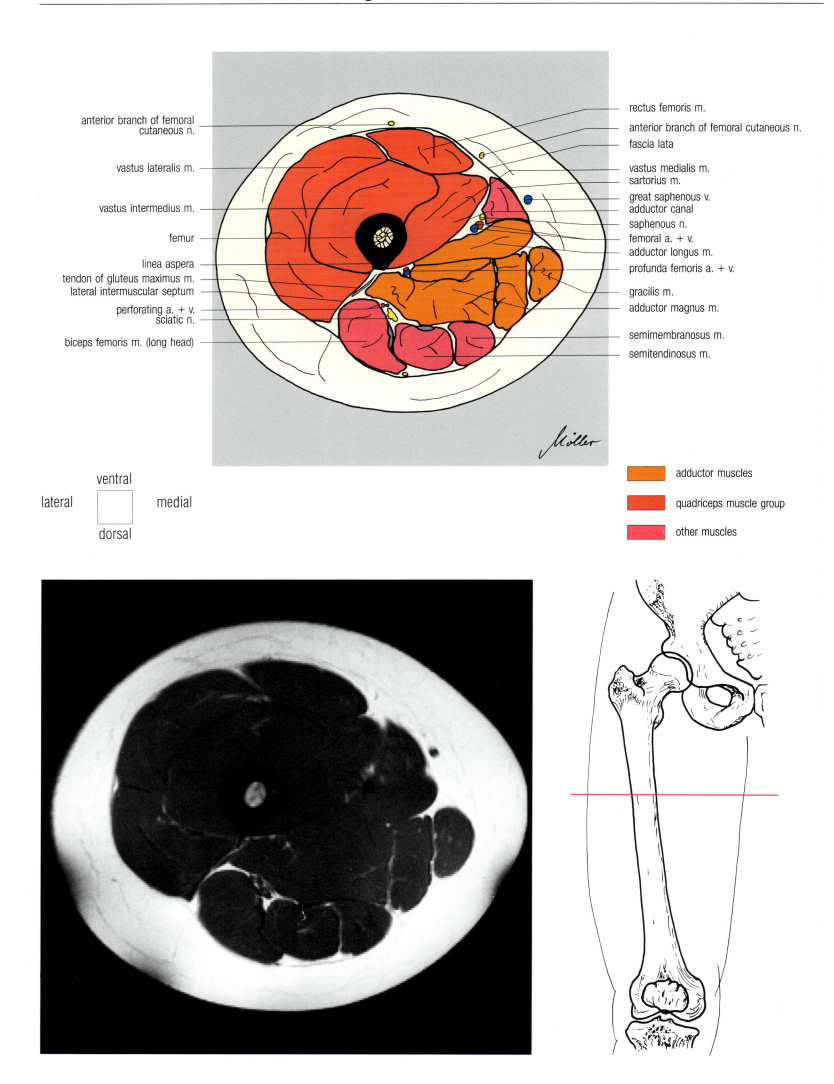

Lower Limbs Axial – Thigh

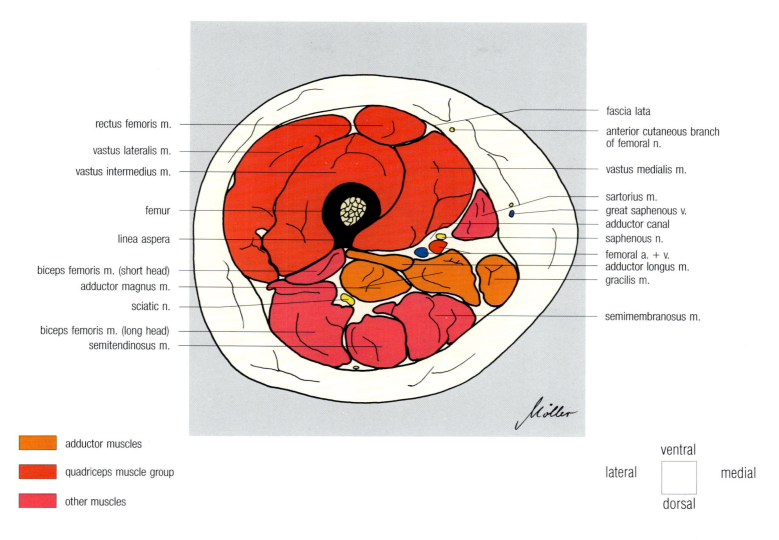

- adductor muscles
- quadriceps muscle group
- other muscles

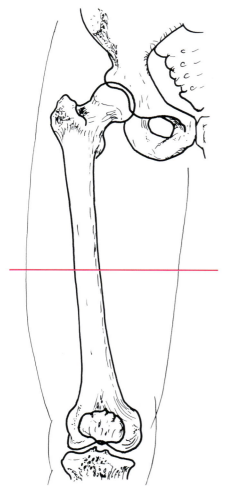
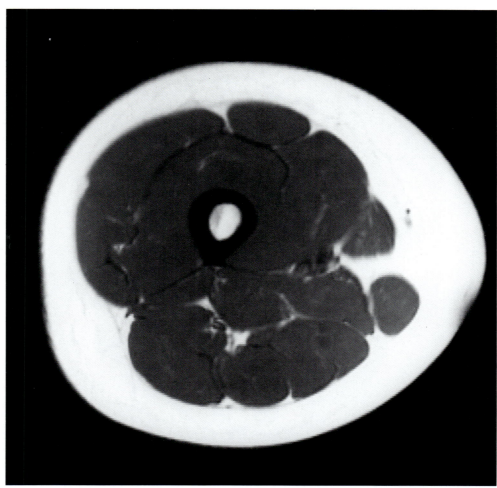

Lower Limbs Axial – Thigh

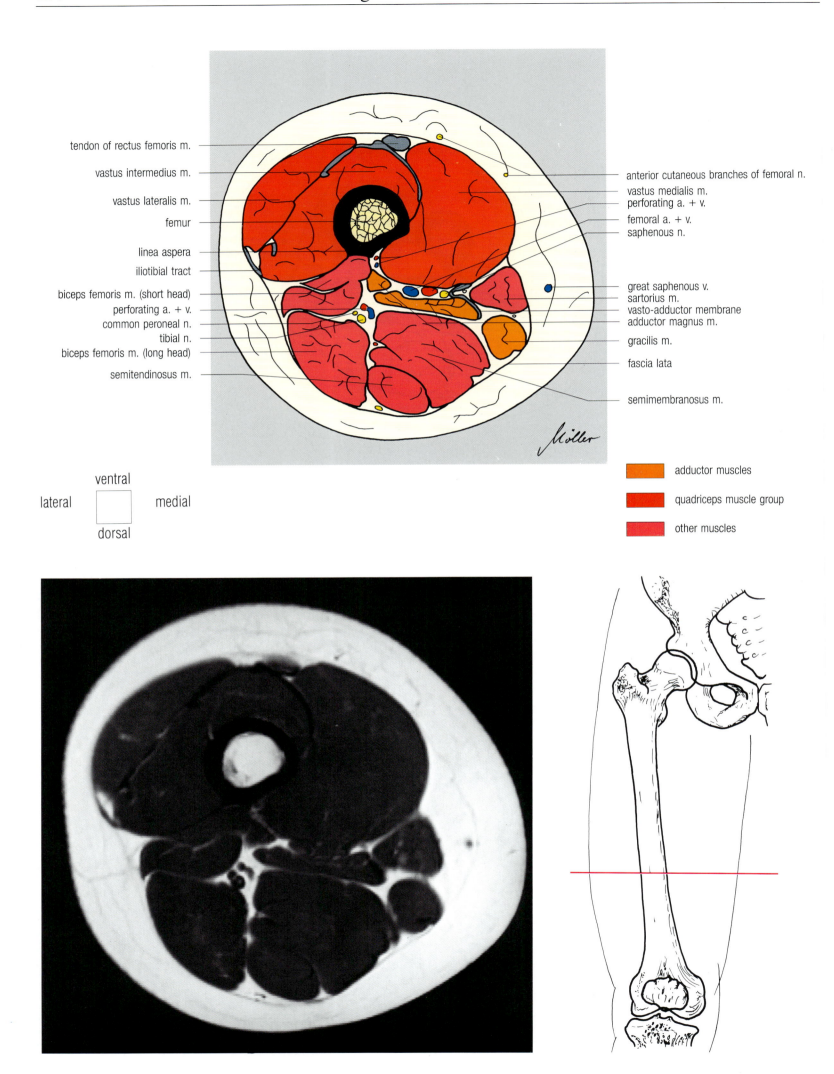

Lower Limbs Axial – Thigh

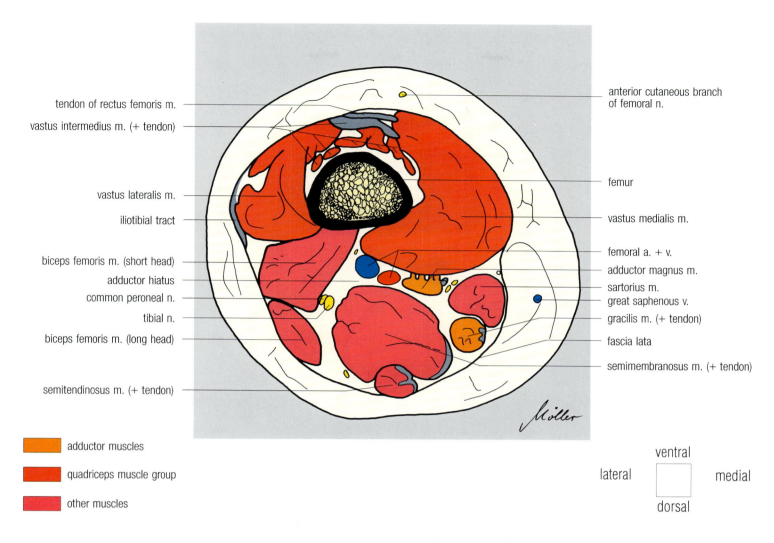

- tendon of rectus femoris m.
- vastus intermedius m. (+ tendon)
- vastus lateralis m.
- iliotibial tract
- biceps femoris m. (short head)
- adductor hiatus
- common peroneal n.
- tibial n.
- biceps femoris m. (long head)
- semitendinosus m. (+ tendon)

- anterior cutaneous branch of femoral n.
- femur
- vastus medialis m.
- femoral a. + v.
- adductor magnus m.
- sartorius m.
- great saphenous v.
- gracilis m. (+ tendon)
- fascia lata
- semimembranosus m. (+ tendon)

- adductor muscles
- quadriceps muscle group
- other muscles

ventral / lateral / medial / dorsal

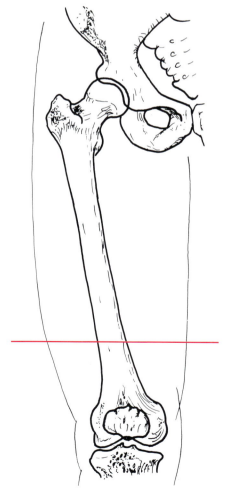
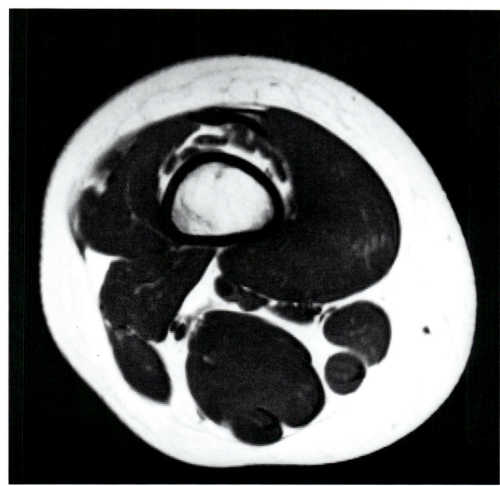

Lower Limbs Axial – Thigh

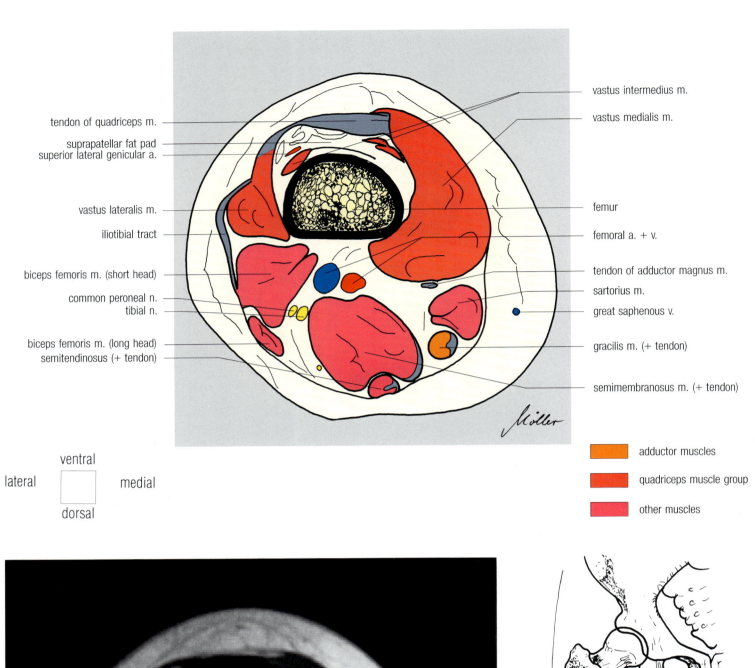

- tendon of quadriceps m.
- suprapatellar fat pad
- superior lateral genicular a.
- vastus lateralis m.
- iliotibial tract
- biceps femoris m. (short head)
- common peroneal n.
- tibial n.
- biceps femoris m. (long head)
- semitendinosus (+ tendon)

- vastus intermedius m.
- vastus medialis m.
- femur
- femoral a. + v.
- tendon of adductor magnus m.
- sartorius m.
- great saphenous v.
- gracilis m. (+ tendon)
- semimembranosus m. (+ tendon)

ventral / dorsal / lateral / medial

- adductor muscles
- quadriceps muscle group
- other muscles

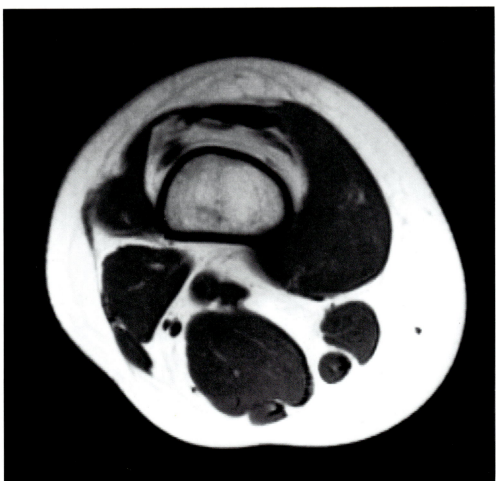
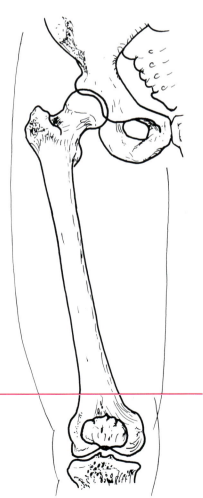

Lower Limbs Axial – Thigh

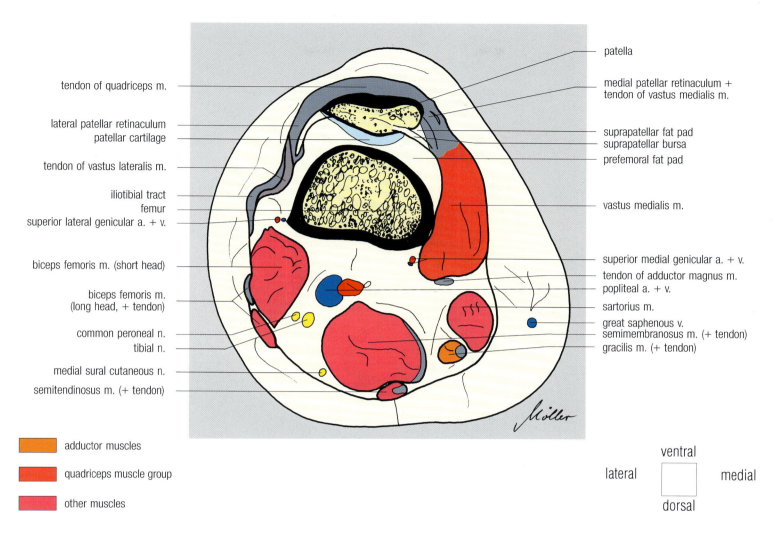

- tendon of quadriceps m.
- lateral patellar retinaculum
- patellar cartilage
- tendon of vastus lateralis m.
- iliotibial tract
- femur
- superior lateral genicular a. + v.
- biceps femoris m. (short head)
- biceps femoris m. (long head, + tendon)
- common peroneal n.
- tibial n.
- medial sural cutaneous n.
- semitendinosus m. (+ tendon)

- patella
- medial patellar retinaculum + tendon of vastus medialis m.
- suprapatellar fat pad
- suprapatellar bursa
- prefemoral fat pad
- vastus medialis m.
- superior medial genicular a. + v.
- tendon of adductor magnus m.
- popliteal a. + v.
- sartorius m.
- great saphenous v.
- semimembranosus m. (+ tendon)
- gracilis m. (+ tendon)

- adductor muscles
- quadriceps muscle group
- other muscles

ventral / lateral / medial / dorsal

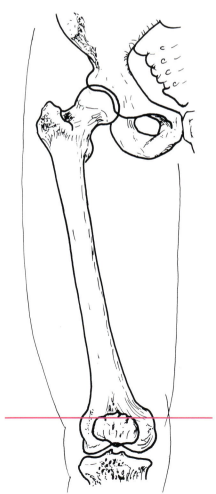
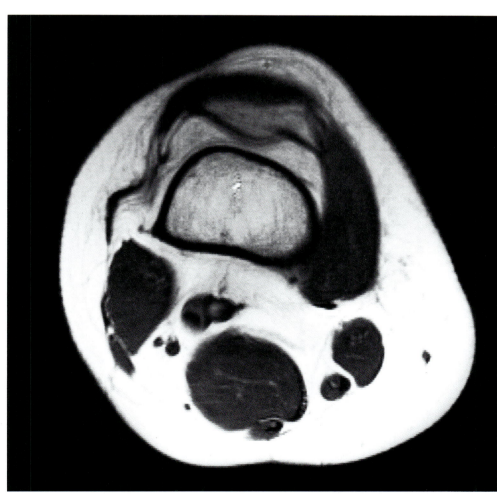

154 Lower Limbs Axial – Thigh

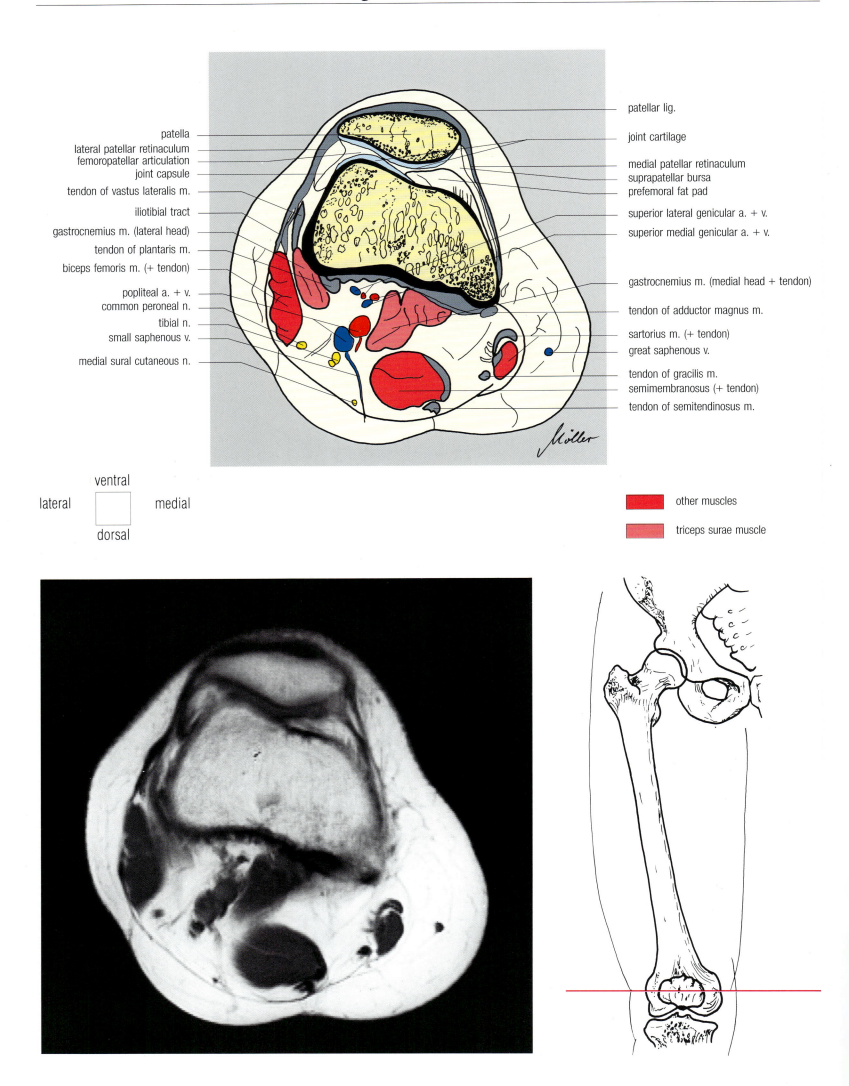

Lower Limbs Axial – Knee 155

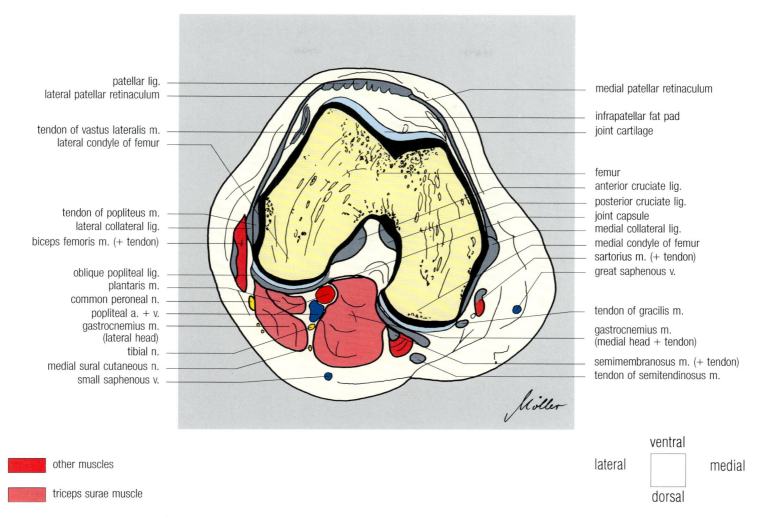

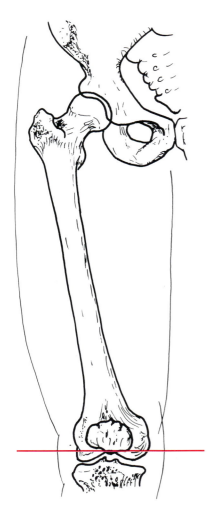
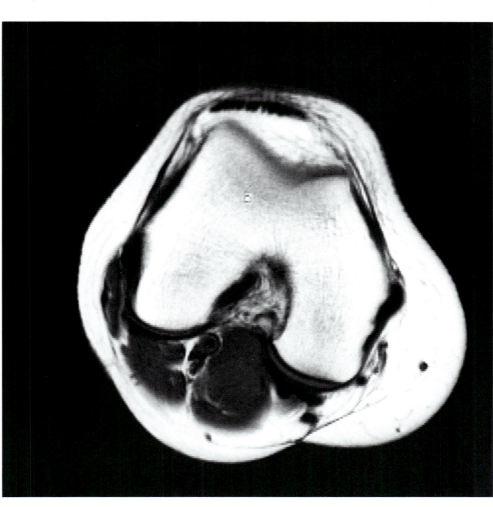

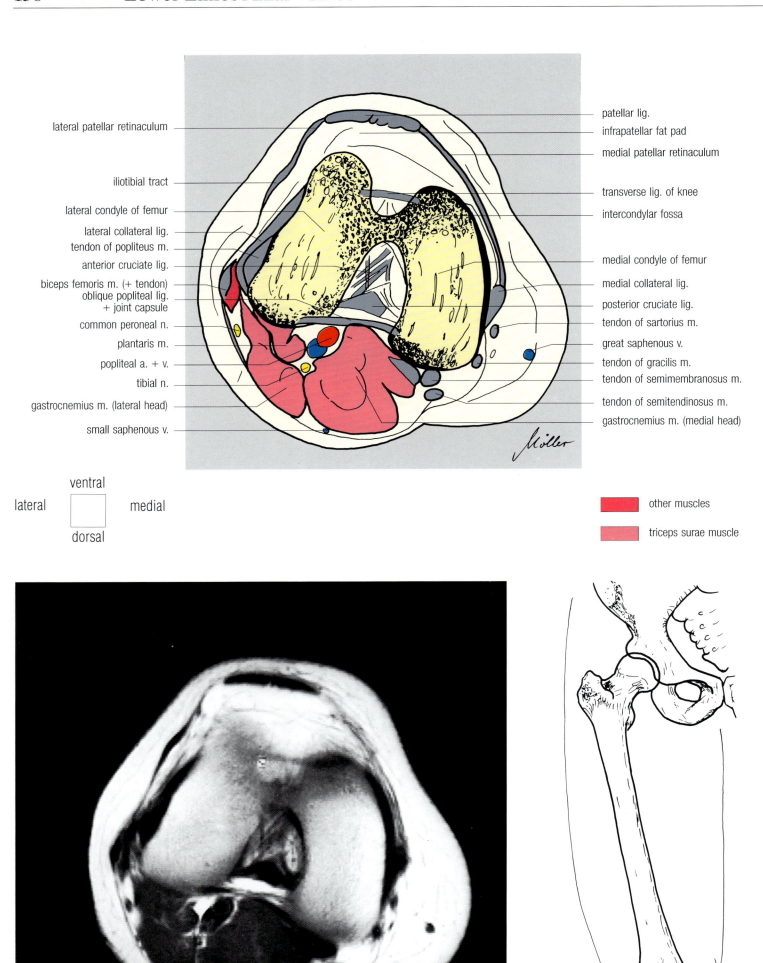

Lower Limbs Axial – Knee

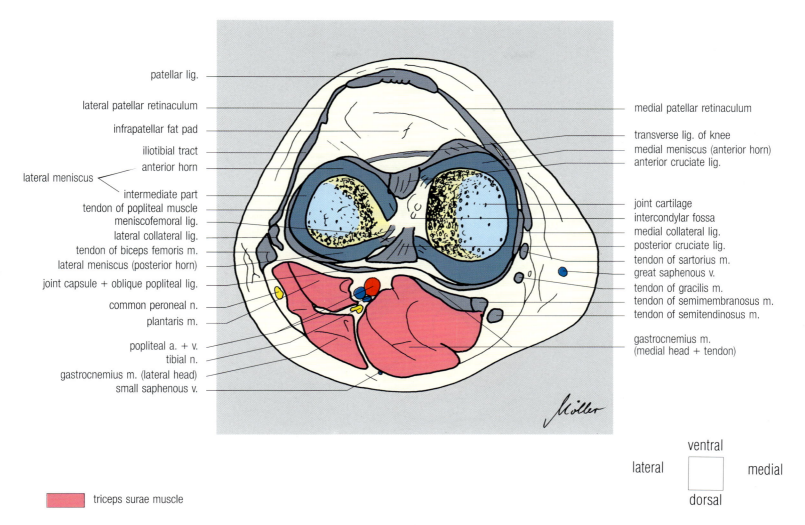

- patellar lig.
- lateral patellar retinaculum
- infrapatellar fat pad
- iliotibial tract
- anterior horn
- lateral meniscus
- intermediate part
- tendon of popliteal muscle
- meniscofemoral lig.
- lateral collateral lig.
- tendon of biceps femoris m.
- lateral meniscus (posterior horn)
- joint capsule + oblique popliteal lig.
- common peroneal n.
- plantaris m.
- popliteal a. + v.
- tibial n.
- gastrocnemius m. (lateral head)
- small saphenous v.

- medial patellar retinaculum
- transverse lig. of knee
- medial meniscus (anterior horn)
- anterior cruciate lig.
- joint cartilage
- intercondylar fossa
- medial collateral lig.
- posterior cruciate lig.
- tendon of sartorius m.
- great saphenous v.
- tendon of gracilis m.
- tendon of semimembranosus m.
- tendon of semitendinosus m.
- gastrocnemius m. (medial head + tendon)

triceps surae muscle

ventral / lateral / medial / dorsal

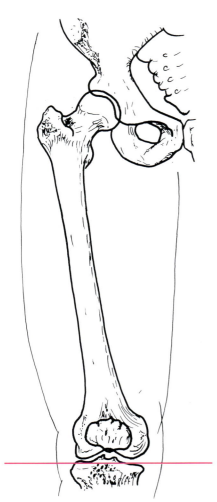

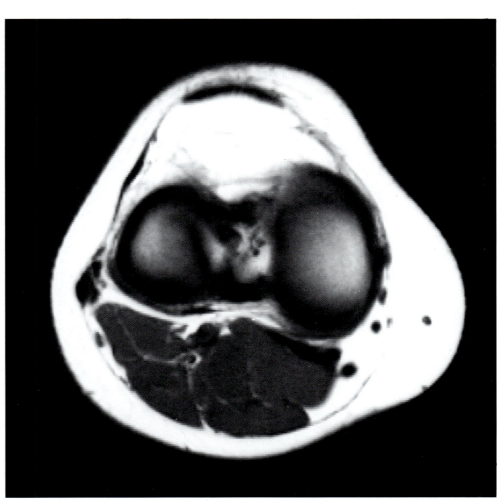

Lower Limbs Axial – Knee

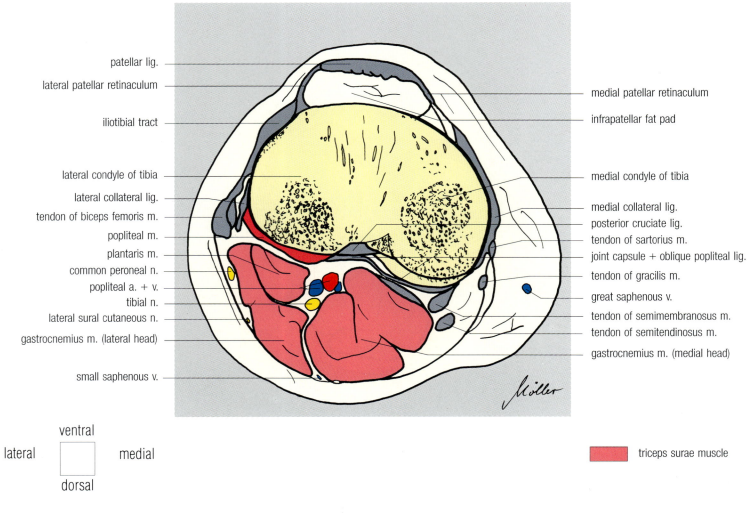

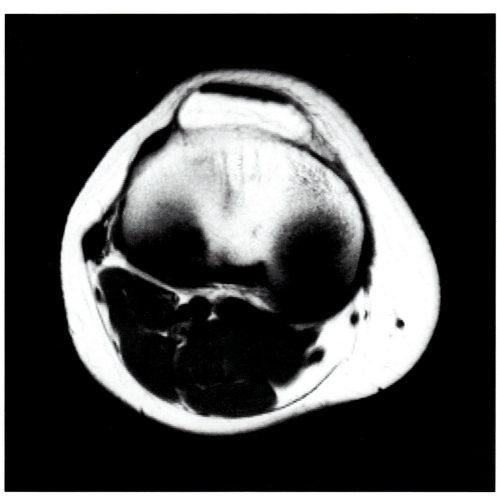
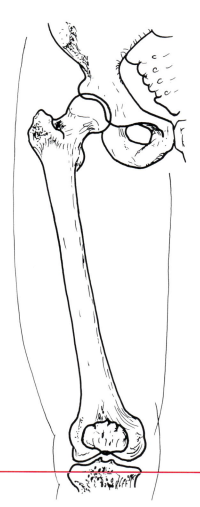

Lower Limbs Axial – Lower Leg

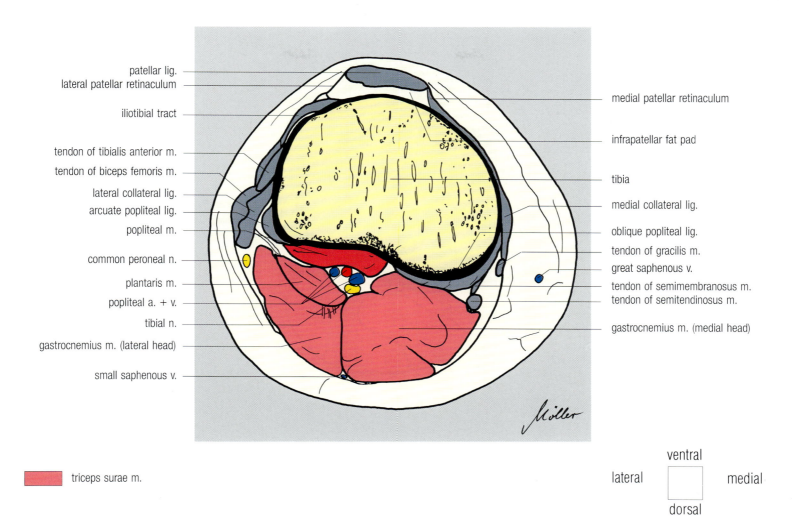

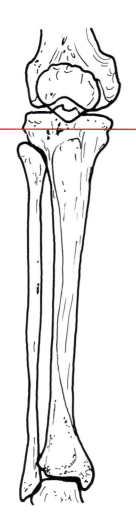
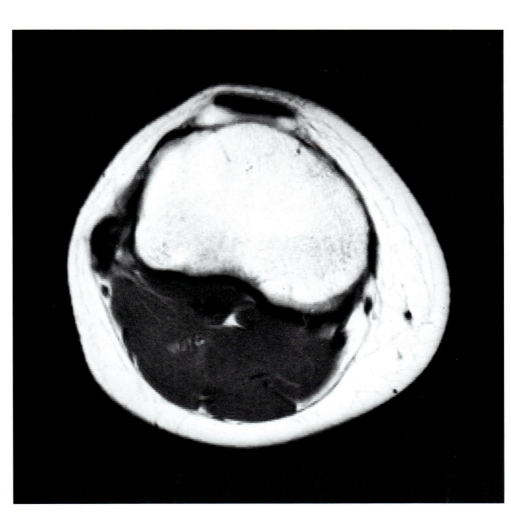

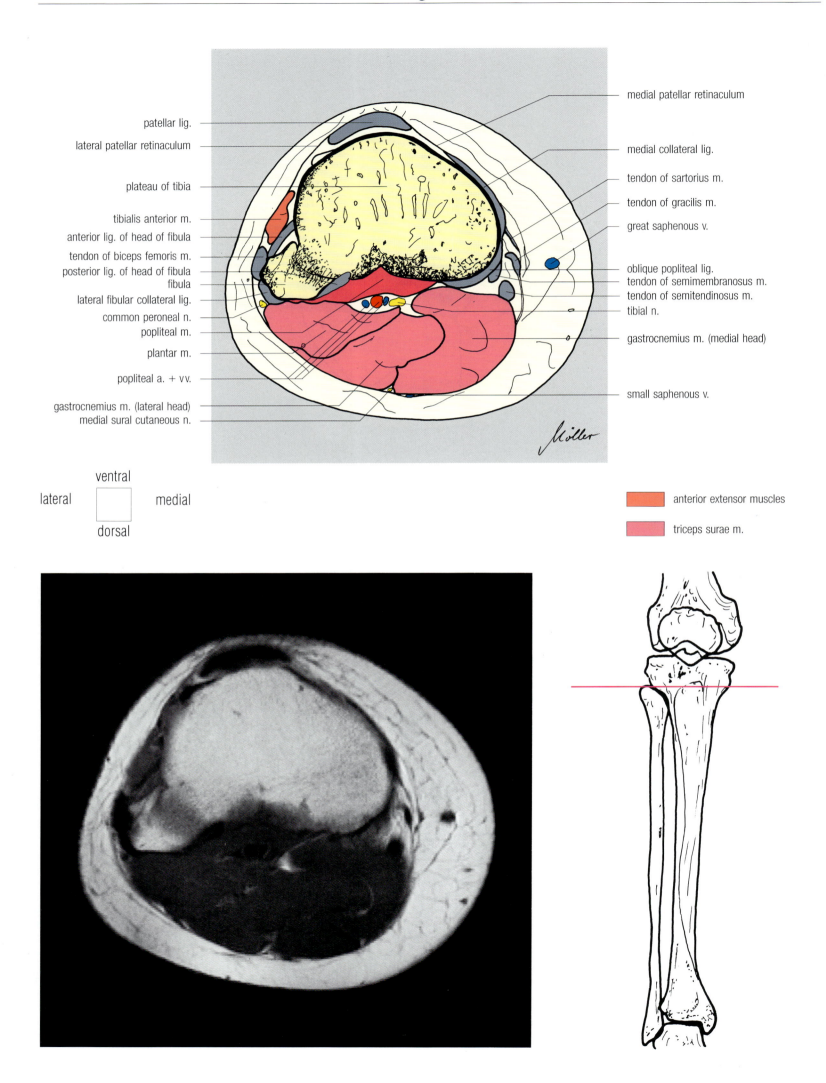

Lower Limbs Axial – Lower Leg

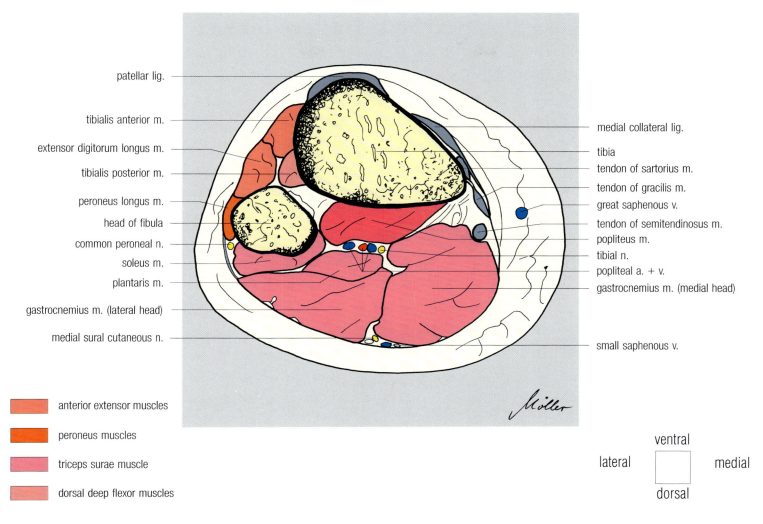

- patellar lig.
- tibialis anterior m.
- extensor digitorum longus m.
- tibialis posterior m.
- peroneus longus m.
- head of fibula
- common peroneal n.
- soleus m.
- plantaris m.
- gastrocnemius m. (lateral head)
- medial sural cutaneous n.

- medial collateral lig.
- tibia
- tendon of sartorius m.
- tendon of gracilis m.
- great saphenous v.
- tendon of semitendinosus m.
- popliteus m.
- tibial n.
- popliteal a. + v.
- gastrocnemius m. (medial head)
- small saphenous v.

- ■ anterior extensor muscles
- ■ peroneus muscles
- ■ triceps surae muscle
- ■ dorsal deep flexor muscles

ventral
lateral — medial
dorsal

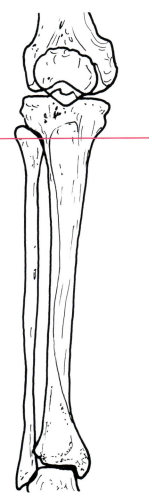
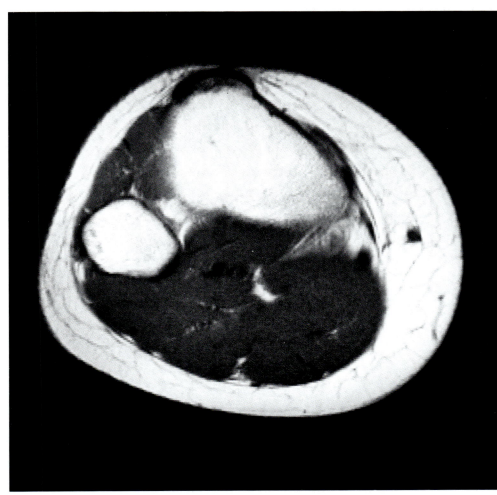

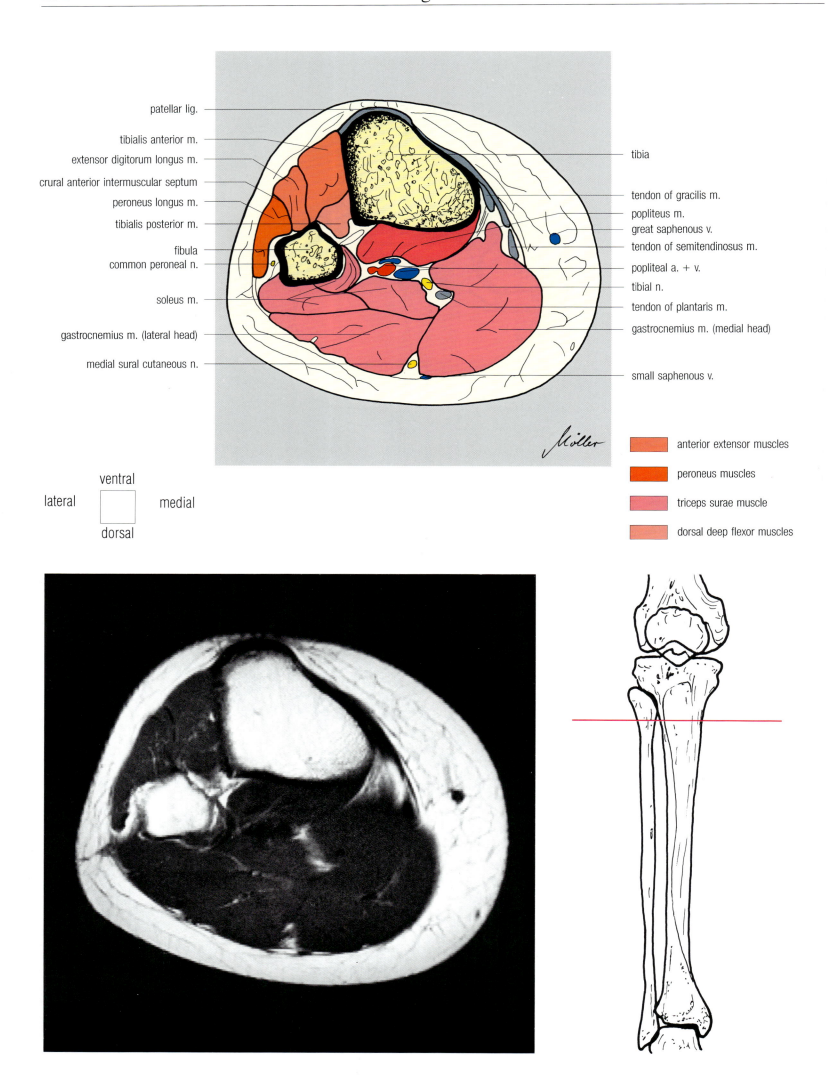

Lower Limbs Axial – Lower Leg

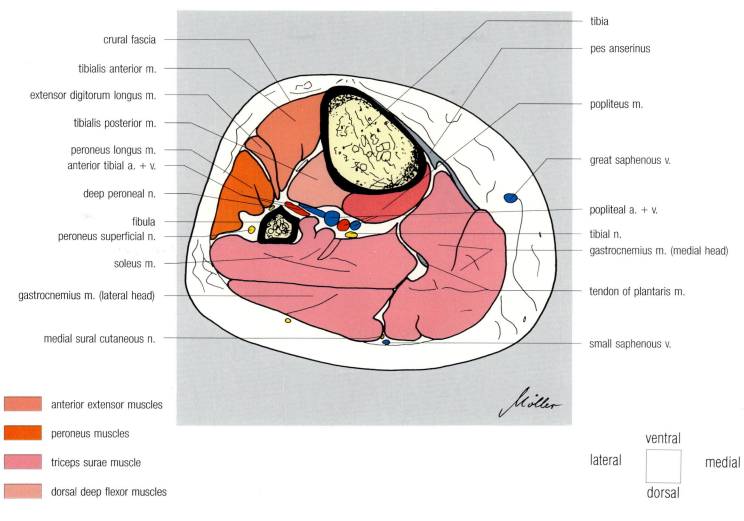

- anterior extensor muscles
- peroneus muscles
- triceps surae muscle
- dorsal deep flexor muscles

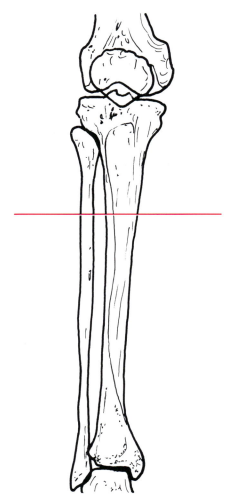

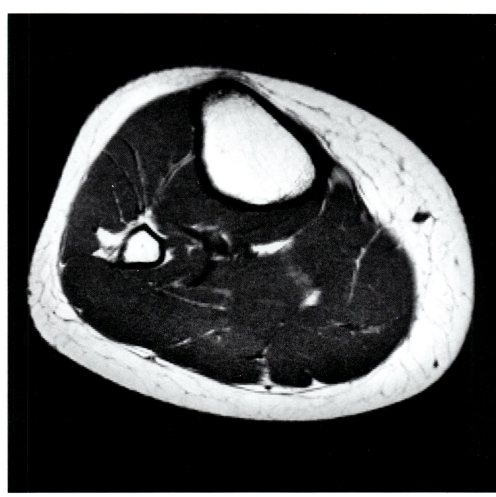

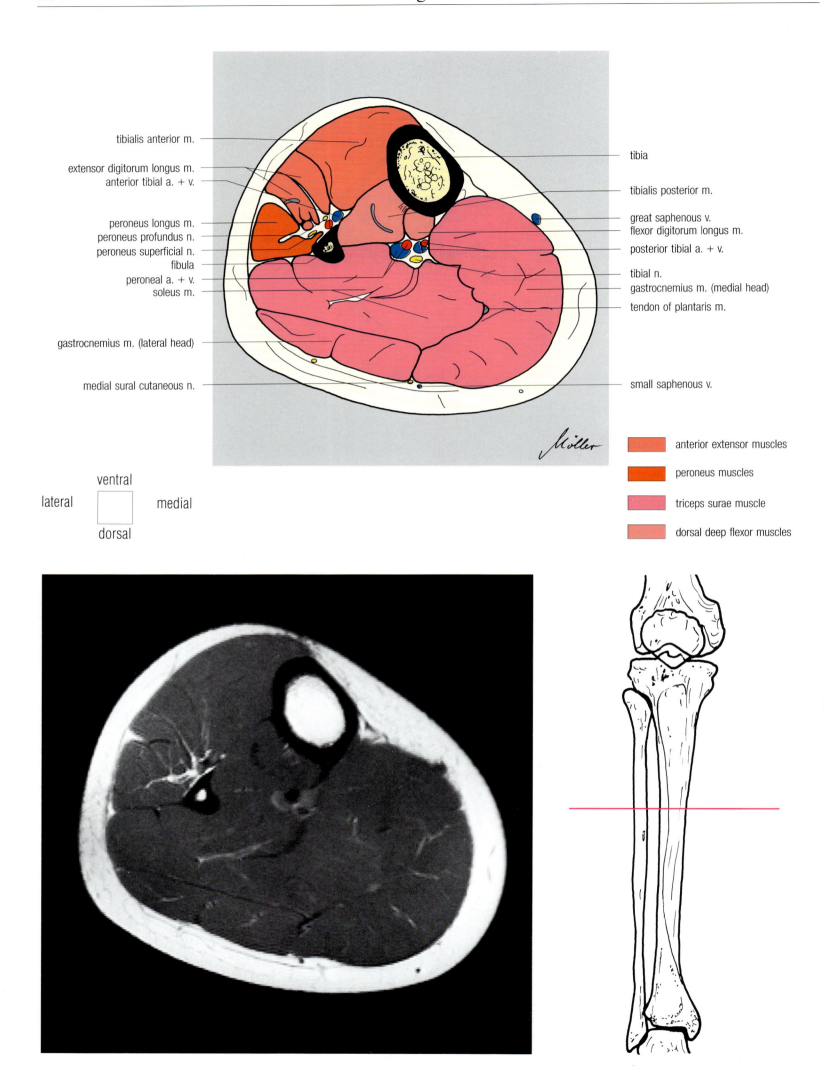

Lower Limbs Axial – Lower Leg

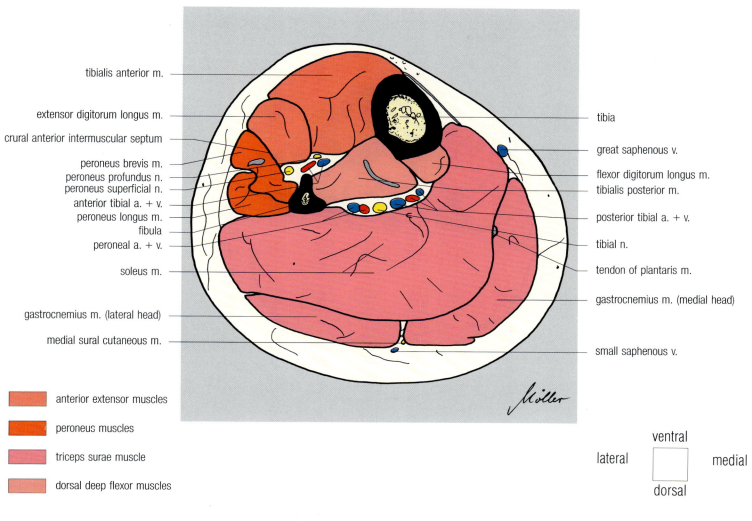

- tibialis anterior m.
- extensor digitorum longus m.
- crural anterior intermuscular septum
- peroneus brevis m.
- peroneus profundus n.
- peroneus superficial n.
- anterior tibial a. + v.
- peroneus longus m.
- fibula
- peroneal a. + v.
- soleus m.
- gastrocnemius m. (lateral head)
- medial sural cutaneous m.

- tibia
- great saphenous v.
- flexor digitorum longus m.
- tibialis posterior m.
- posterior tibial a. + v.
- tibial n.
- tendon of plantaris m.
- gastrocnemius m. (medial head)
- small saphenous v.

- anterior extensor muscles
- peroneus muscles
- triceps surae muscle
- dorsal deep flexor muscles

ventral
lateral — medial
dorsal

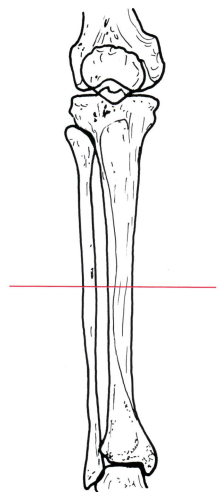
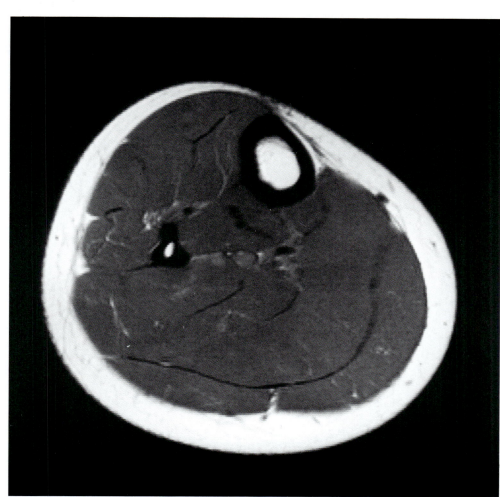

Lower Limbs Axial – Lower Leg

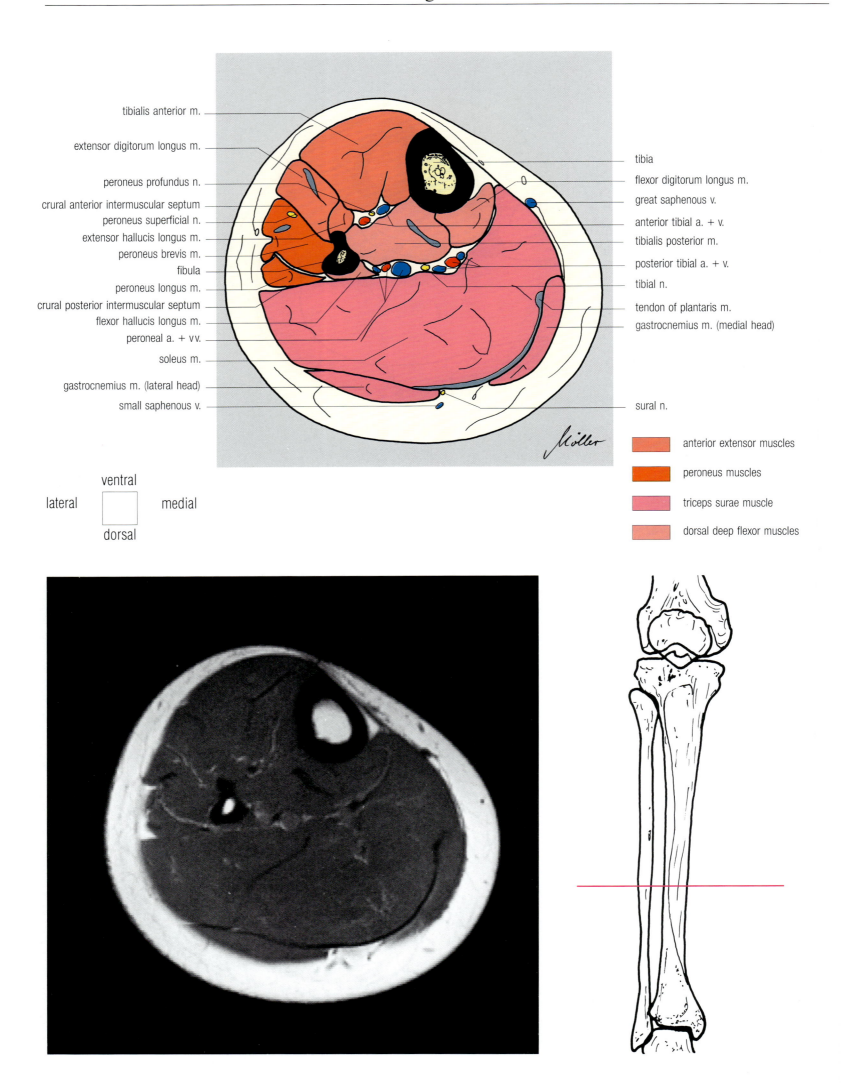

Lower Limbs Axial – Lower Leg

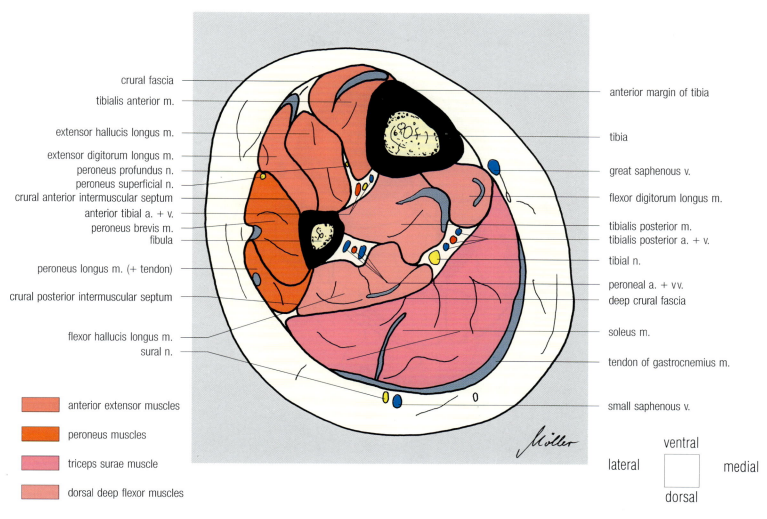

- crural fascia
- tibialis anterior m.
- extensor hallucis longus m.
- extensor digitorum longus m.
- peroneus profundus n.
- peroneus superficial n.
- crural anterior intermuscular septum
- anterior tibial a. + v.
- peroneus brevis m.
- fibula
- peroneus longus m. (+ tendon)
- crural posterior intermuscular septum
- flexor hallucis longus m.
- sural n.

- anterior margin of tibia
- tibia
- great saphenous v.
- flexor digitorum longus m.
- tibialis posterior m.
- tibialis posterior a. + v.
- tibial n.
- peroneal a. + vv.
- deep crural fascia
- soleus m.
- tendon of gastrocnemius m.
- small saphenous v.

Legend:
- anterior extensor muscles
- peroneus muscles
- triceps surae muscle
- dorsal deep flexor muscles

ventral / lateral / medial / dorsal

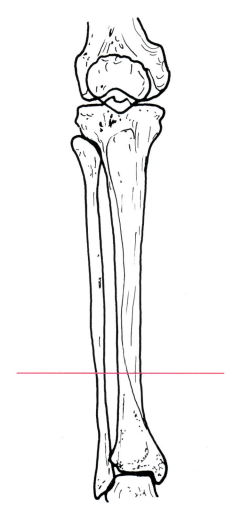

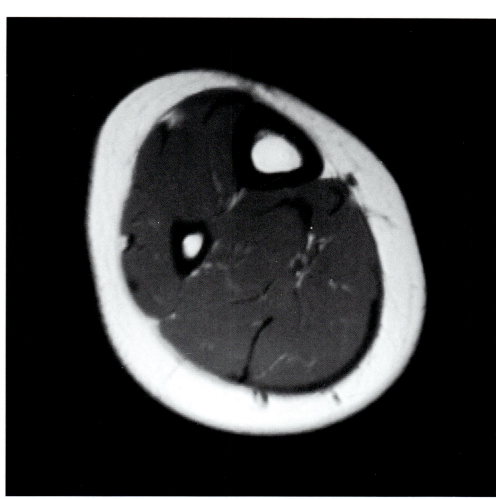

167

Lower Limbs Axial – Lower Leg

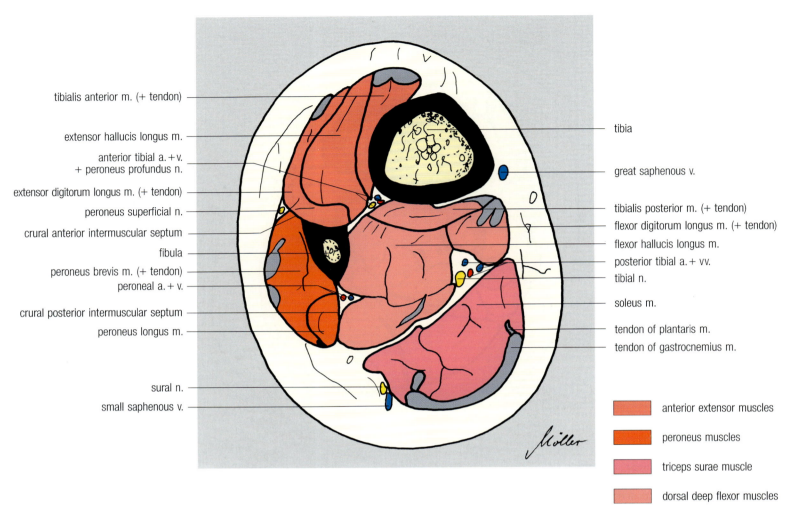

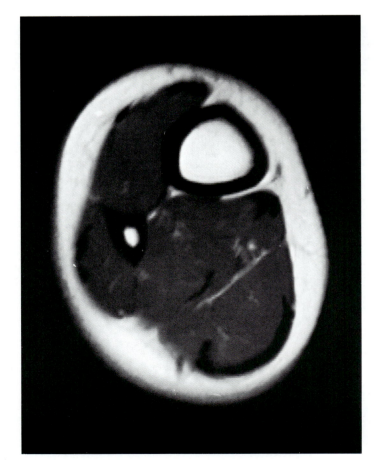

ventral
lateral | | medial
dorsal

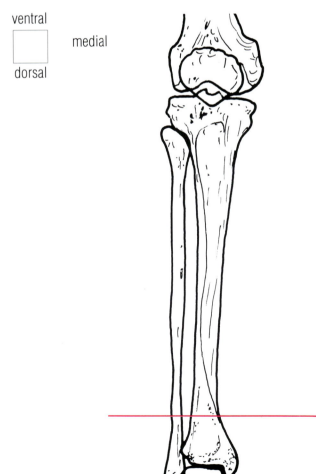

Lower Limbs Axial – Lower Leg

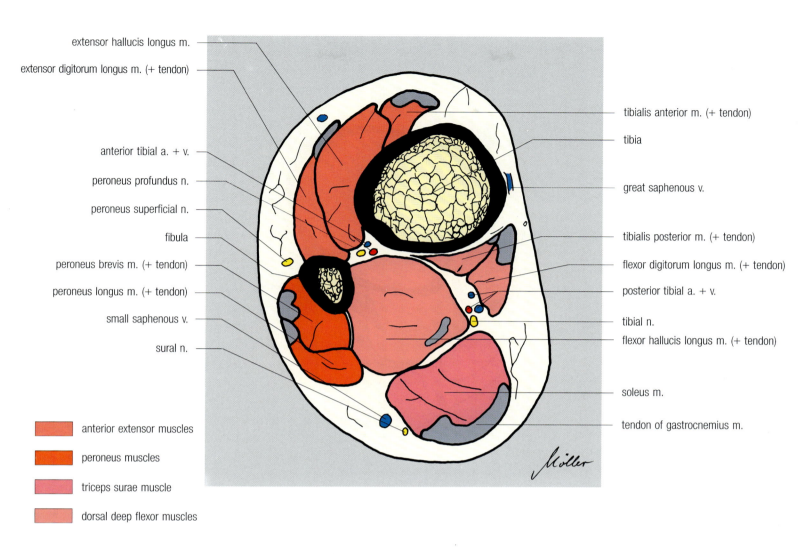

- extensor hallucis longus m.
- extensor digitorum longus m. (+ tendon)
- anterior tibial a. + v.
- peroneus profundus n.
- peroneus superficial n.
- fibula
- peroneus brevis m. (+ tendon)
- peroneus longus m. (+ tendon)
- small saphenous v.
- sural n.
- tibialis anterior m. (+ tendon)
- tibia
- great saphenous v.
- tibialis posterior m. (+ tendon)
- flexor digitorum longus m. (+ tendon)
- posterior tibial a. + v.
- tibial n.
- flexor hallucis longus m. (+ tendon)
- soleus m.
- tendon of gastrocnemius m.

■ anterior extensor muscles
■ peroneus muscles
■ triceps surae muscle
■ dorsal deep flexor muscles

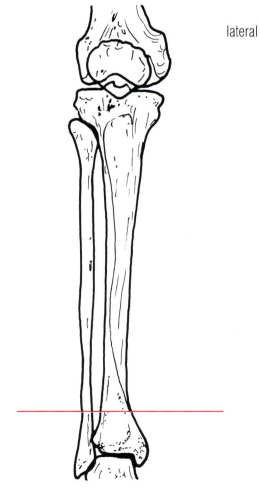

ventral / lateral / medial / dorsal

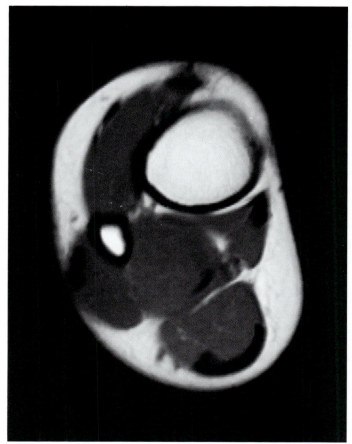

Lower Limbs Axial – Lower Leg

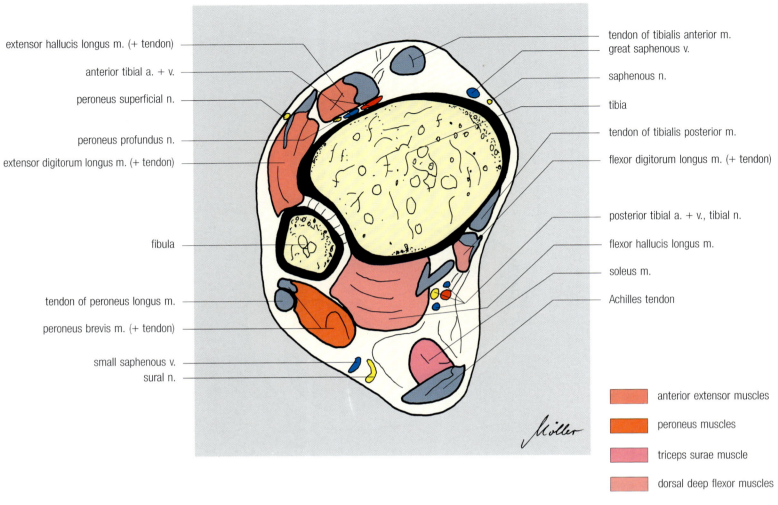

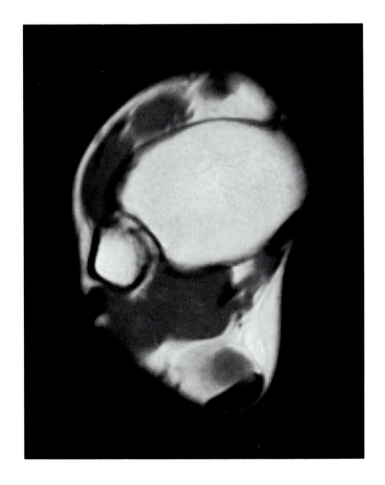
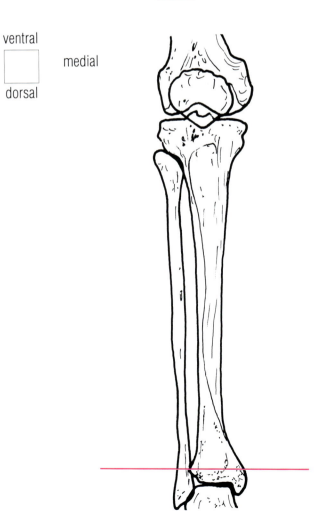

Lower Limbs Axial – Ankle and Foot

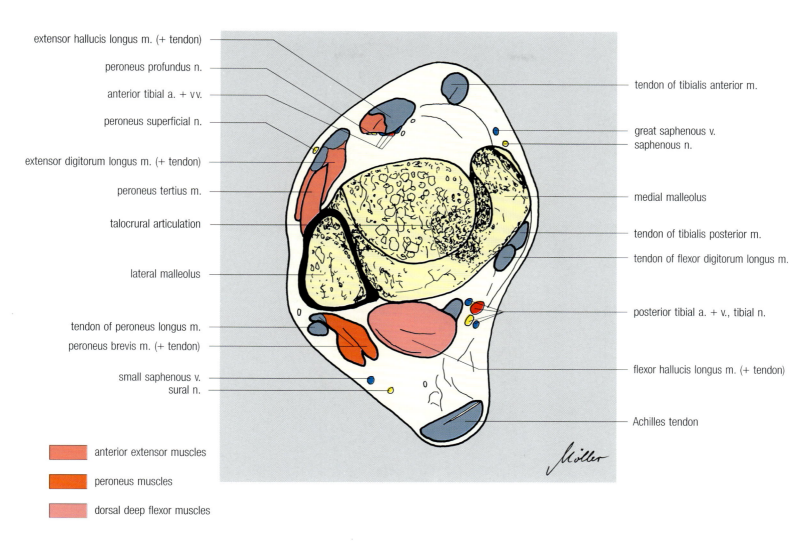

- extensor hallucis longus m. (+ tendon)
- peroneus profundus n.
- anterior tibial a. + vv.
- peroneus superficial n.
- extensor digitorum longus m. (+ tendon)
- peroneus tertius m.
- talocrural articulation
- lateral malleolus
- tendon of peroneus longus m.
- peroneus brevis m. (+ tendon)
- small saphenous v.
- sural n.

- tendon of tibialis anterior m.
- great saphenous v.
- saphenous n.
- medial malleolus
- tendon of tibialis posterior m.
- tendon of flexor digitorum longus m.
- posterior tibial a. + v., tibial n.
- flexor hallucis longus m. (+ tendon)
- Achilles tendon

■ anterior extensor muscles
■ peroneus muscles
■ dorsal deep flexor muscles

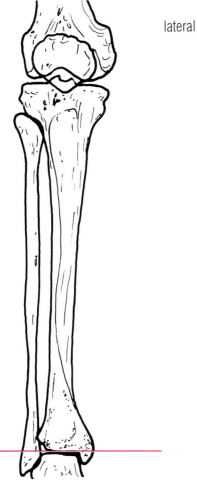

ventral
lateral — medial
dorsal

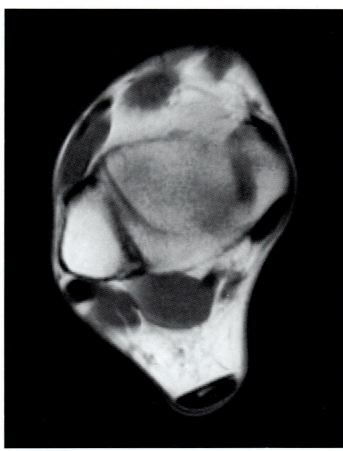

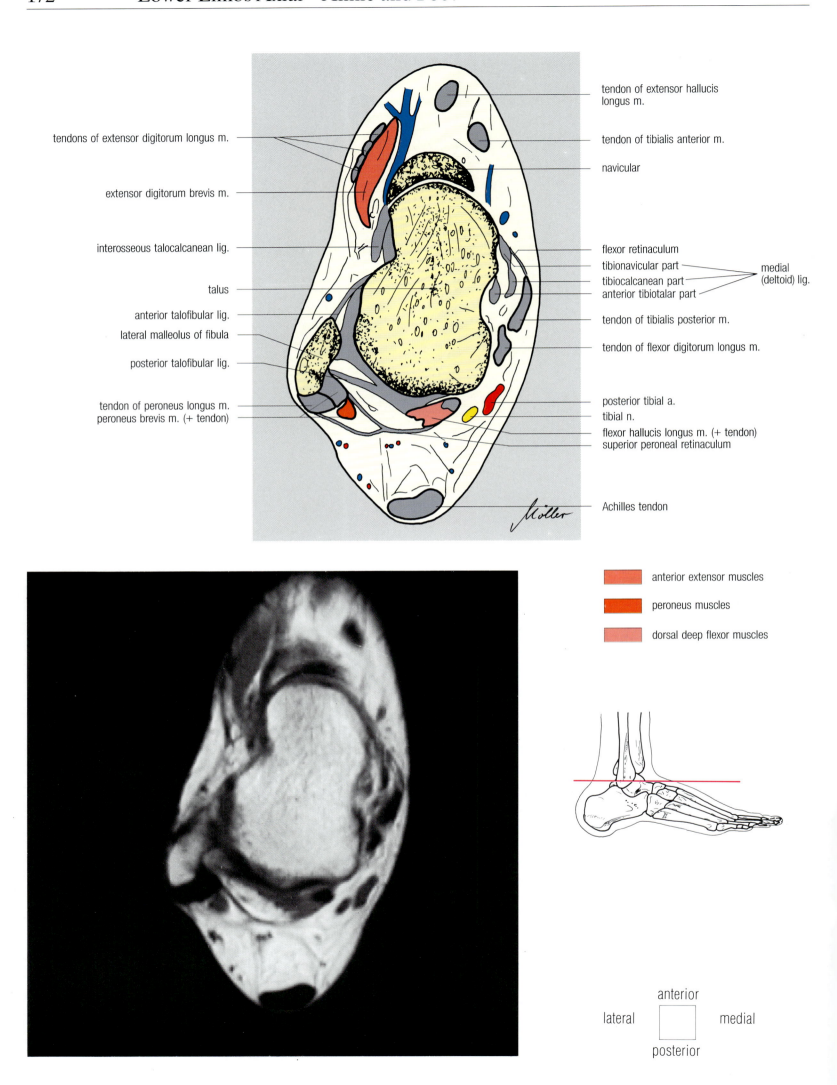

Lower Limbs Axial – Ankle and Foot

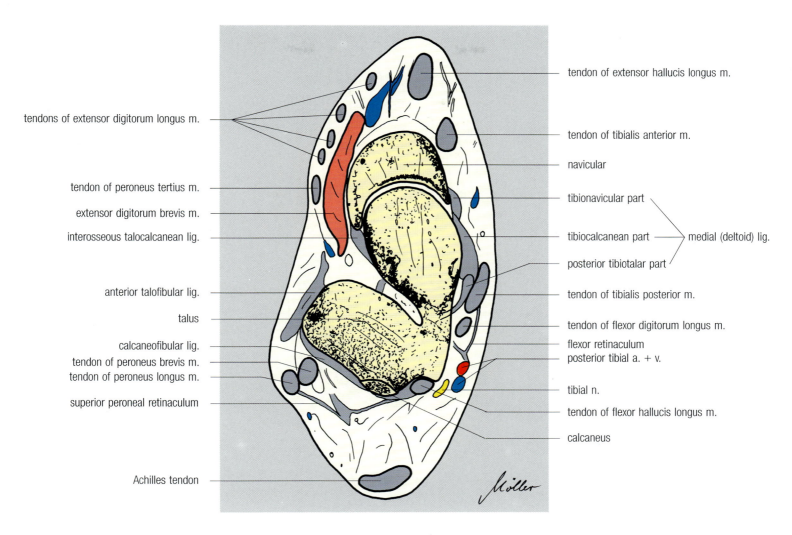

- tendons of extensor digitorum longus m.
- tendon of peroneus tertius m.
- extensor digitorum brevis m.
- interosseous talocalcanean lig.
- anterior talofibular lig.
- talus
- calcaneofibular lig.
- tendon of peroneus brevis m.
- tendon of peroneus longus m.
- superior peroneal retinaculum
- Achilles tendon

- tendon of extensor hallucis longus m.
- tendon of tibialis anterior m.
- navicular
- tibionavicular part
- tibiocalcanean part ⟶ medial (deltoid) lig.
- posterior tibiotalar part
- tendon of tibialis posterior m.
- tendon of flexor digitorum longus m.
- flexor retinaculum
- posterior tibial a. + v.
- tibial n.
- tendon of flexor hallucis longus m.
- calcaneus

■ extensor muscles group

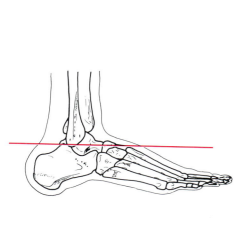

anterior
lateral □ medial
posterior

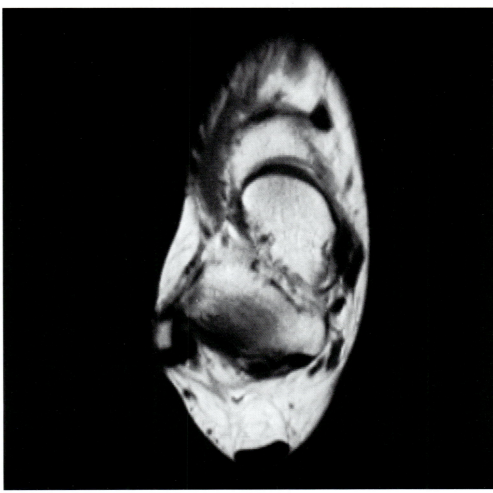

Lower Limbs Axial – Ankle and Foot

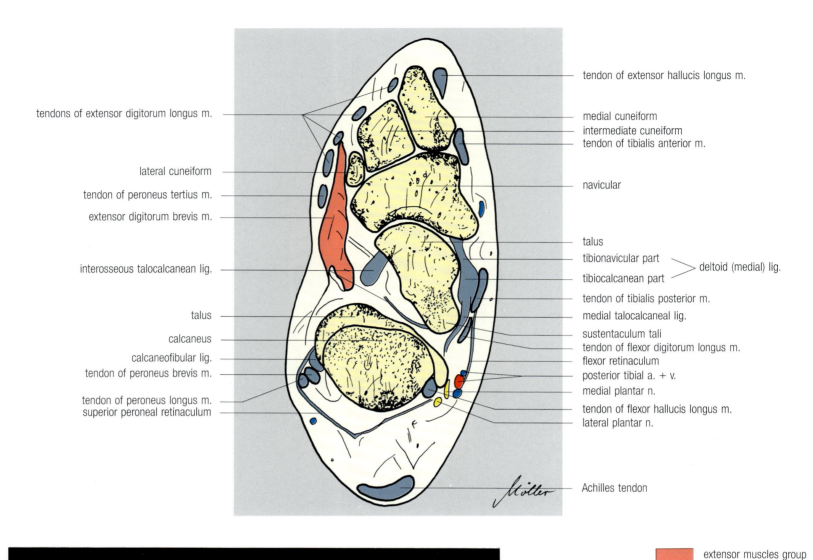

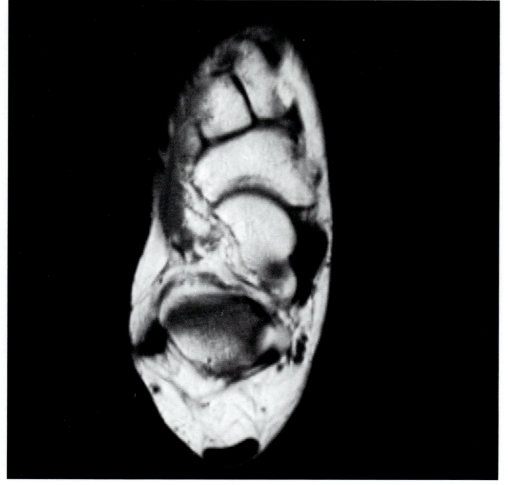

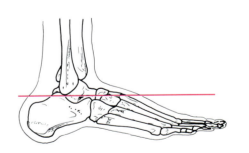

Lower Limbs Axial – Ankle and Foot

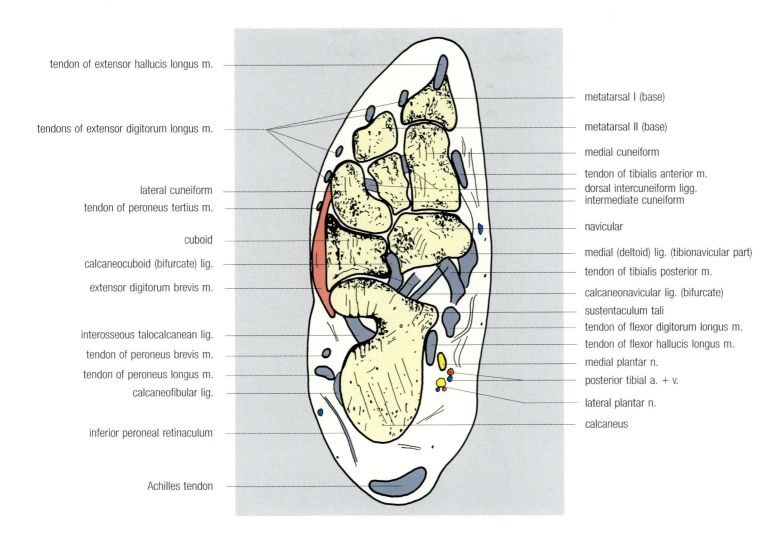

- tendon of extensor hallucis longus m.
- tendons of extensor digitorum longus m.
- lateral cuneiform
- tendon of peroneus tertius m.
- cuboid
- calcaneocuboid (bifurcate) lig.
- extensor digitorum brevis m.
- interosseous talocalcanean lig.
- tendon of peroneus brevis m.
- tendon of peroneus longus m.
- calcaneofibular lig.
- inferior peroneal retinaculum
- Achilles tendon

- metatarsal I (base)
- metatarsal II (base)
- medial cuneiform
- tendon of tibialis anterior m.
- dorsal intercuneiform ligg.
- intermediate cuneiform
- navicular
- medial (deltoid) lig. (tibionavicular part)
- tendon of tibialis posterior m.
- calcaneonavicular lig. (bifurcate)
- sustentaculum tali
- tendon of flexor digitorum longus m.
- tendon of flexor hallucis longus m.
- medial plantar n.
- posterior tibial a. + v.
- lateral plantar n.
- calcaneus

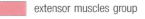 extensor muscles group

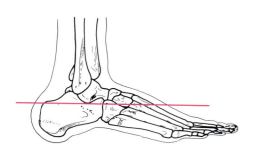

anterior — lateral / medial — posterior

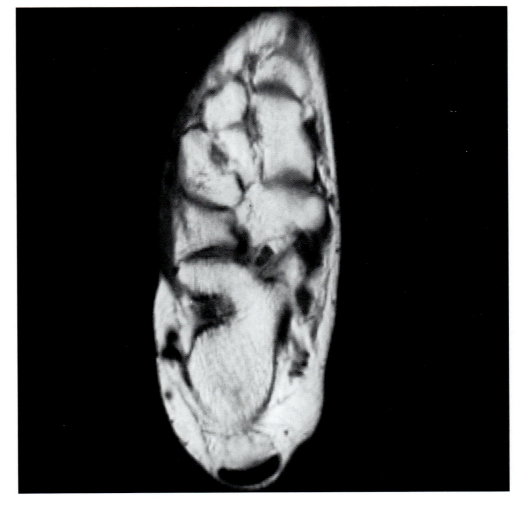

176 Lower Limbs Axial – Ankle and Foot

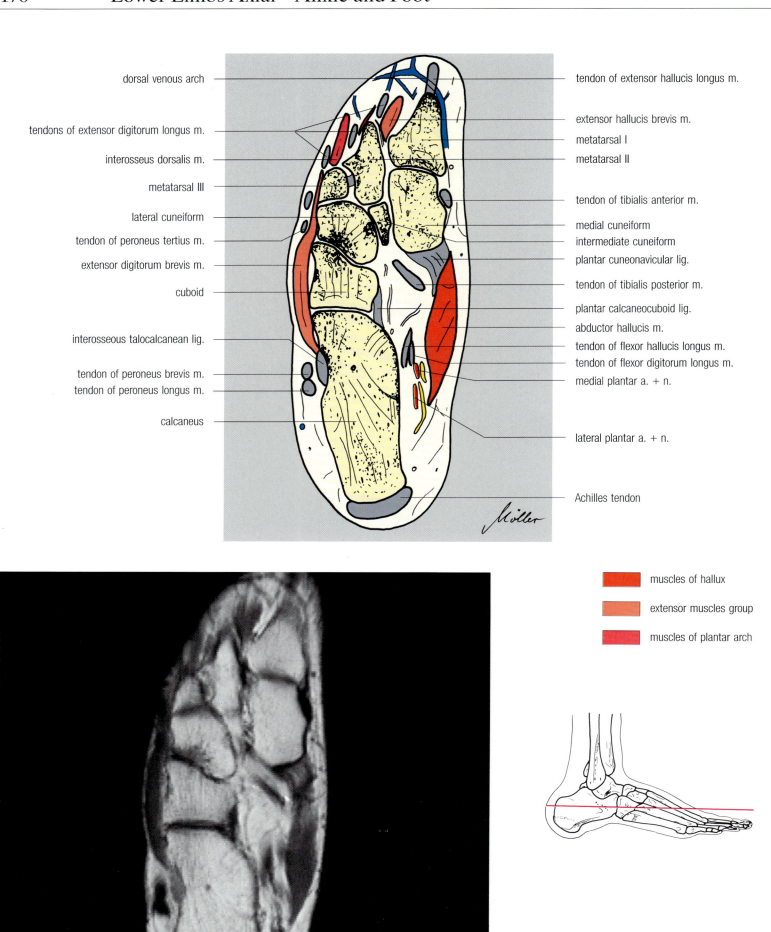

Lower Limbs Axial – Ankle and Foot

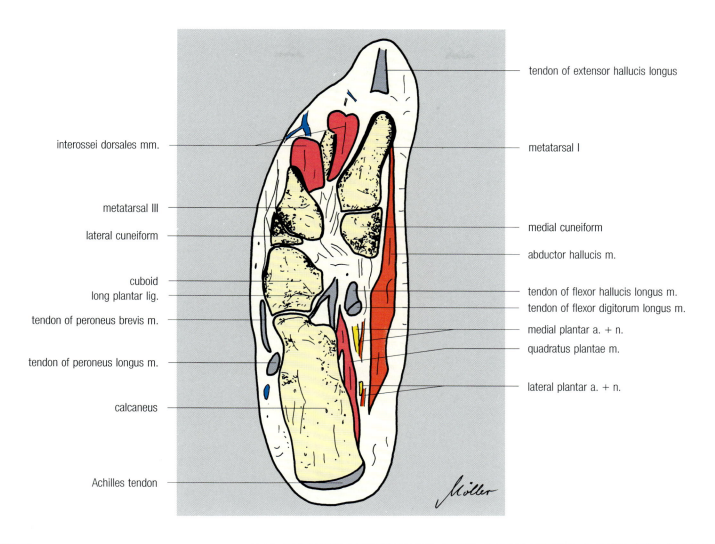

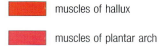
muscles of hallux

muscles of plantar arch

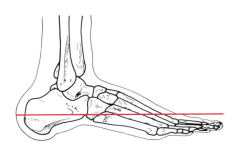

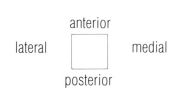

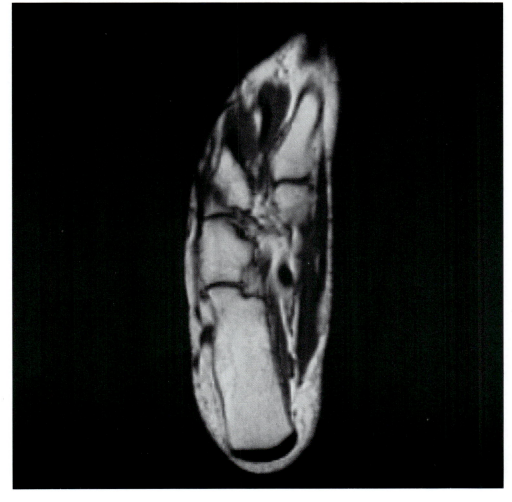

178 Lower Limbs Axial – Ankle and Foot

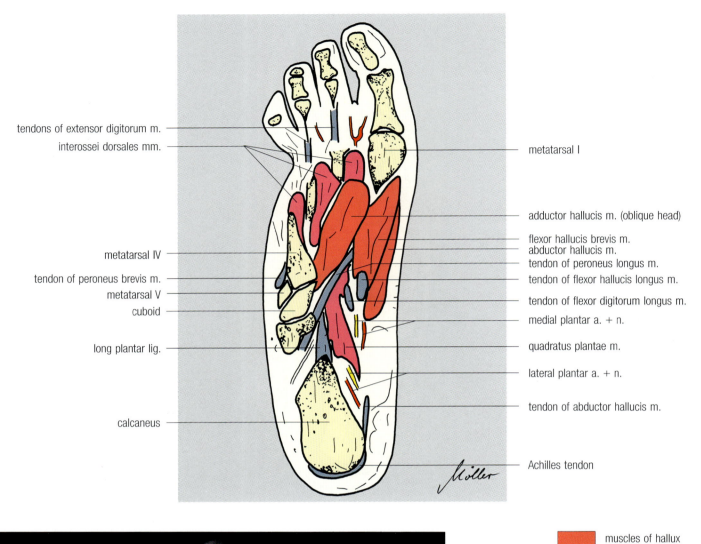

- tendons of extensor digitorum m.
- interossei dorsales mm.
- metatarsal I
- metatarsal IV
- adductor hallucis m. (oblique head)
- flexor hallucis brevis m.
- abductor hallucis m.
- tendon of peroneus longus m.
- tendon of peroneus brevis m.
- metatarsal V
- tendon of flexor hallucis longus m.
- cuboid
- tendon of flexor digitorum longus m.
- medial plantar a. + n.
- long plantar lig.
- quadratus plantae m.
- lateral plantar a. + n.
- calcaneus
- tendon of abductor hallucis m.
- Achilles tendon

■ muscles of hallux
■ muscles of plantar arch

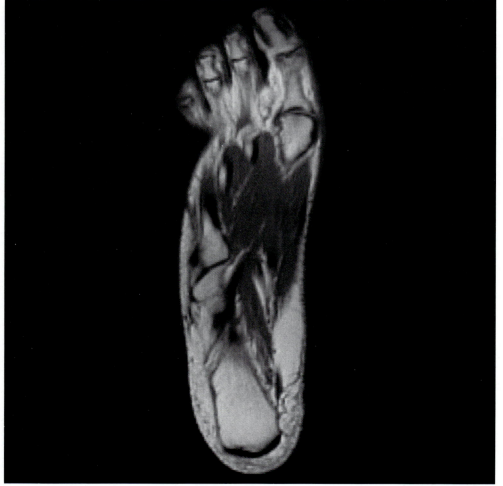

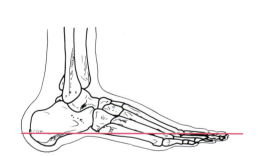

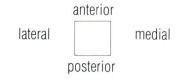

Lower Limbs Axial – Ankle and Foot 179

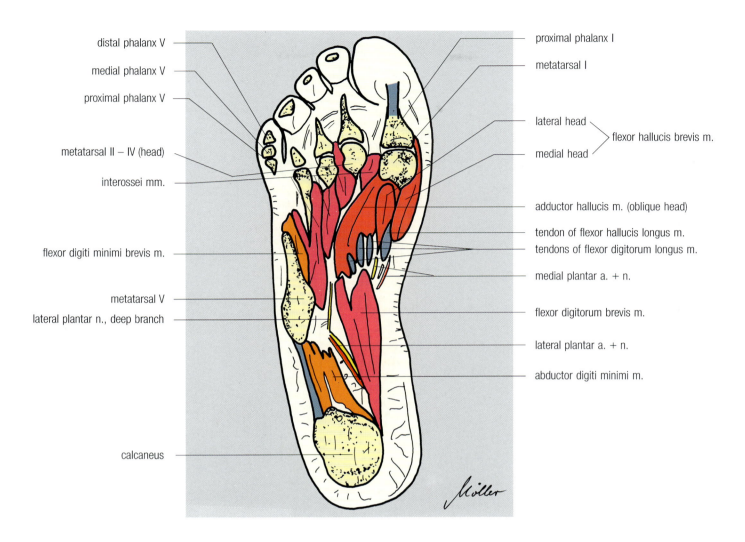

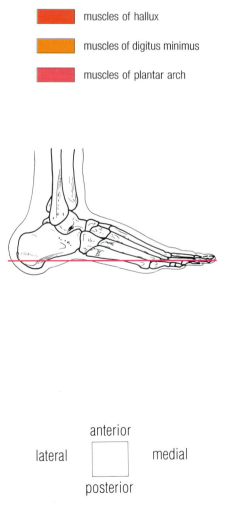

- muscles of hallux
- muscles of digitus minimus
- muscles of plantar arch

anterior
lateral — medial
posterior

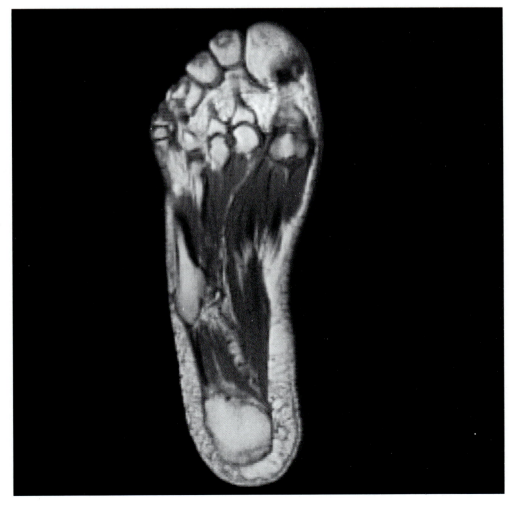

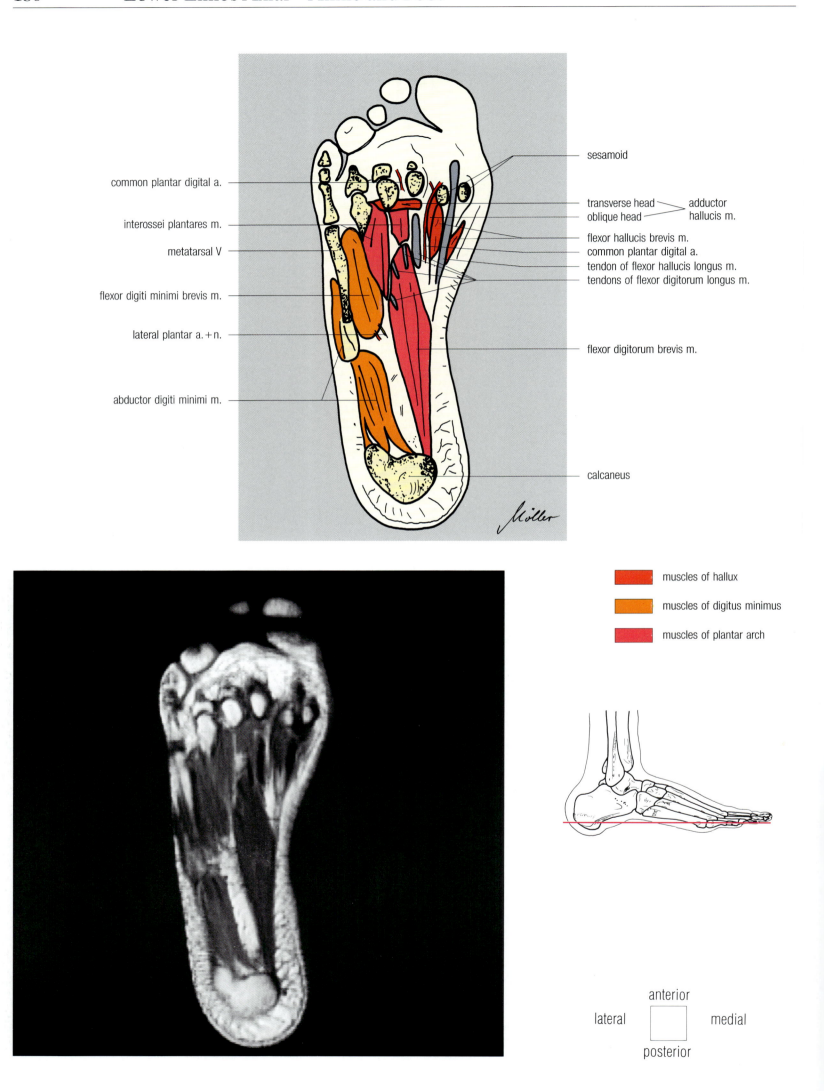

Lower Limbs Axial – Ankle and Foot

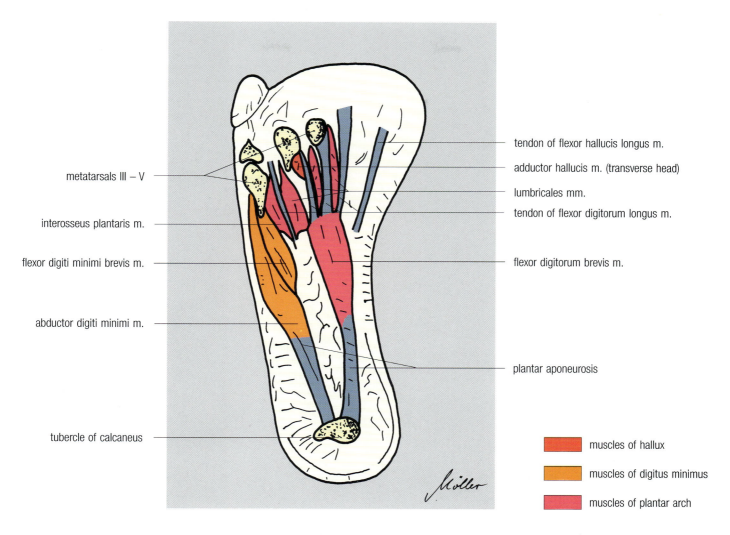

- tendon of flexor hallucis longus m.
- adductor hallucis m. (transverse head)
- lumbricales mm.
- tendon of flexor digitorum longus m.
- metatarsals III – V
- interosseus plantaris m.
- flexor digiti minimi brevis m.
- flexor digitorum brevis m.
- abductor digiti minimi m.
- plantar aponeurosis
- tubercle of calcaneus

■ muscles of hallux
■ muscles of digitus minimus
■ muscles of plantar arch

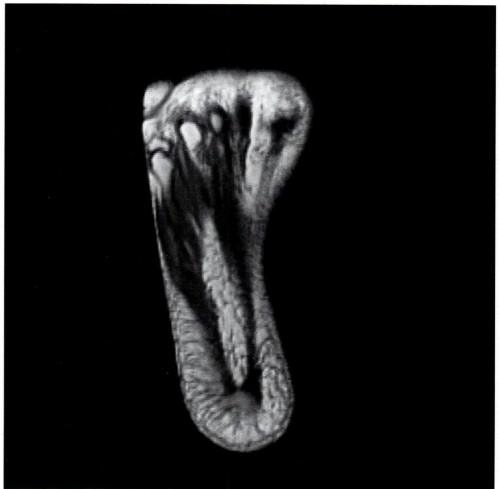

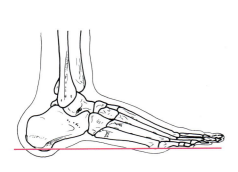

anterior
lateral — medial
posterior

181

Hip

Coronal

Sagittal

Hip – Coronal

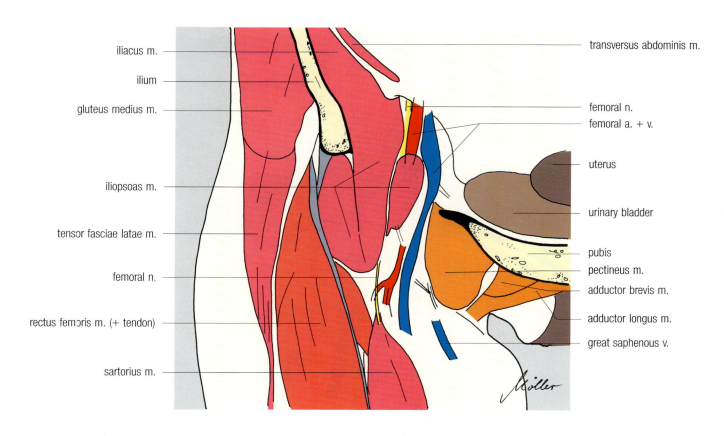

- adductor muscles
- quadriceps muscle group
- other muscles

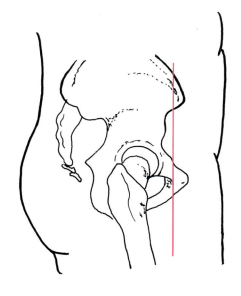

proximal | lateral — medial | distal

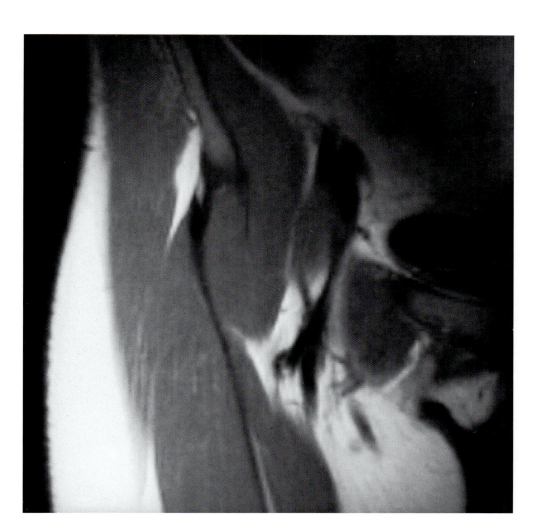

Hip – Coronal

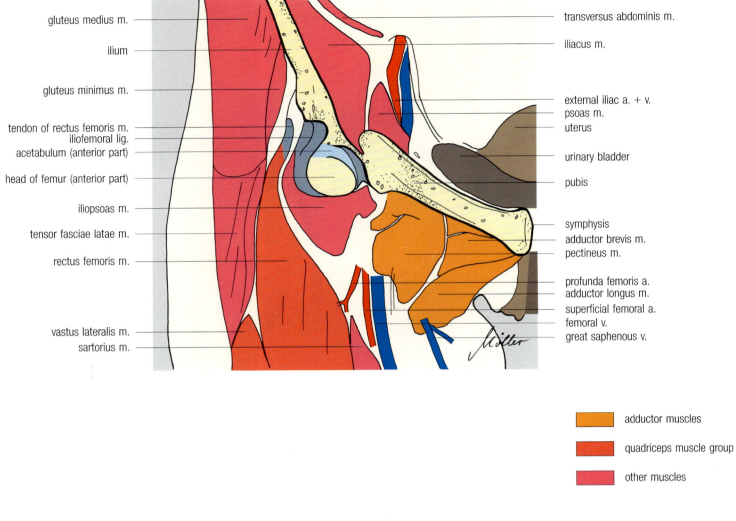

- gluteus medius m.
- ilium
- gluteus minimus m.
- tendon of rectus femoris m.
- iliofemoral lig.
- acetabulum (anterior part)
- head of femur (anterior part)
- iliopsoas m.
- tensor fasciae latae m.
- rectus femoris m.
- vastus lateralis m.
- sartorius m.
- transversus abdominis m.
- iliacus m.
- external iliac a. + v.
- psoas m.
- uterus
- urinary bladder
- pubis
- symphysis
- adductor brevis m.
- pectineus m.
- profunda femoris a.
- adductor longus m.
- superficial femoral a.
- femoral v.
- great saphenous v.

■ adductor muscles
■ quadriceps muscle group
■ other muscles

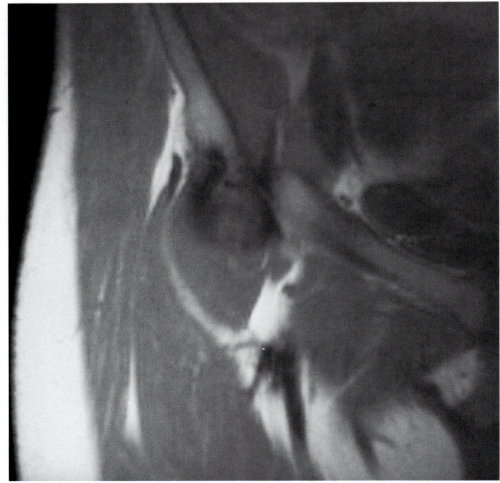

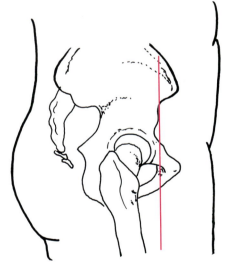

proximal

lateral   medial

distal

Hip – Coronal

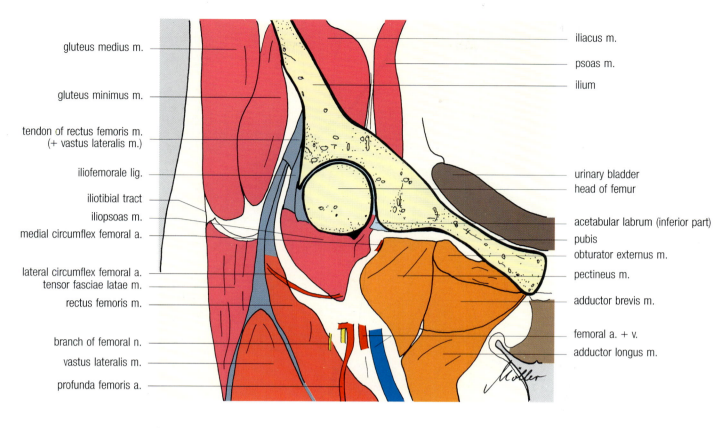

- adductor muscles
- quadriceps muscle group
- other muscles

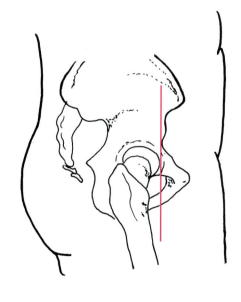

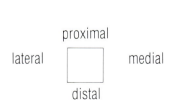

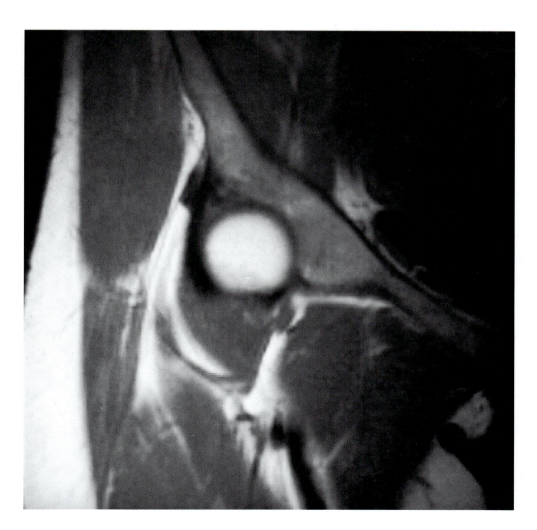

Hip – Coronal

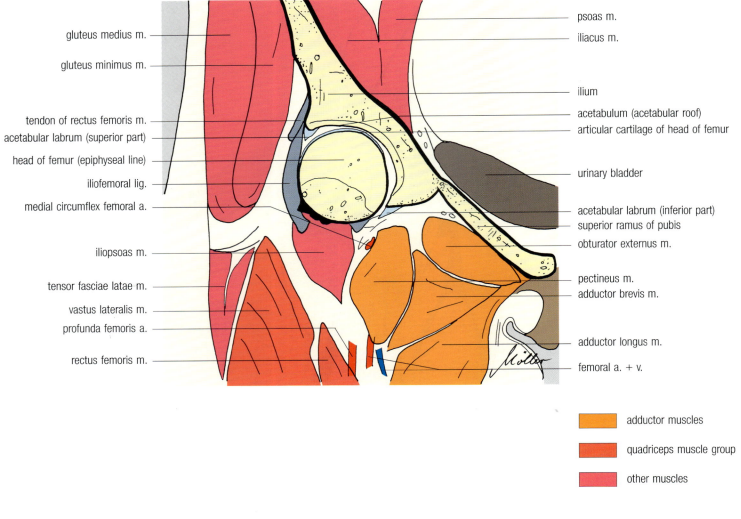

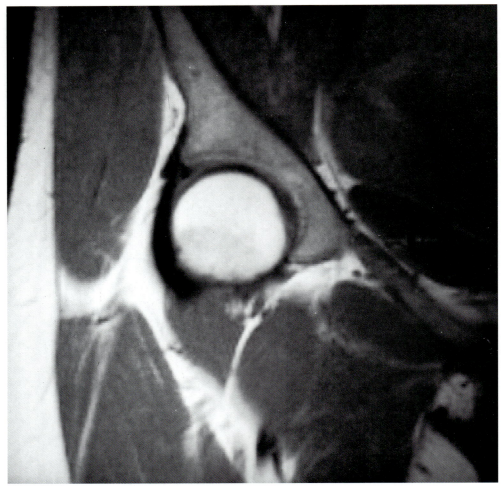

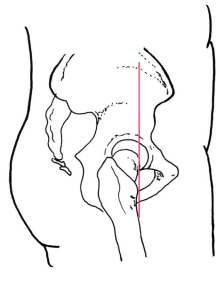

Hip – Coronal

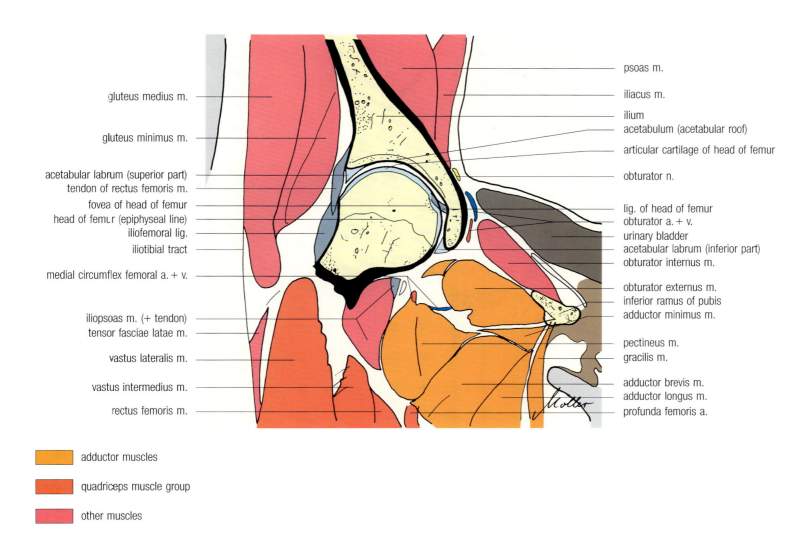

- gluteus medius m.
- gluteus minimus m.
- acetabular labrum (superior part)
- tendon of rectus femoris m.
- fovea of head of femur
- head of femur (epiphyseal line)
- iliofemoral lig.
- iliotibial tract
- medial circumflex femoral a. + v.
- iliopsoas m. (+ tendon)
- tensor fasciae latae m.
- vastus lateralis m.
- vastus intermedius m.
- rectus femoris m.
- psoas m.
- iliacus m.
- ilium
- acetabulum (acetabular roof)
- articular cartilage of head of femur
- obturator n.
- lig. of head of femur
- obturator a. + v.
- urinary bladder
- acetabular labrum (inferior part)
- obturator internus m.
- obturator externus m.
- inferior ramus of pubis
- adductor minimus m.
- pectineus m.
- gracilis m.
- adductor brevis m.
- adductor longus m.
- profunda femoris a.

■ adductor muscles
■ quadriceps muscle group
■ other muscles

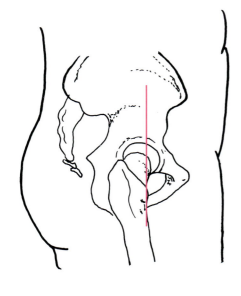

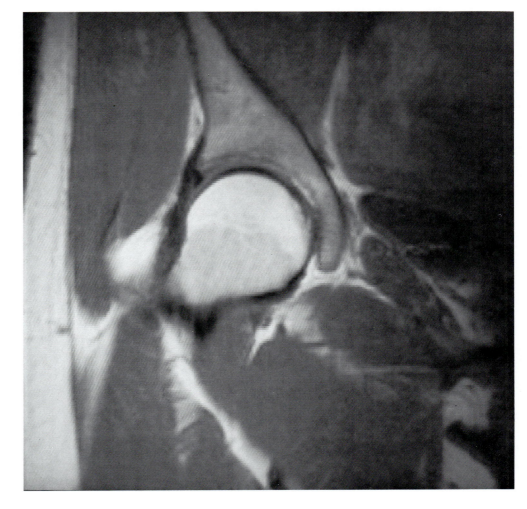

proximal / lateral / medial / distal

Hip – Coronal

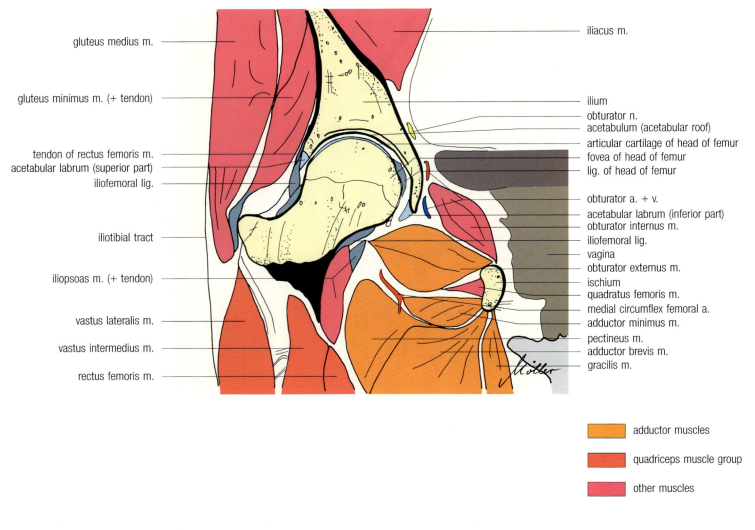

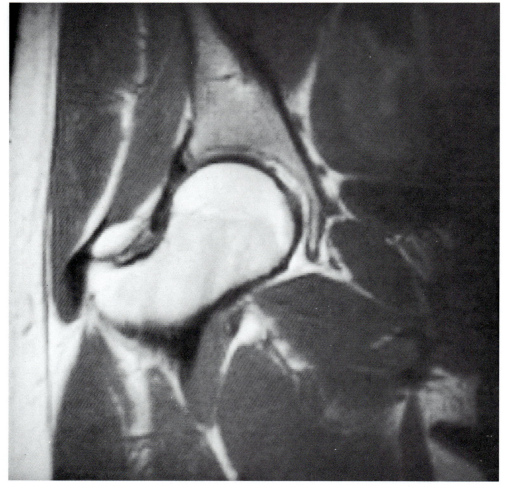

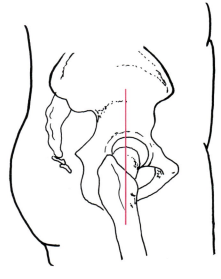

Hip – Coronal

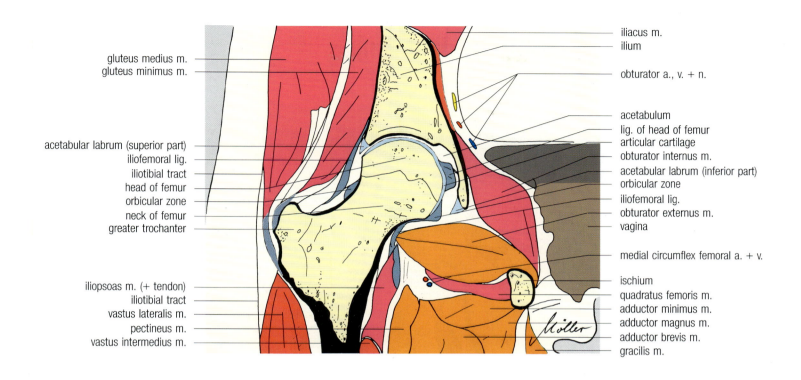

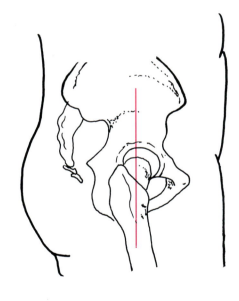

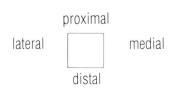

- adductor muscles
- quadriceps muscle group
- other muscles

proximal
lateral — medial
distal

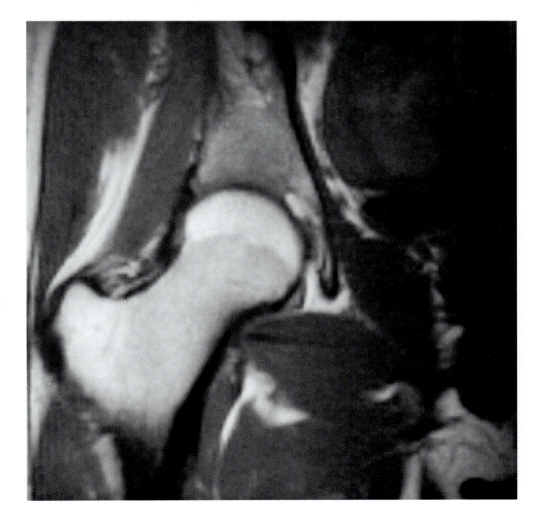

Hip – Coronal

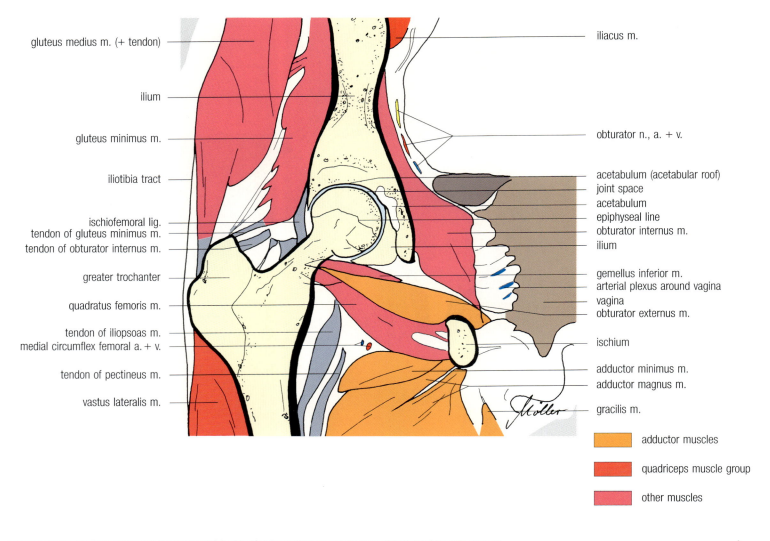

- gluteus medius m. (+ tendon)
- ilium
- gluteus minimus m.
- iliotibia tract
- ischiofemoral lig.
- tendon of gluteus minimus m.
- tendon of obturator internus m.
- greater trochanter
- quadratus femoris m.
- tendon of iliopsoas m.
- medial circumflex femoral a. + v.
- tendon of pectineus m.
- vastus lateralis m.

- iliacus m.
- obturator n., a. + v.
- acetabulum (acetabular roof)
- joint space
- acetabulum
- epiphyseal line
- obturator internus m.
- ilium
- gemellus inferior m.
- arterial plexus around vagina
- vagina
- obturator externus m.
- ischium
- adductor minimus m.
- adductor magnus m.
- gracilis m.

■ adductor muscles
■ quadriceps muscle group
■ other muscles

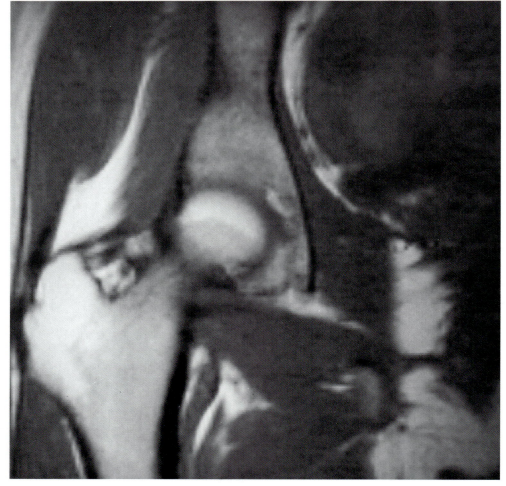

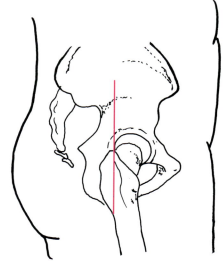

proximal
lateral — medial
distal

Hip – Coronal

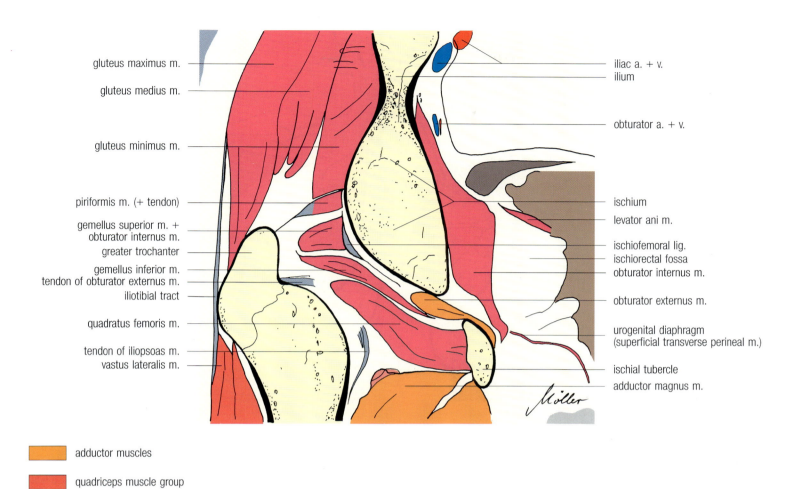

- adductor muscles
- quadriceps muscle group
- other muscles

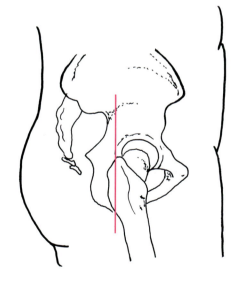

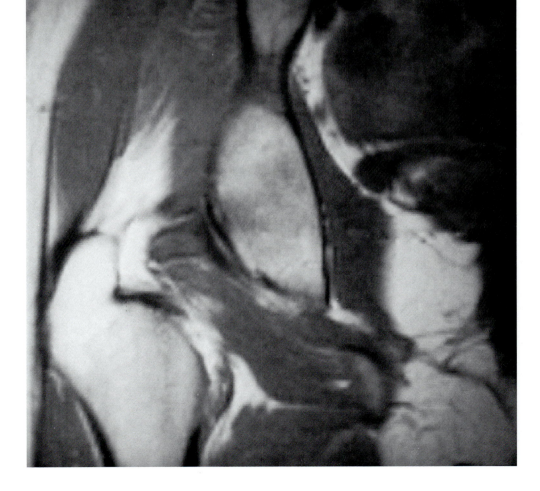

Hip – Coronal

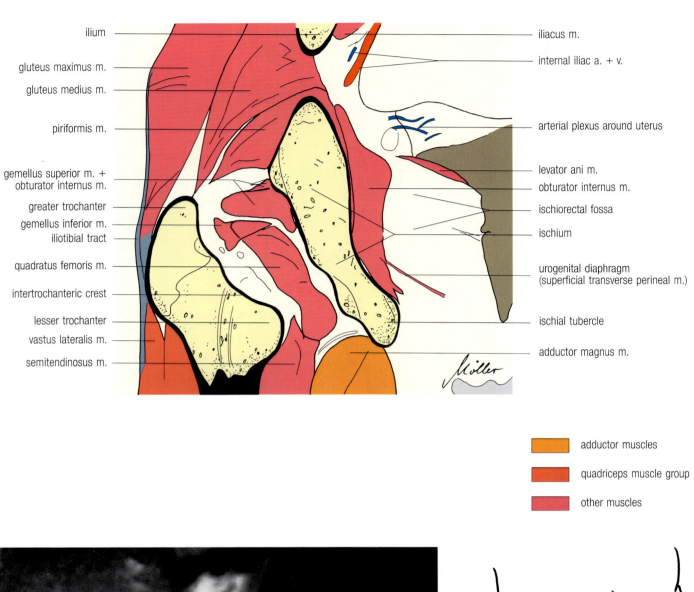

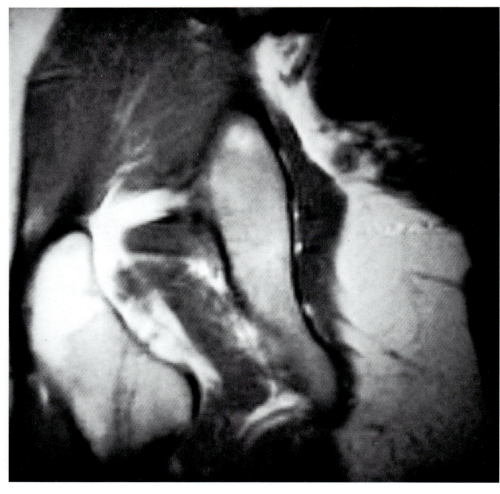

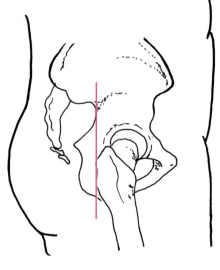

Hip – Sagittal

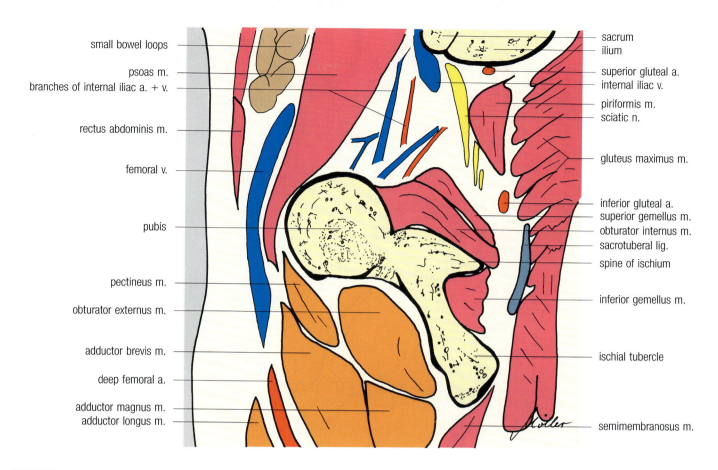

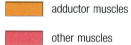

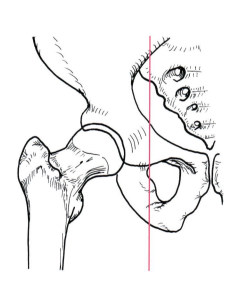

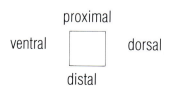

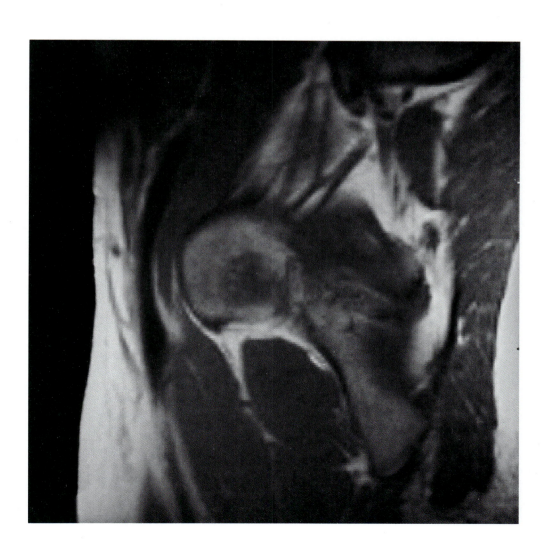

Hip – Sagittal

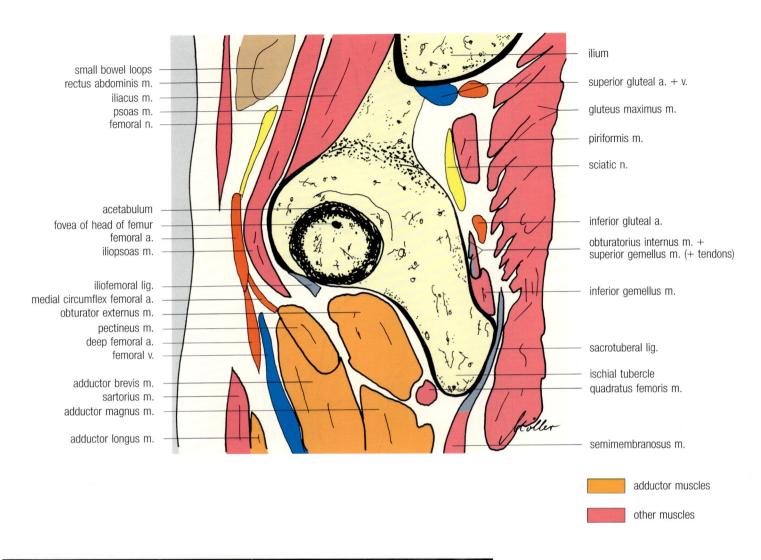

- small bowel loops
- rectus abdominis m.
- iliacus m.
- psoas m.
- femoral n.
- acetabulum
- fovea of head of femur
- femoral a.
- iliopsoas m.
- iliofemoral lig.
- medial circumflex femoral a.
- obturator externus m.
- pectineus m.
- deep femoral a.
- femoral v.
- adductor brevis m.
- sartorius m.
- adductor magnus m.
- adductor longus m.

- ilium
- superior gluteal a. + v.
- gluteus maximus m.
- piriformis m.
- sciatic n.
- inferior gluteal a.
- obturatorius internus m. + superior gemellus m. (+ tendons)
- inferior gemellus m.
- sacrotuberal lig.
- ischial tubercle
- quadratus femoris m.
- semimembranosus m.

■ adductor muscles
■ other muscles

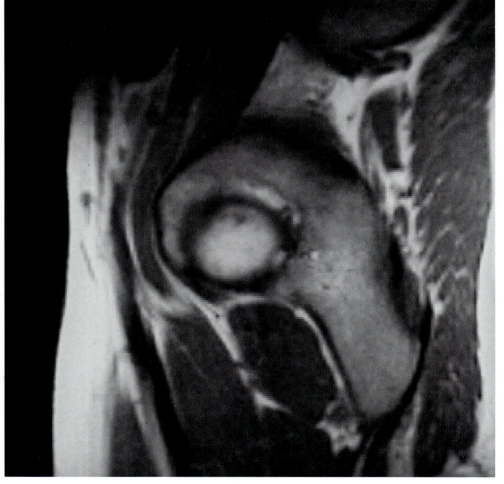

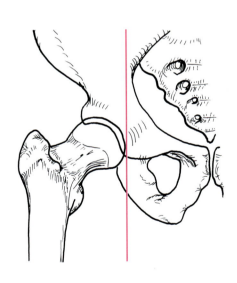

proximal
ventral ☐ dorsal
distal

Hip – Sagittal

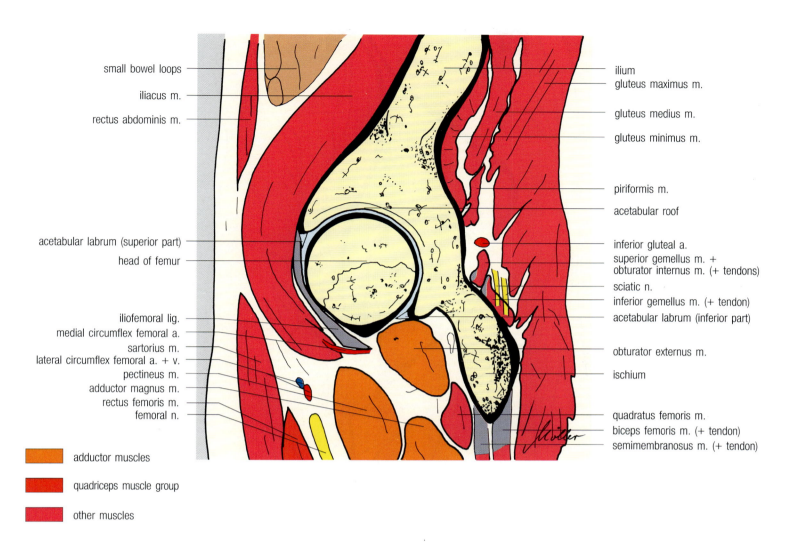

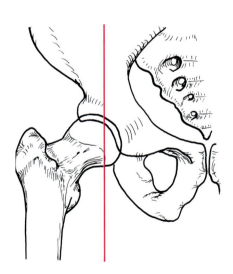

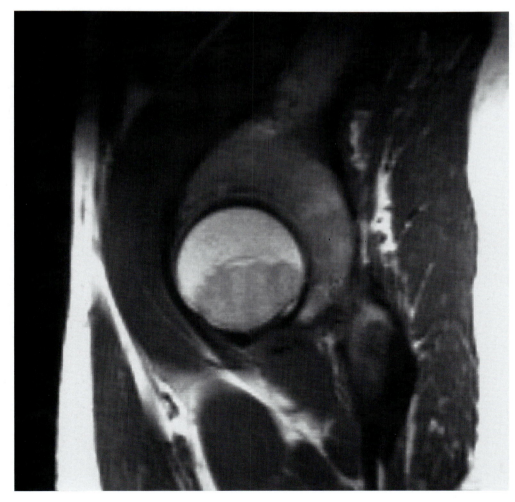

Hip – Sagittal

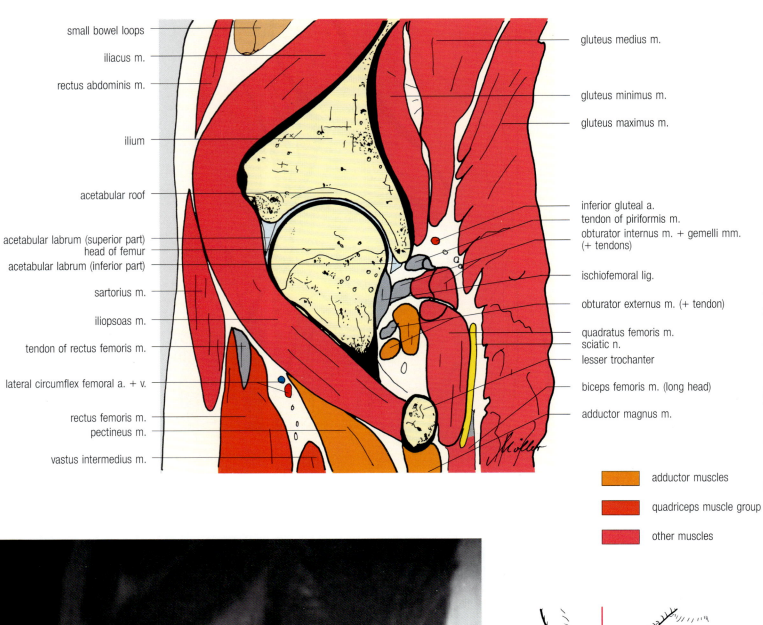

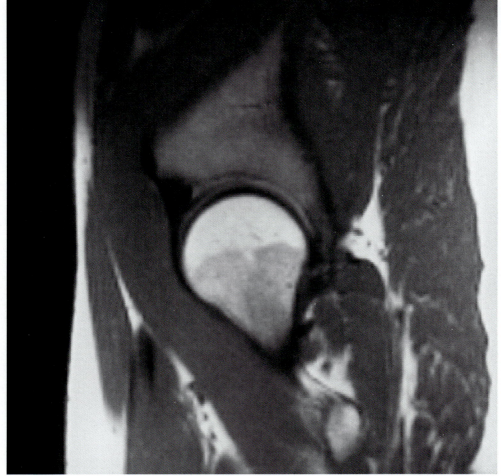

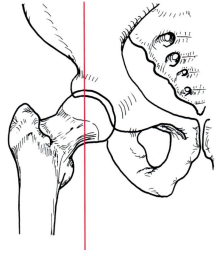

Hip – Sagittal 199

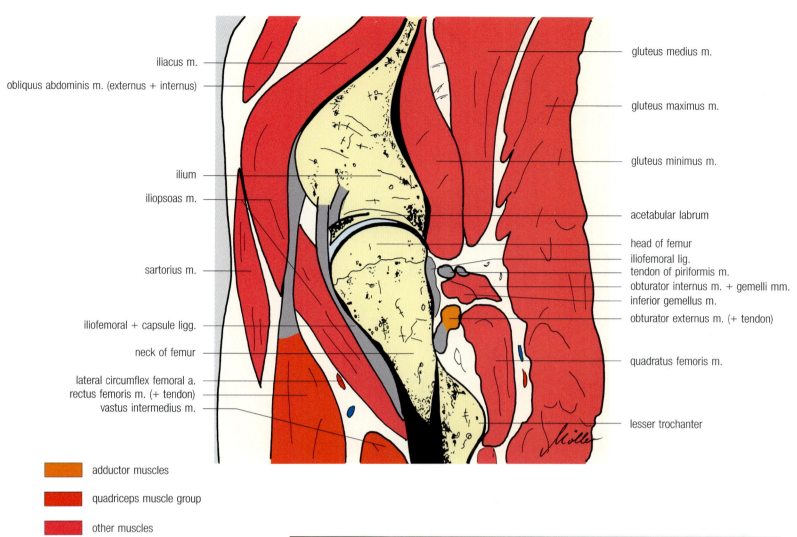

- iliacus m.
- obliquus abdominis m. (externus + internus)
- ilium
- iliopsoas m.
- sartorius m.
- iliofemoral + capsule ligg.
- neck of femur
- lateral circumflex femoral a.
- rectus femoris m. (+ tendon)
- vastus intermedius m.
- gluteus medius m.
- gluteus maximus m.
- gluteus minimus m.
- acetabular labrum
- head of femur
- iliofemoral lig.
- tendon of piriformis m.
- obturator internus m. + gemelli mm.
- inferior gemellus m.
- obturator externus m. (+ tendon)
- quadratus femoris m.
- lesser trochanter

- adductor muscles
- quadriceps muscle group
- other muscles

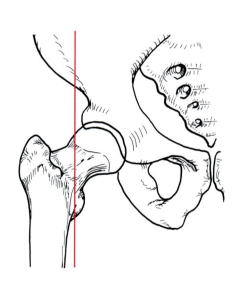

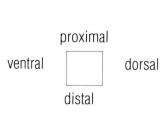

proximal / ventral – dorsal / distal

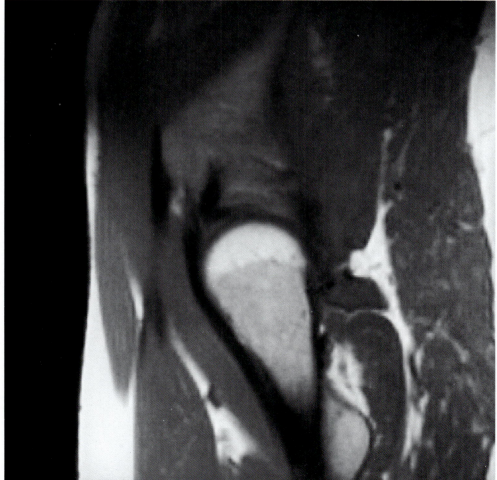

Hip – Sagittal

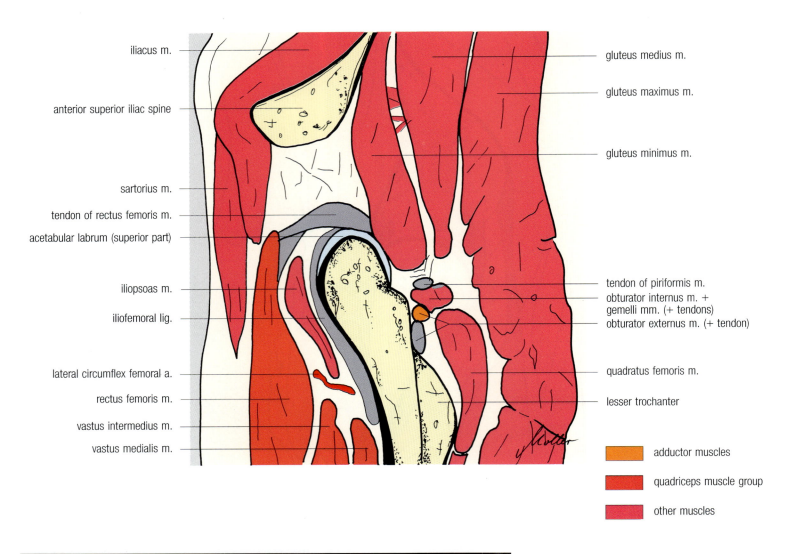

- iliacus m.
- anterior superior iliac spine
- sartorius m.
- tendon of rectus femoris m.
- acetabular labrum (superior part)
- iliopsoas m.
- iliofemoral lig.
- lateral circumflex femoral a.
- rectus femoris m.
- vastus intermedius m.
- vastus medialis m.
- gluteus medius m.
- gluteus maximus m.
- gluteus minimus m.
- tendon of piriformis m.
- obturator internus m. + gemelli mm. (+ tendons)
- obturator externus m. (+ tendon)
- quadratus femoris m.
- lesser trochanter

■ adductor muscles
■ quadriceps muscle group
■ other muscles

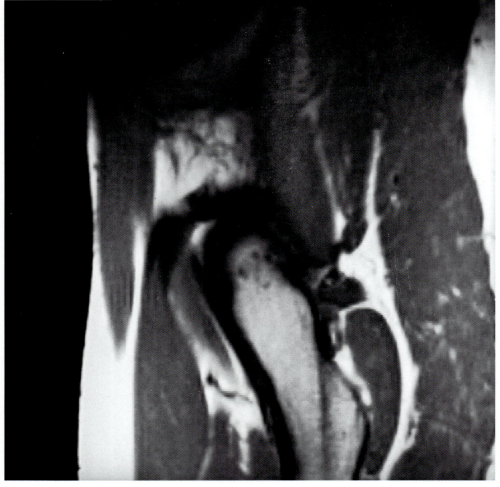

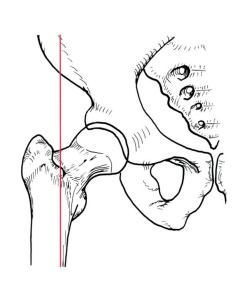

proximal
ventral □ dorsal
distal

Hip – Sagittal

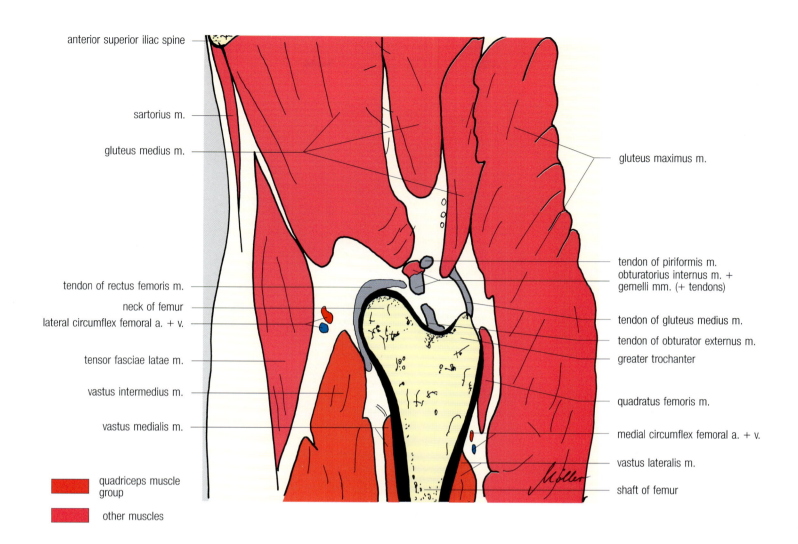

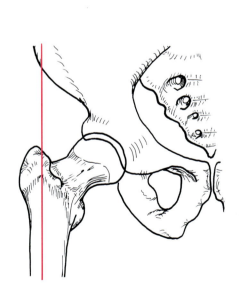

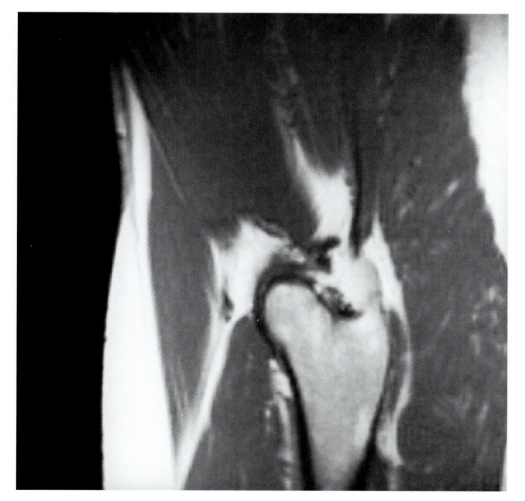

Thigh

Coronal

Sagittal

Thigh – Coronal

205

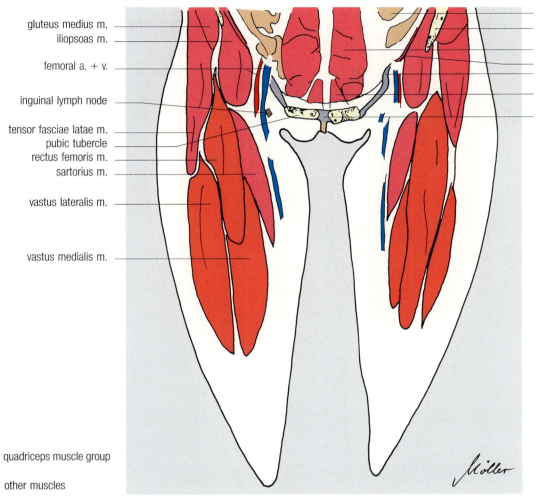

quadriceps muscle group
other muscles

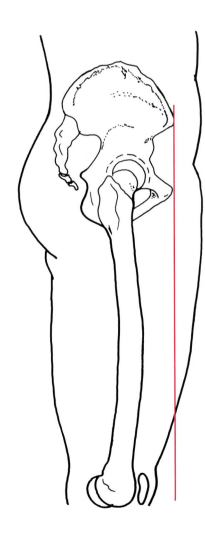
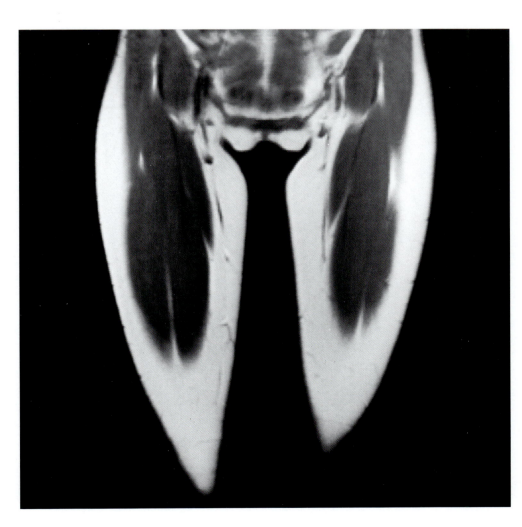

206 Thigh – Coronal

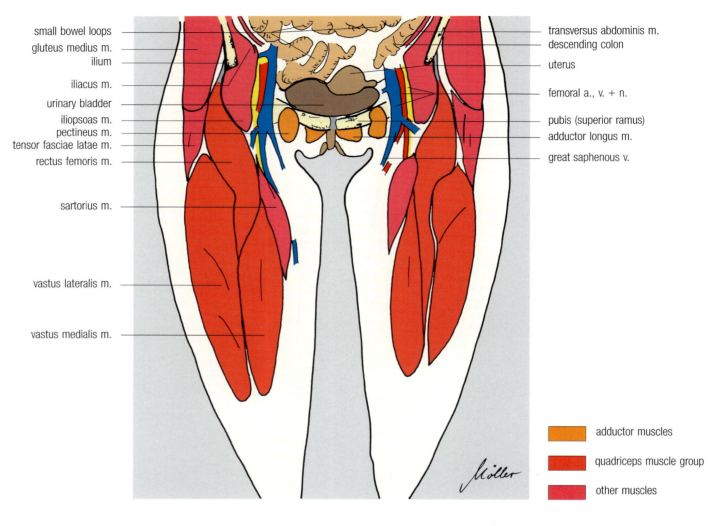
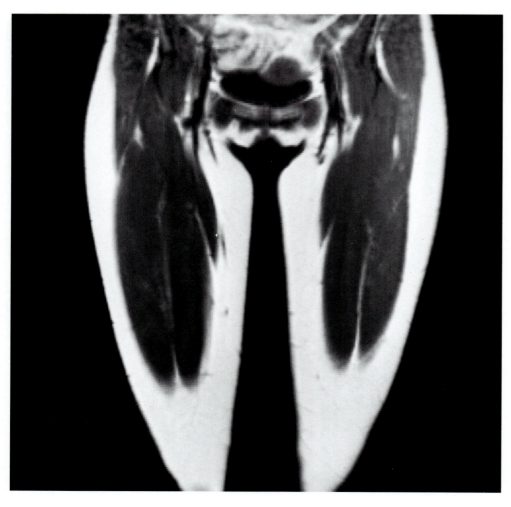
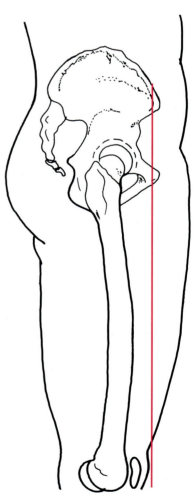

Thigh – Coronal 207

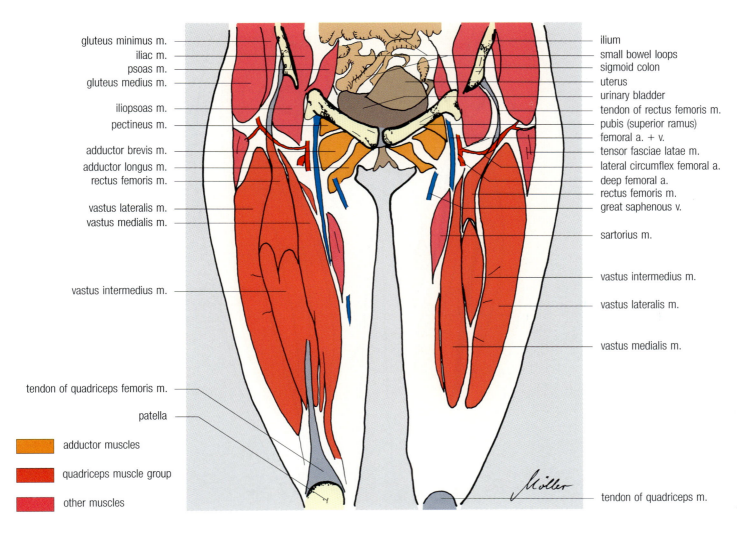
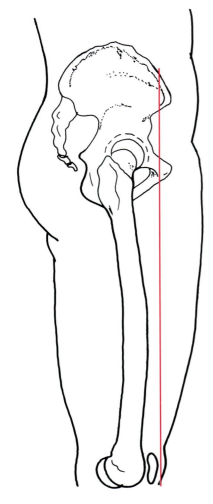
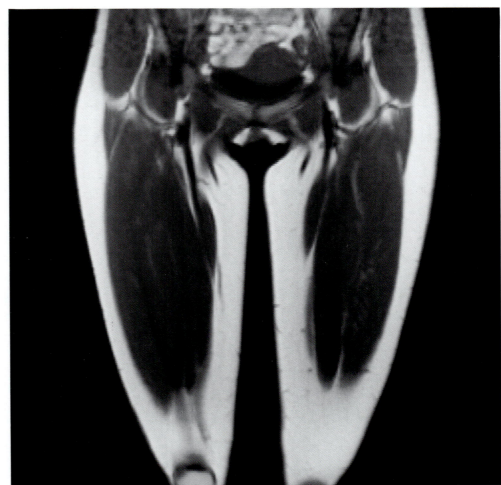

208 Thigh – Coronal

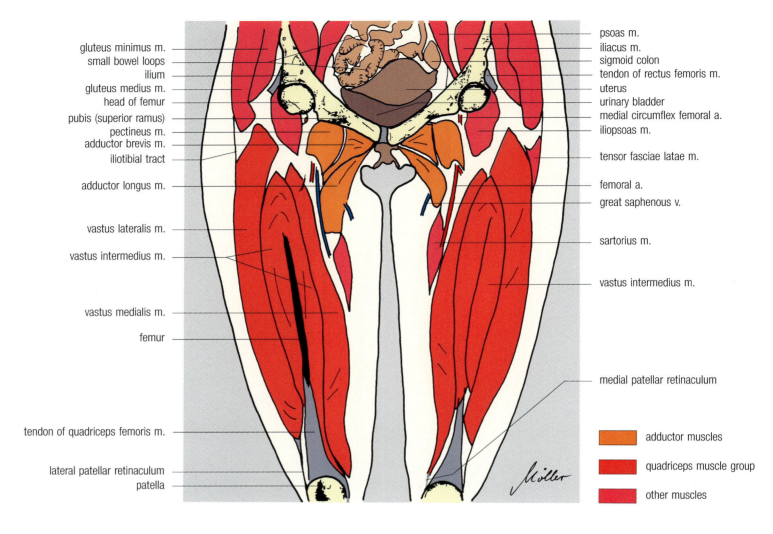

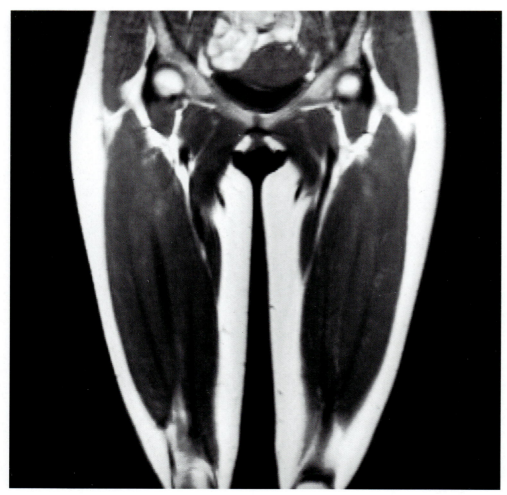
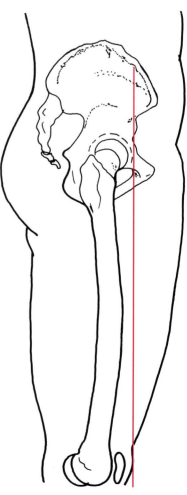

Thigh – Coronal

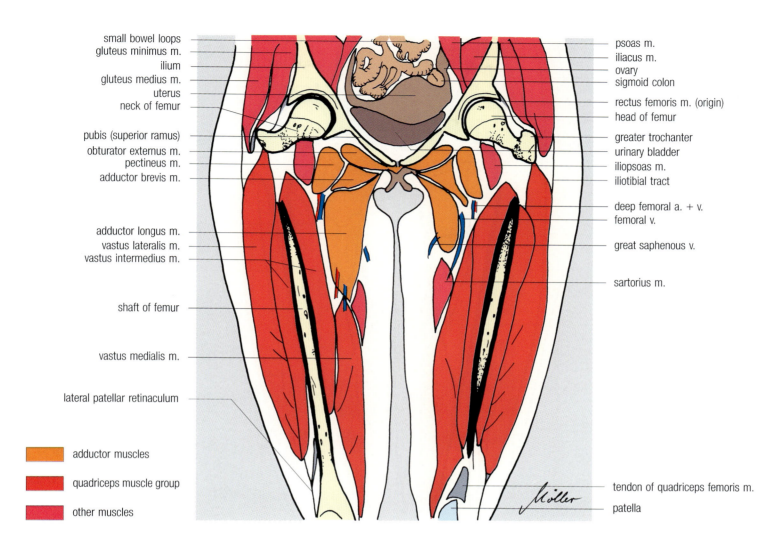

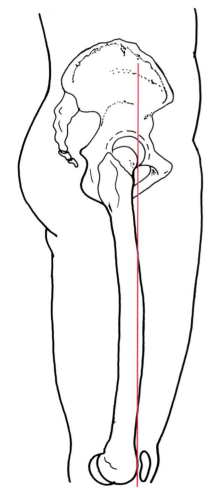
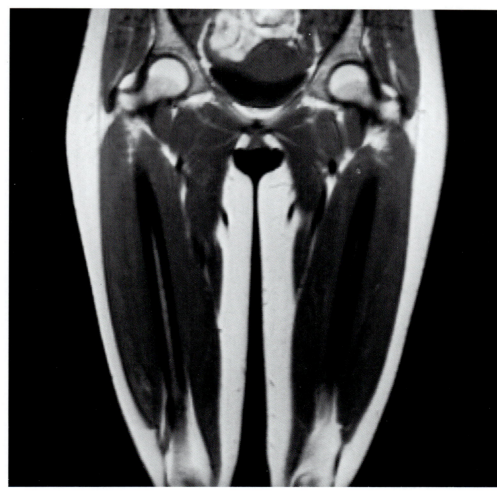

210 Thigh – Coronal

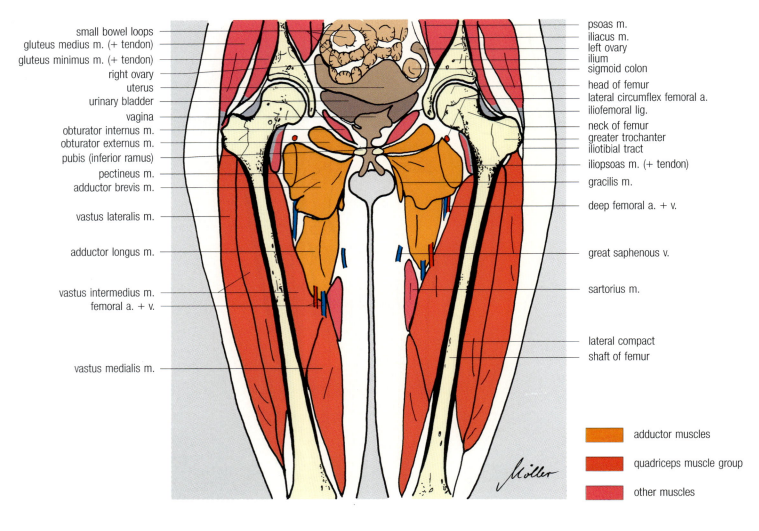

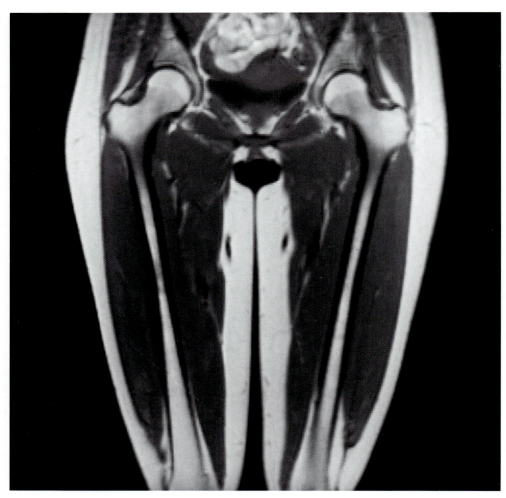
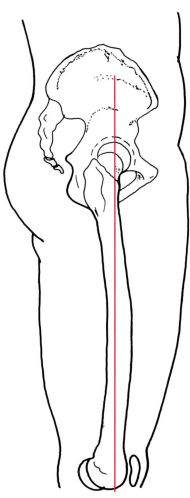

Thigh – Coronal

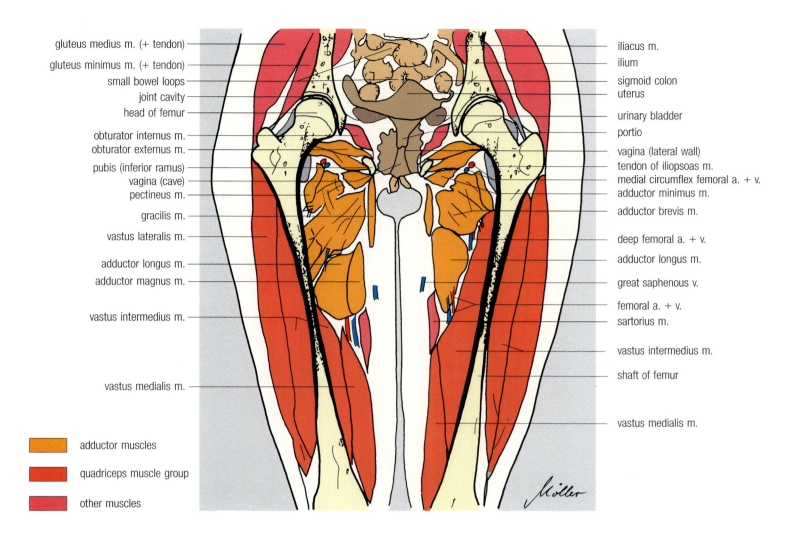

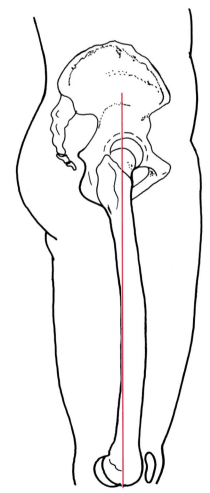

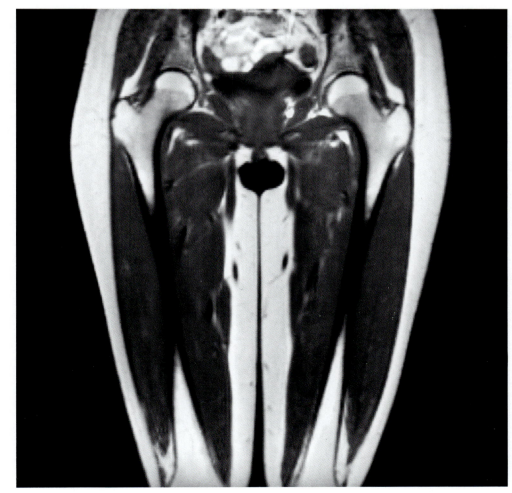

Thigh – Coronal

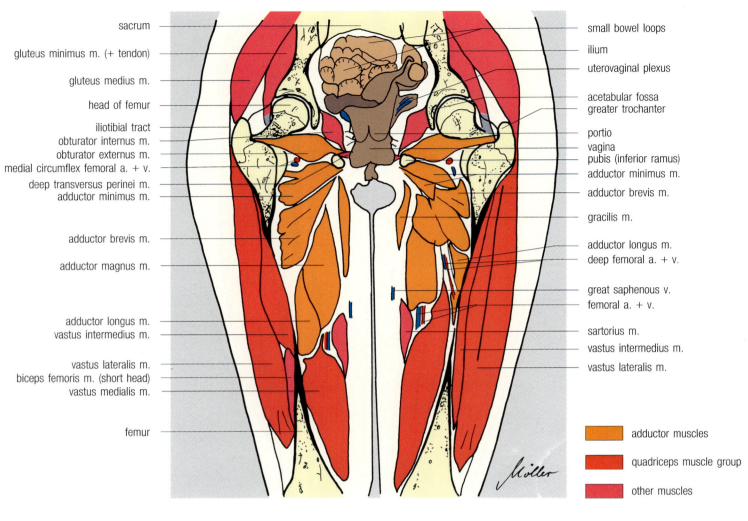
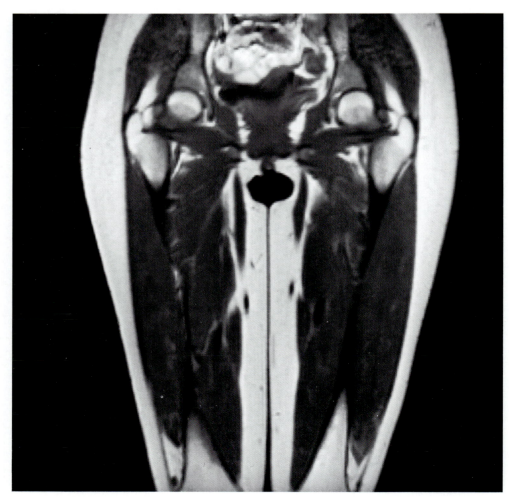
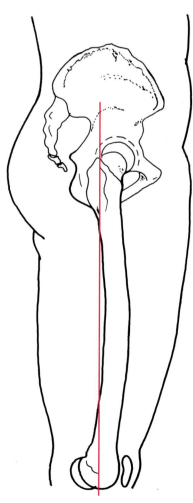

Thigh – Coronal

213

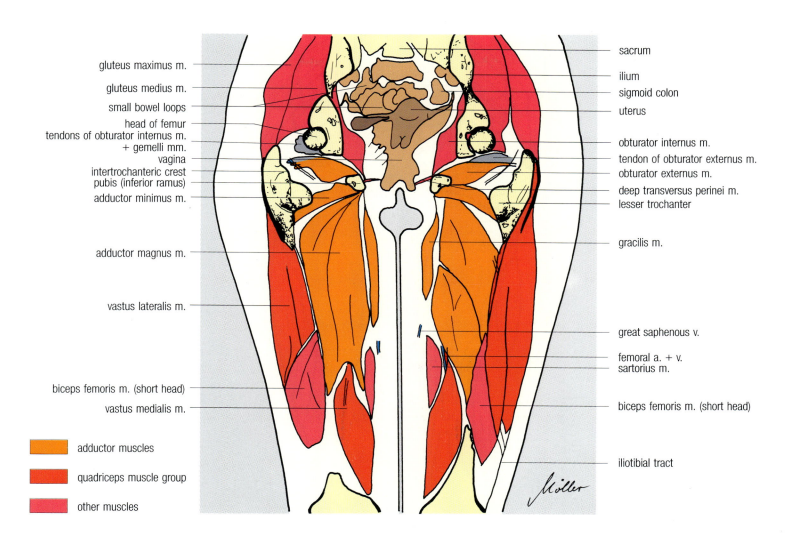

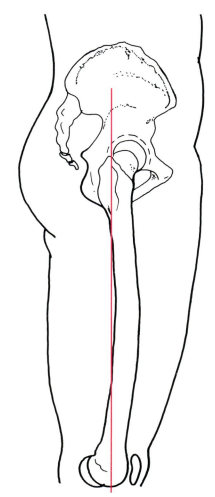
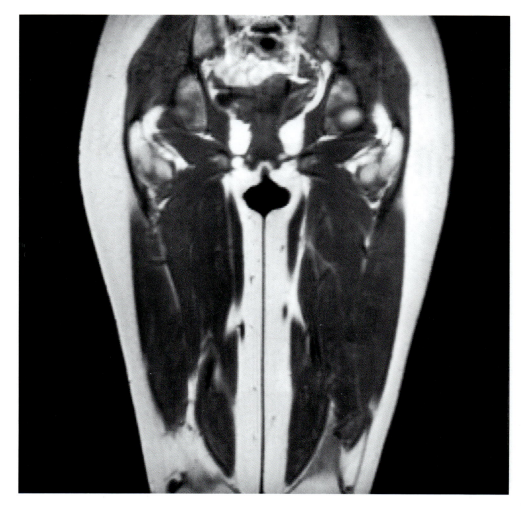

214 Thigh – Coronal

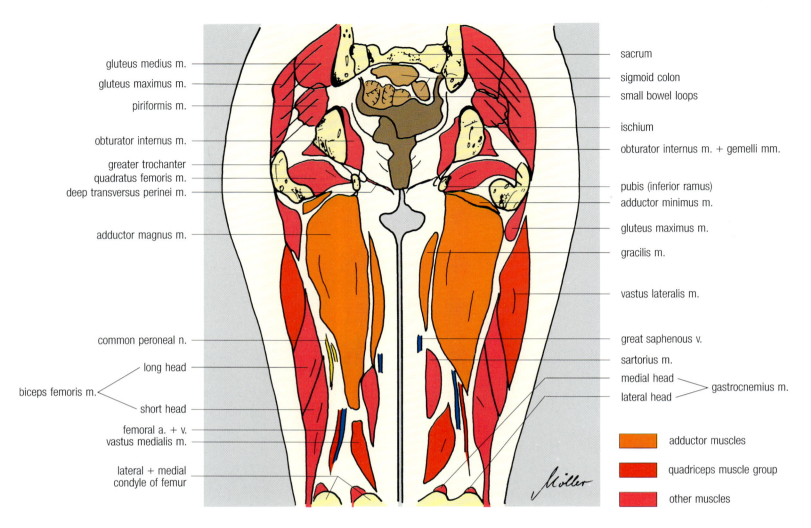

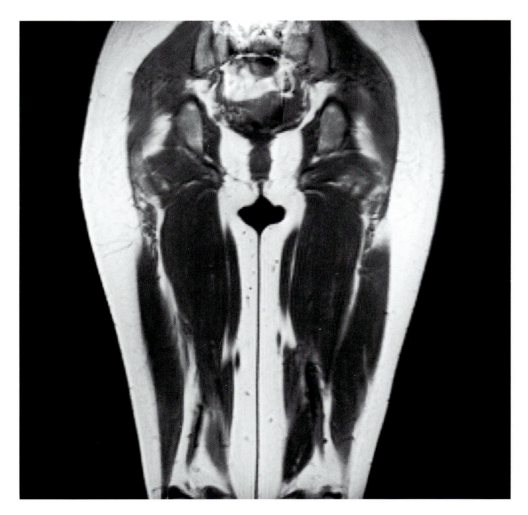
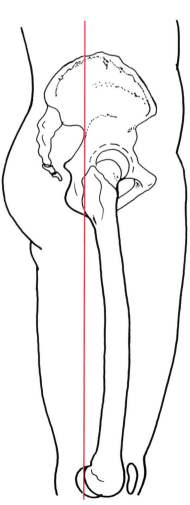

Thigh – Coronal

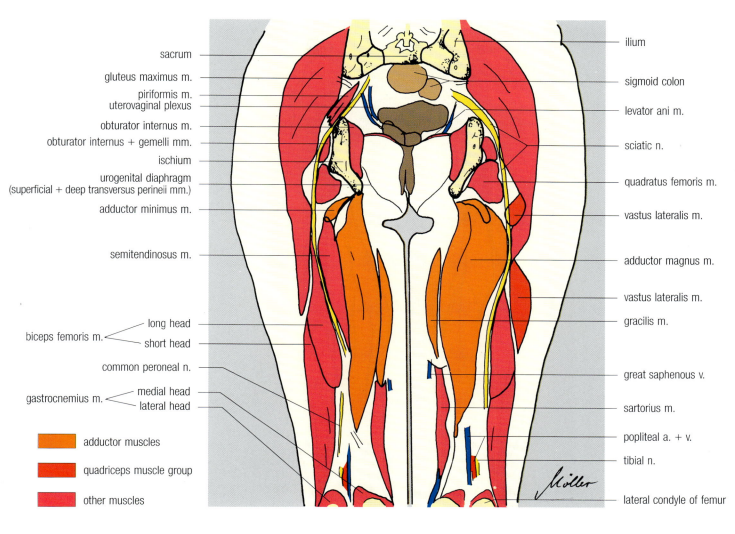
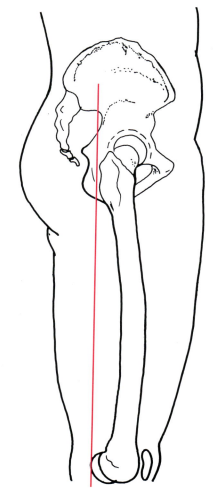
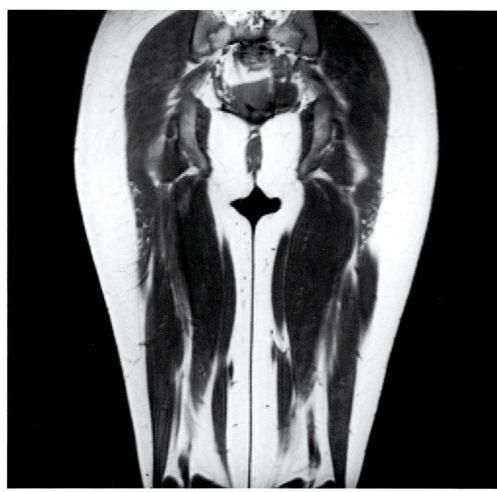

216 Thigh – Coronal

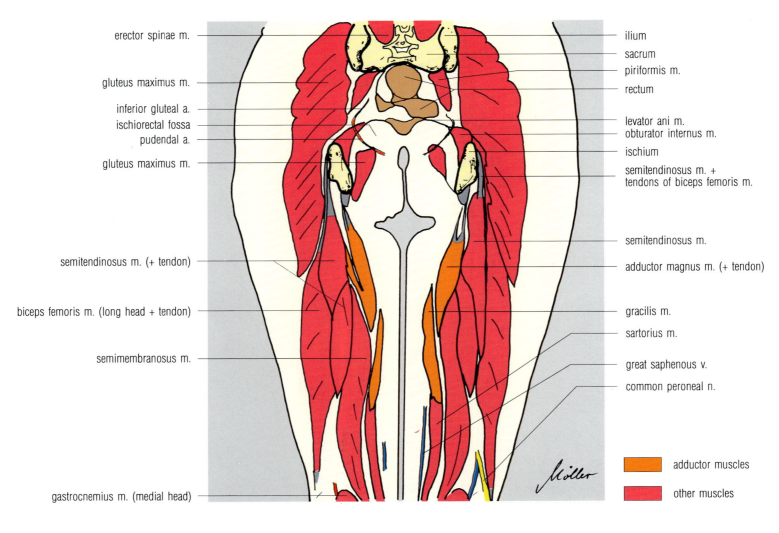

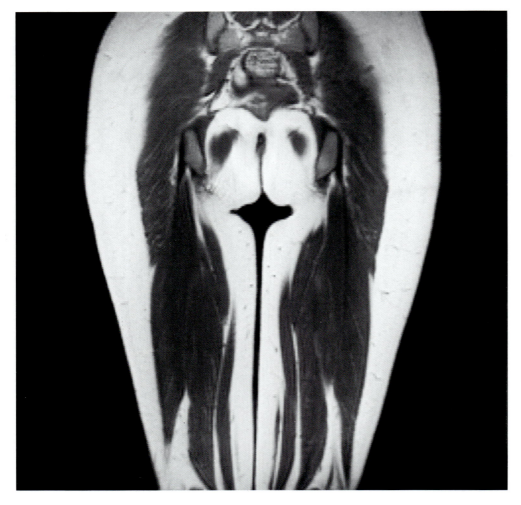
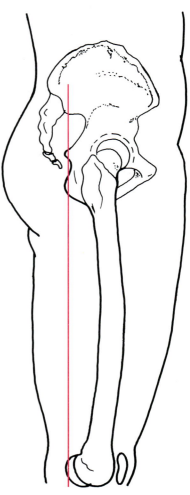

Thigh – Coronal 217

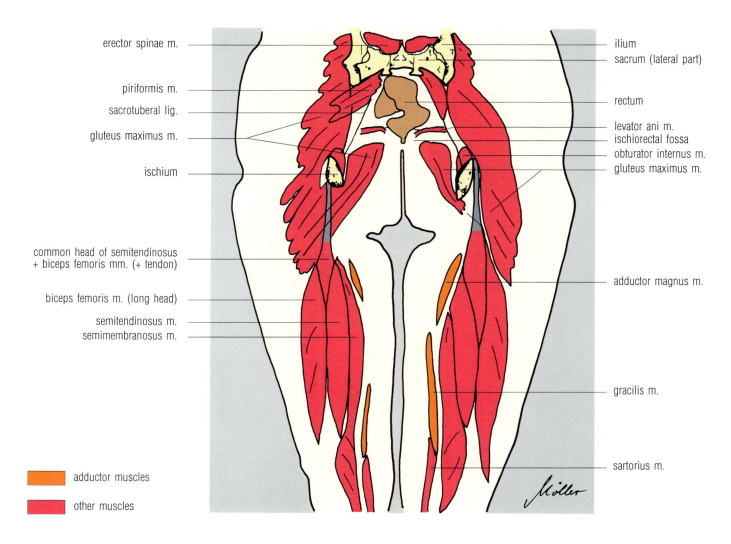

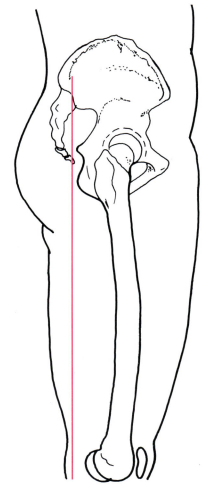
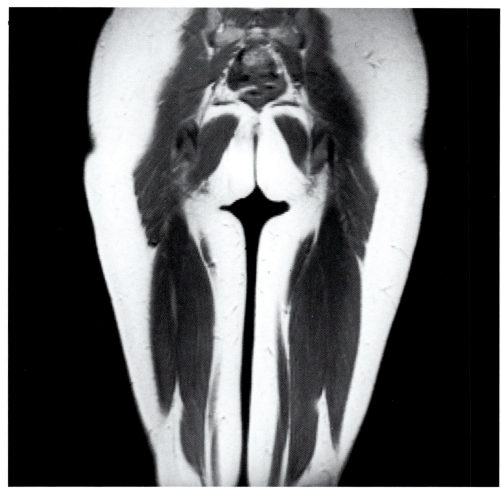

Thigh – Sagittal

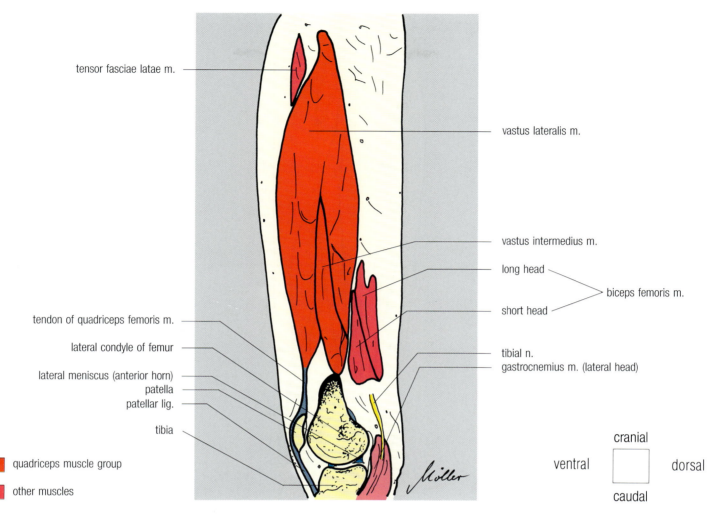

- tensor fasciae latae m.
- vastus lateralis m.
- vastus intermedius m.
- long head
- short head
- biceps femoris m.
- tendon of quadriceps femoris m.
- lateral condyle of femur
- lateral meniscus (anterior horn)
- patella
- patellar lig.
- tibia
- tibial n.
- gastrocnemius m. (lateral head)

■ quadriceps muscle group
▨ other muscles

cranial
ventral — dorsal
caudal

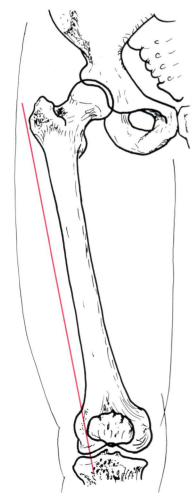
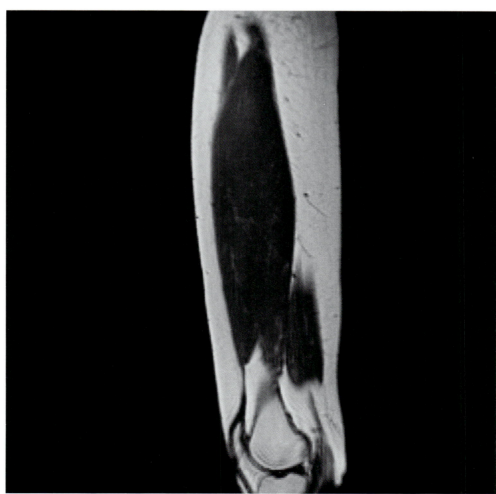

220 Thigh – Sagittal

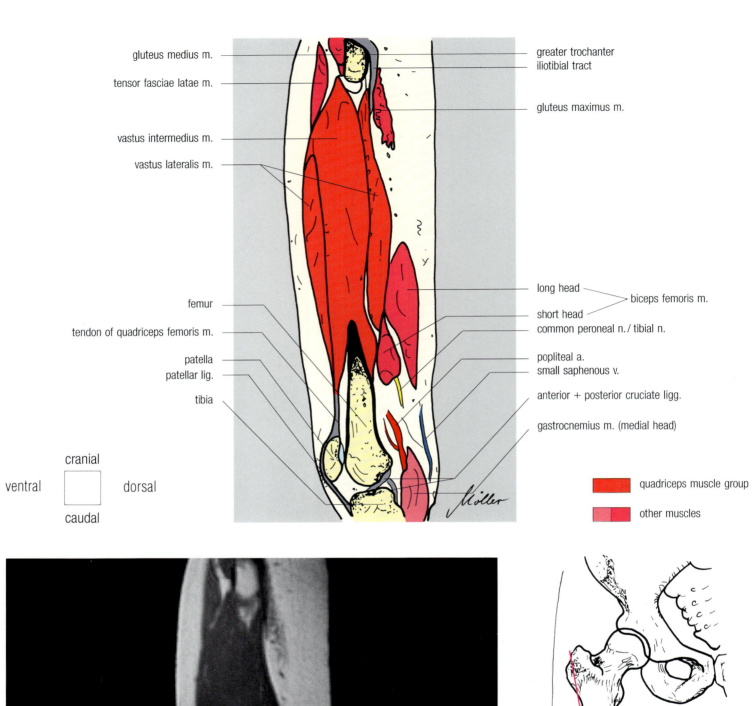

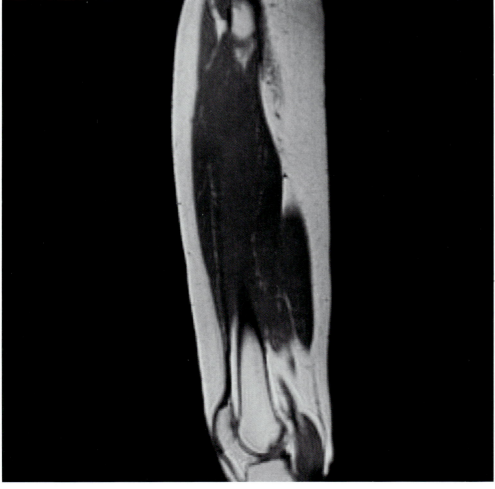
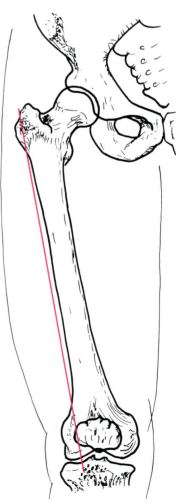

Thigh – Sagittal

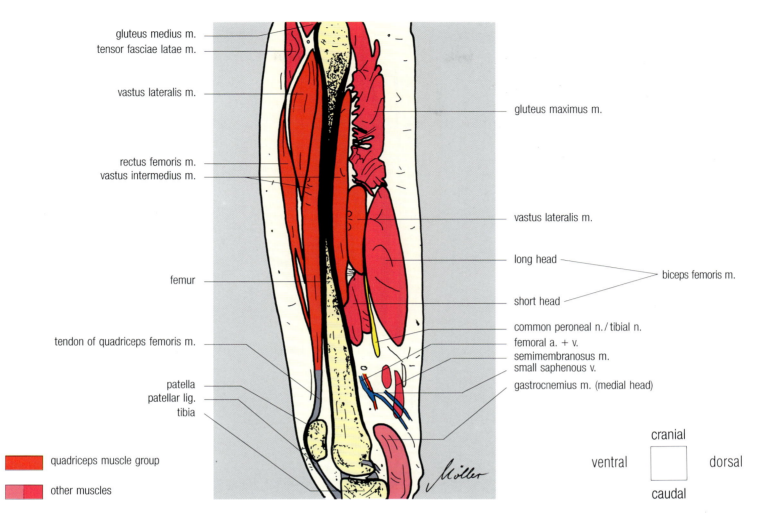

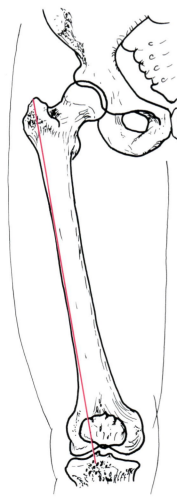
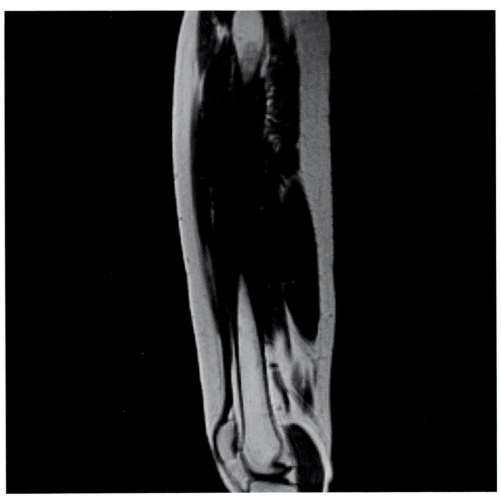

Thigh – Sagittal

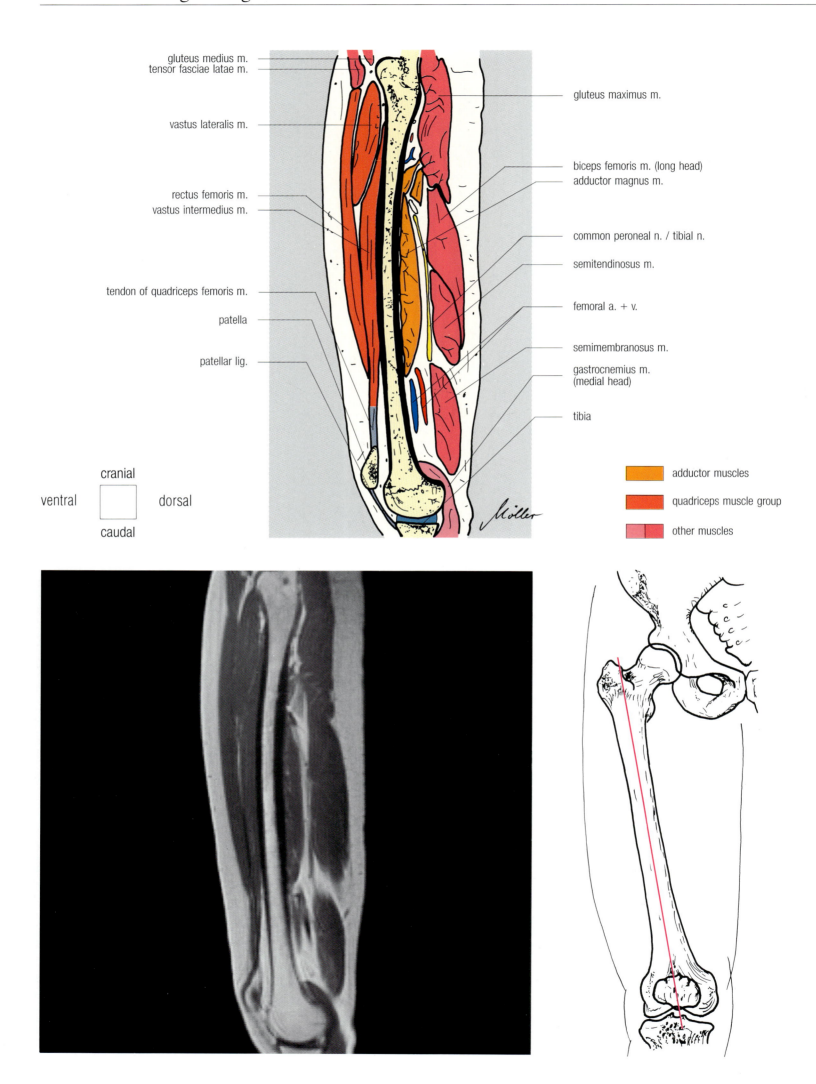

Thigh – Sagittal

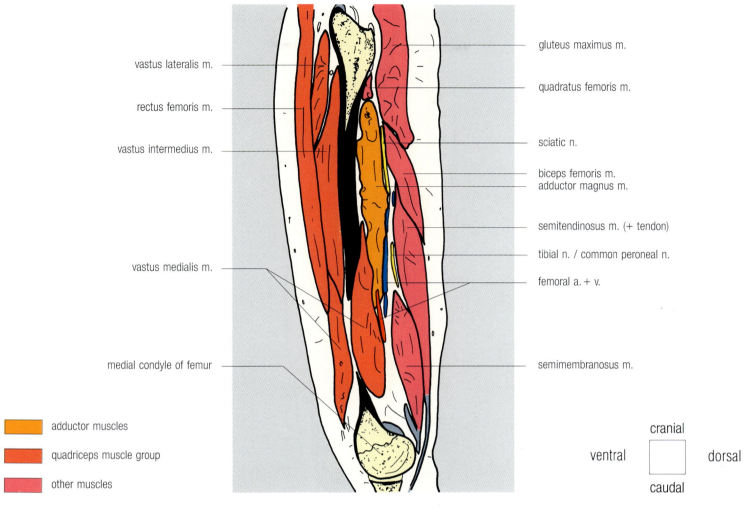

- vastus lateralis m.
- rectus femoris m.
- vastus intermedius m.
- vastus medialis m.
- medial condyle of femur
- gluteus maximus m.
- quadratus femoris m.
- sciatic n.
- biceps femoris m.
- adductor magnus m.
- semitendinosus m. (+ tendon)
- tibial n. / common peroneal n.
- femoral a. + v.
- semimembranosus m.

■ adductor muscles
■ quadriceps muscle group
■ other muscles

cranial
ventral — dorsal
caudal

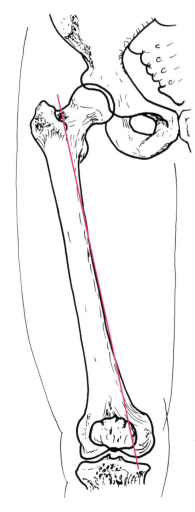

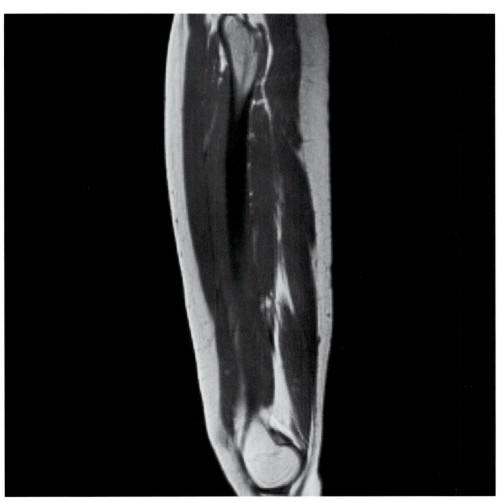

224 Thigh – Sagittal

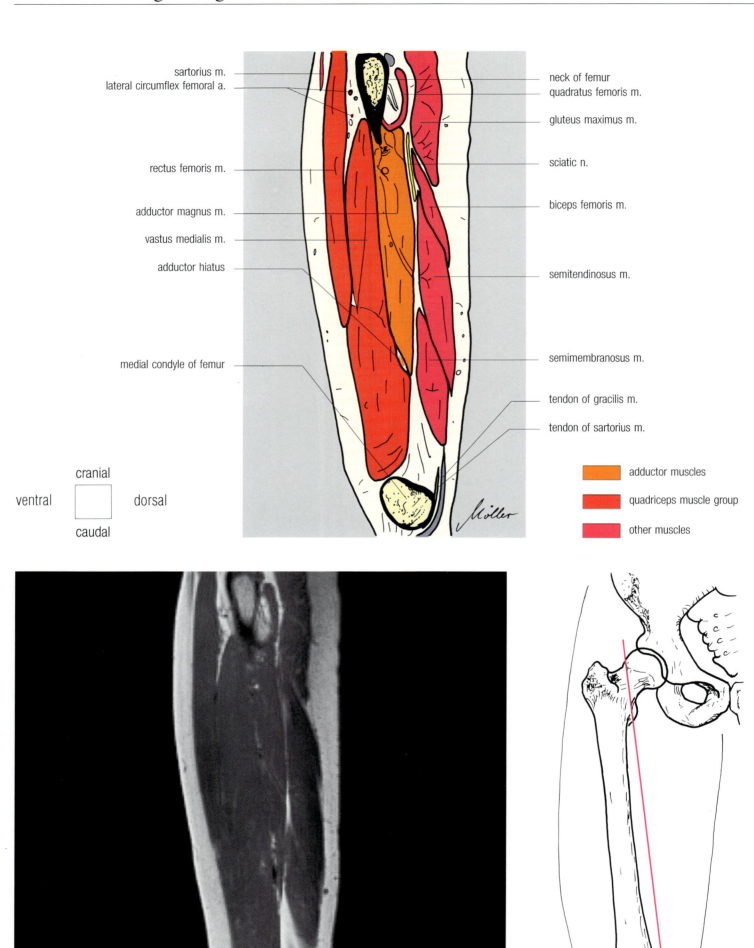

Thigh – Sagittal

225

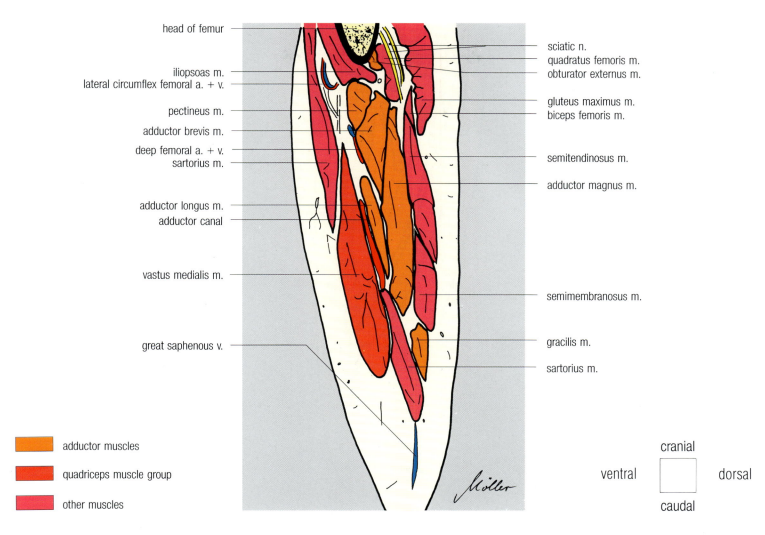

- head of femur
- iliopsoas m.
- lateral circumflex femoral a. + v.
- pectineus m.
- adductor brevis m.
- deep femoral a. + v.
- sartorius m.
- adductor longus m.
- adductor canal
- vastus medialis m.
- great saphenous v.

- sciatic n.
- quadratus femoris m.
- obturator externus m.
- gluteus maximus m.
- biceps femoris m.
- semitendinosus m.
- adductor magnus m.
- semimembranosus m.
- gracilis m.
- sartorius m.

■ adductor muscles
■ quadriceps muscle group
■ other muscles

cranial
ventral □ dorsal
caudal

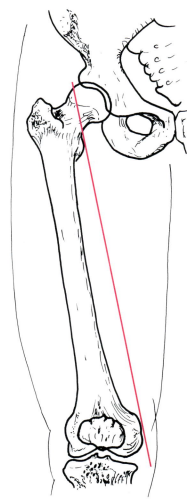
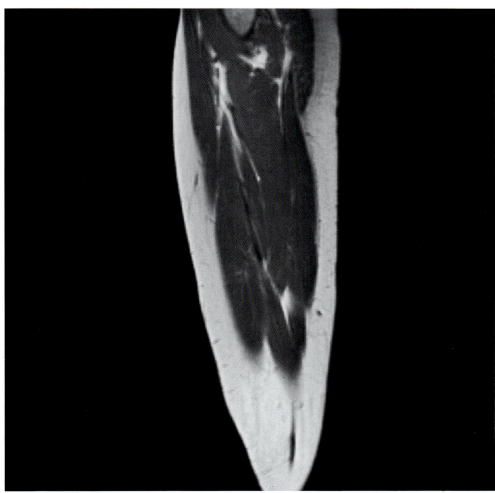

226 Thigh – Sagittal

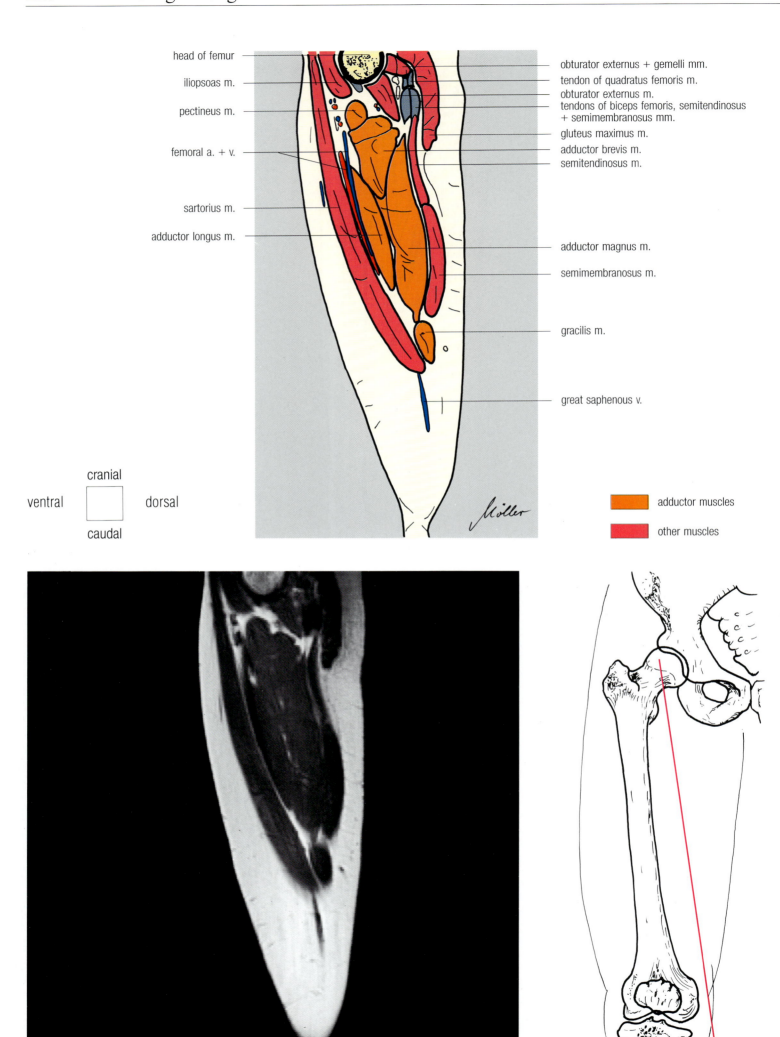

Knee

Coronal

Sagittal

Knee – Coronal

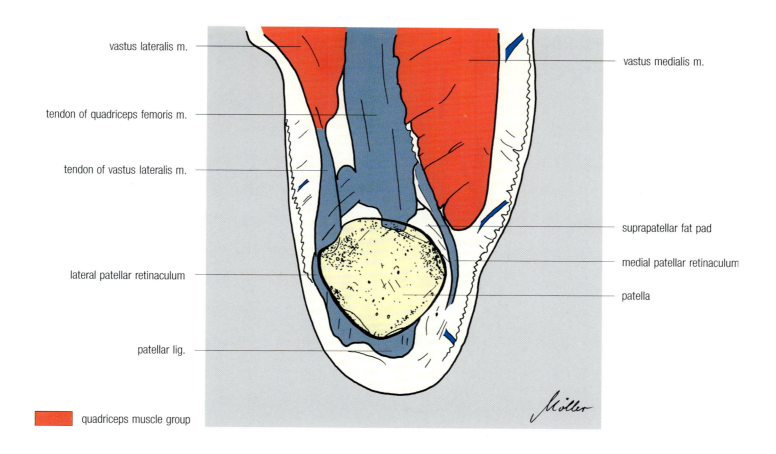

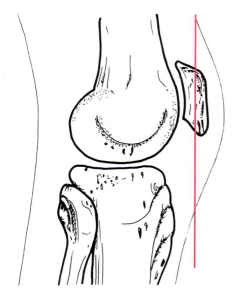
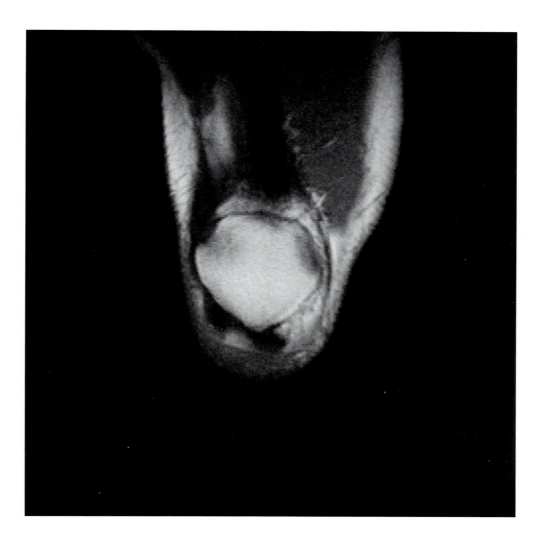

Knee – Coronal

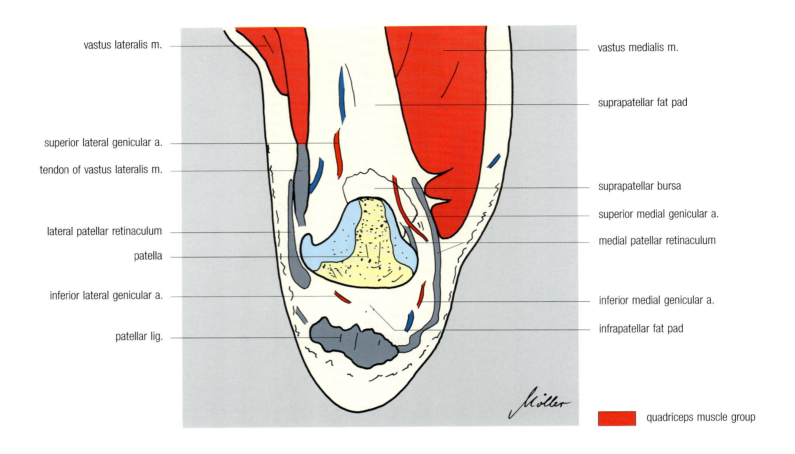

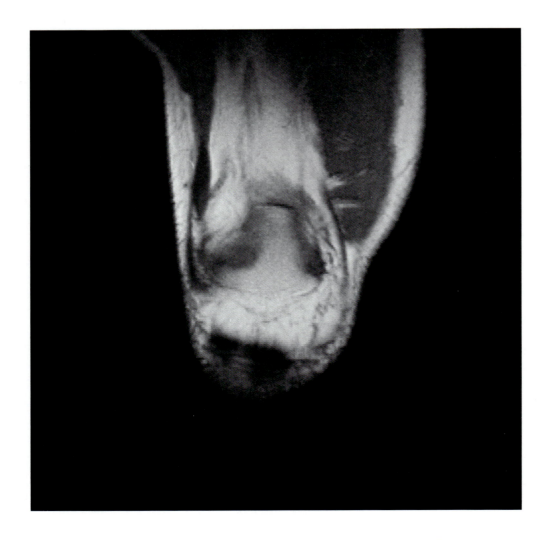

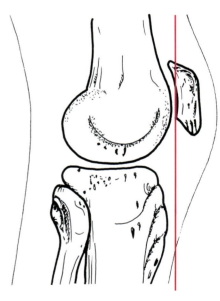

cranial
lateral medial
caudal

Knee – Coronal

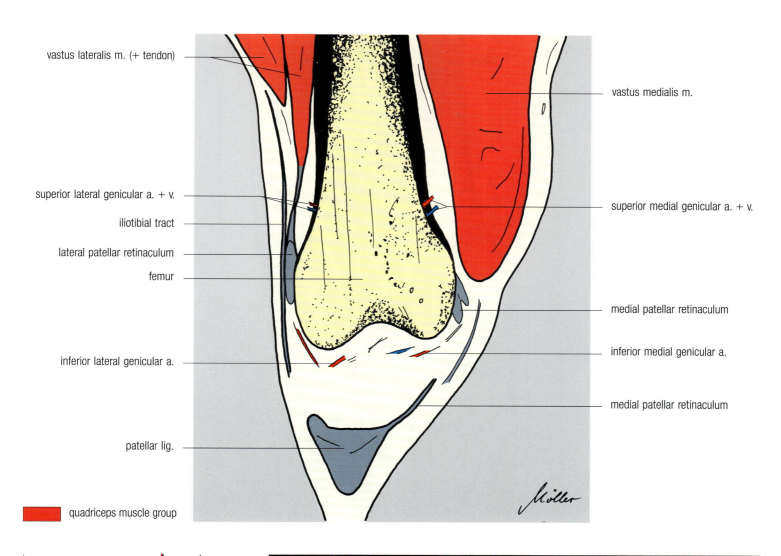

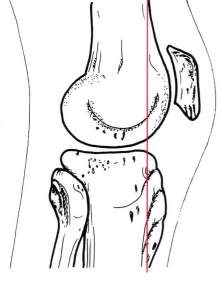
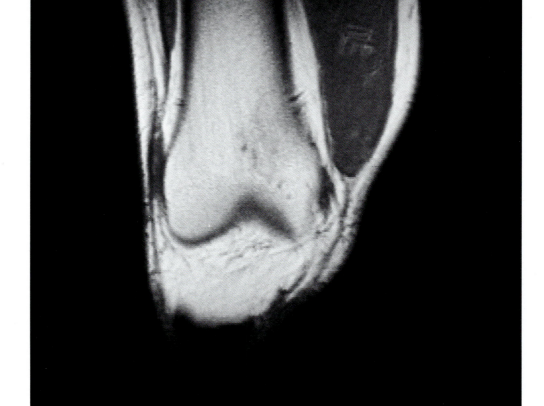

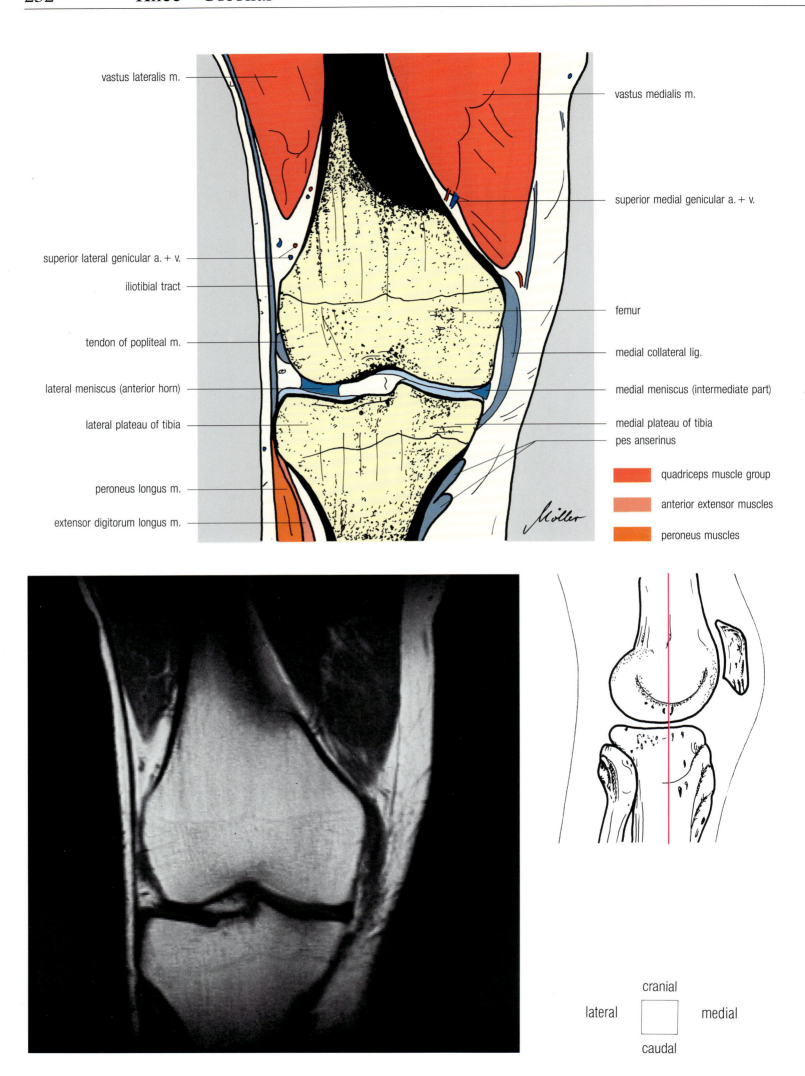

Knee – Coronal 233

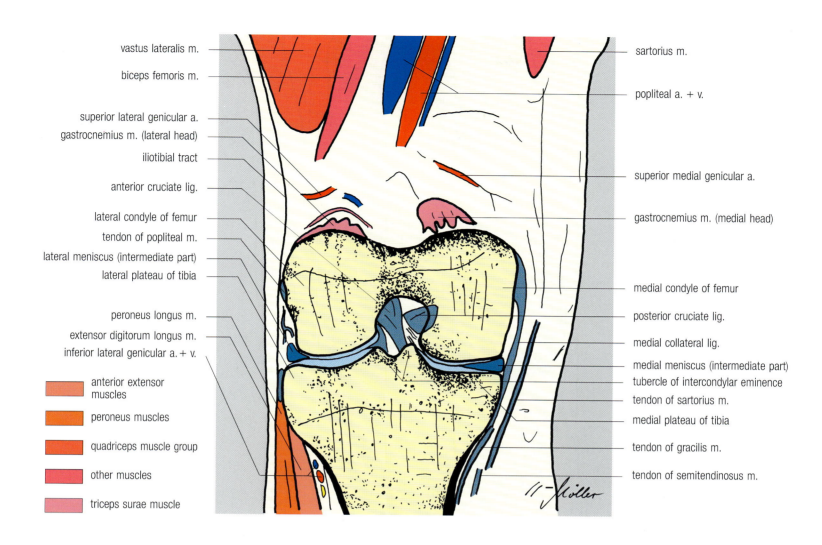

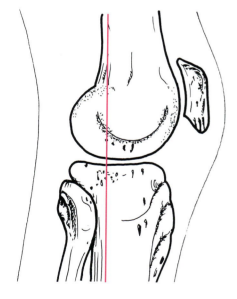

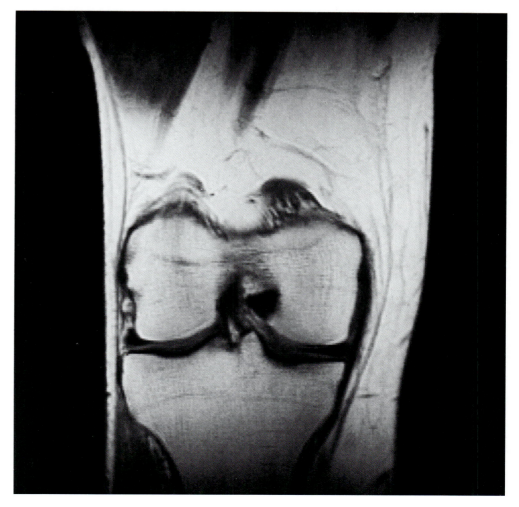

Knee – Coronal

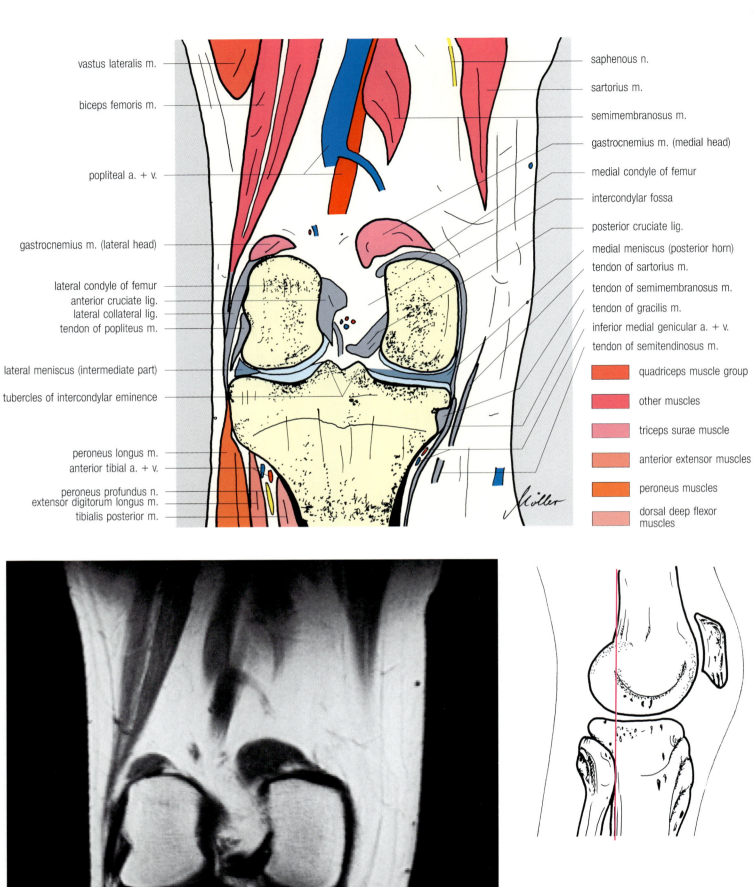

Knee – Coronal 235

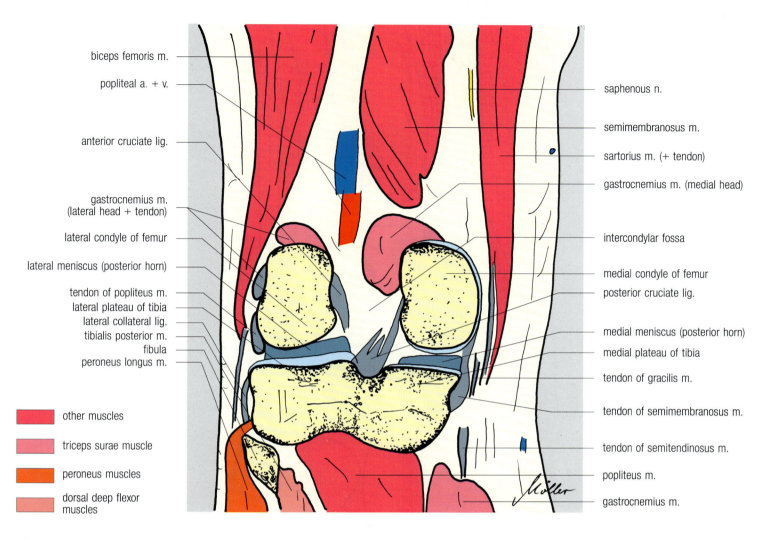

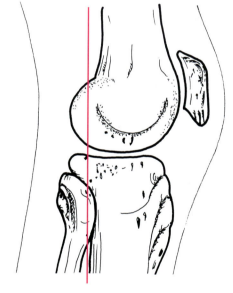

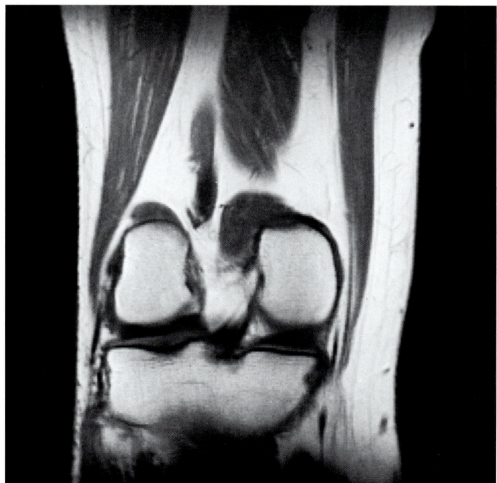

236 Knee – Coronal

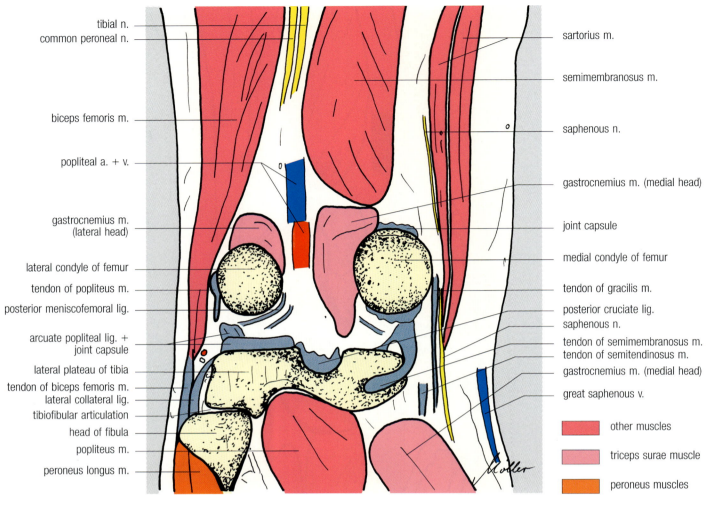
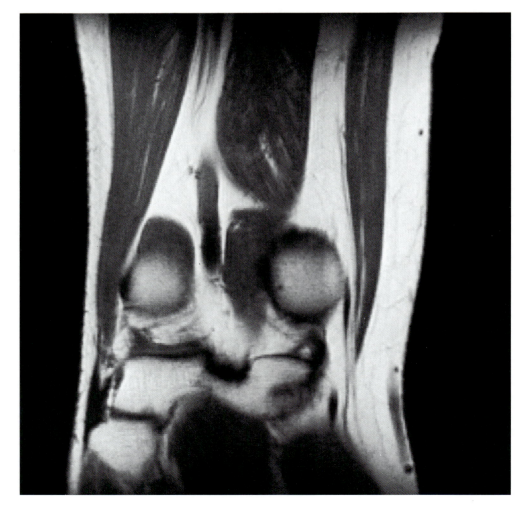
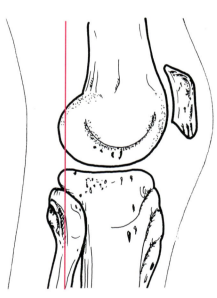

Knee – Coronal

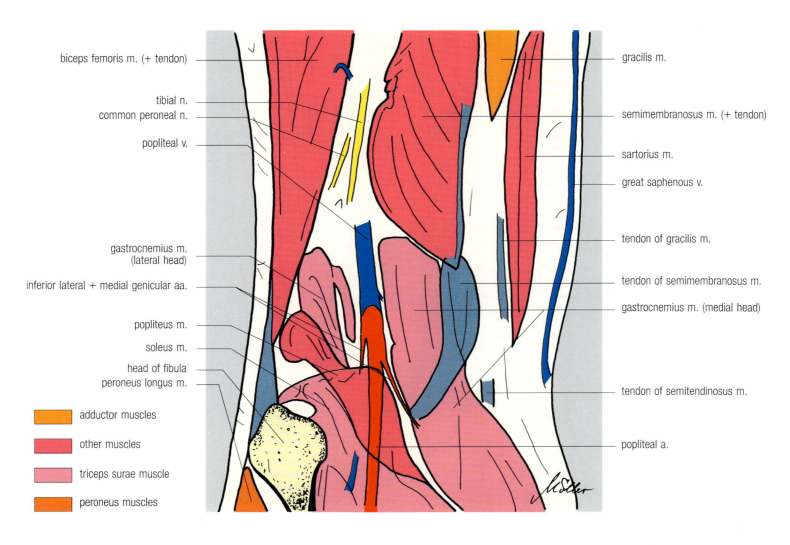

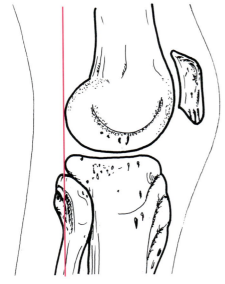

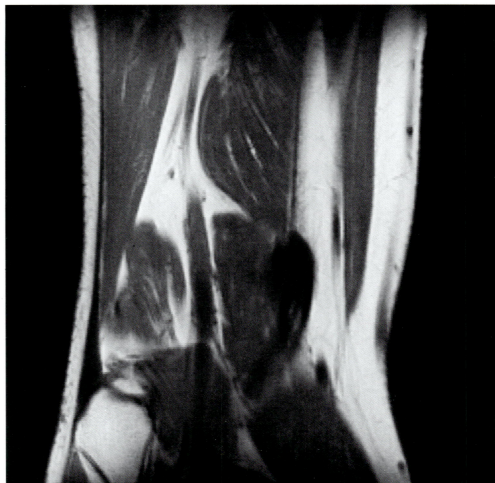

Knee – Coronal

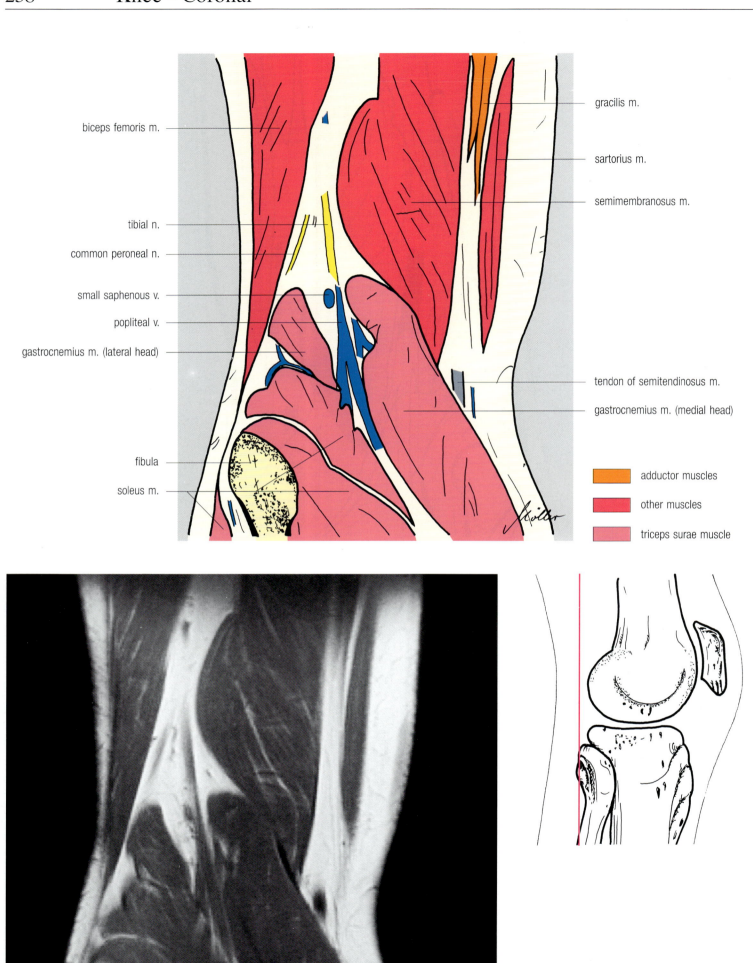

Knee – Coronal

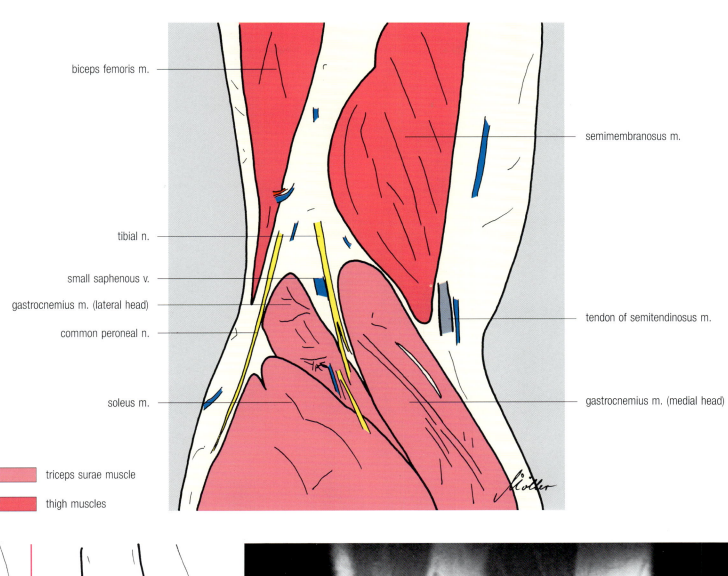

- biceps femoris m.
- semimembranosus m.
- tibial n.
- small saphenous v.
- gastrocnemius m. (lateral head)
- tendon of semitendinosus m.
- common peroneal n.
- soleus m.
- gastrocnemius m. (medial head)

triceps surae muscle
thigh muscles

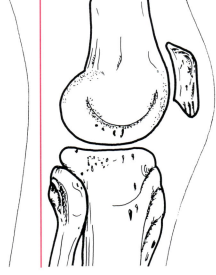

cranial
lateral — medial
caudal

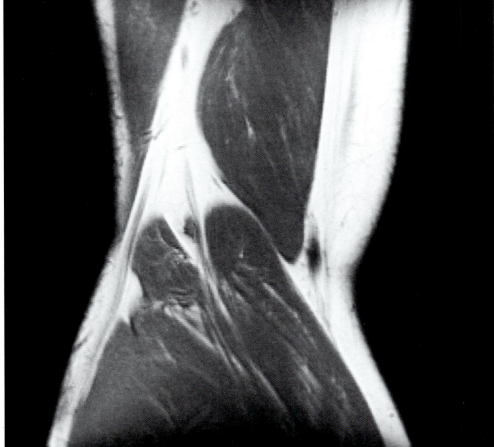

Knee – Sagittal

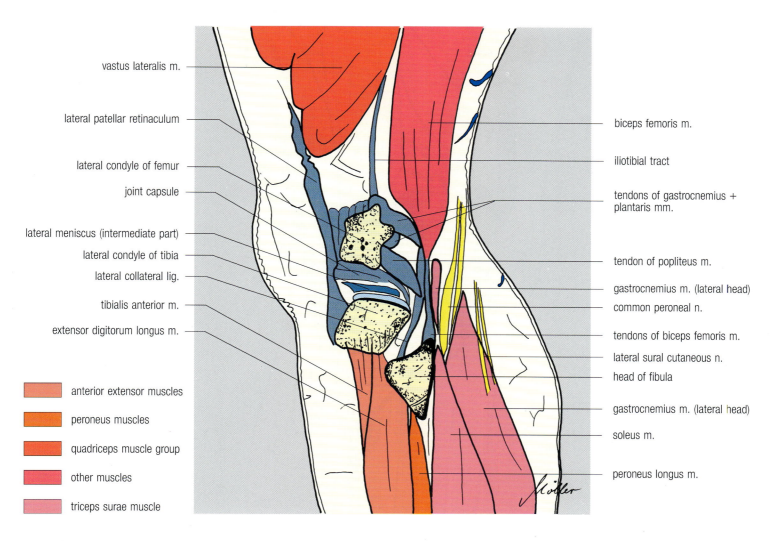

- vastus lateralis m.
- lateral patellar retinaculum
- lateral condyle of femur
- joint capsule
- lateral meniscus (intermediate part)
- lateral condyle of tibia
- lateral collateral lig.
- tibialis anterior m.
- extensor digitorum longus m.

- biceps femoris m.
- iliotibial tract
- tendons of gastrocnemius + plantaris mm.
- tendon of popliteus m.
- gastrocnemius m. (lateral head)
- common peroneal n.
- tendons of biceps femoris m.
- lateral sural cutaneous n.
- head of fibula
- gastrocnemius m. (lateral head)
- soleus m.
- peroneus longus m.

Legend:
- anterior extensor muscles
- peroneus muscles
- quadriceps muscle group
- other muscles
- triceps surae muscle

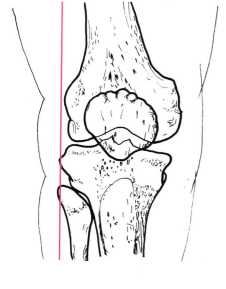

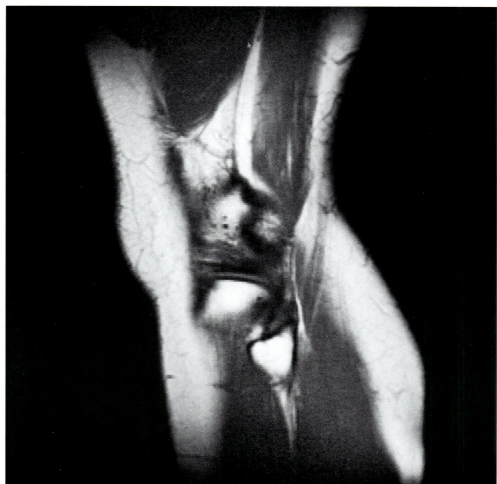

cranial / ventral / dorsal / caudal

Knee – Sagittal

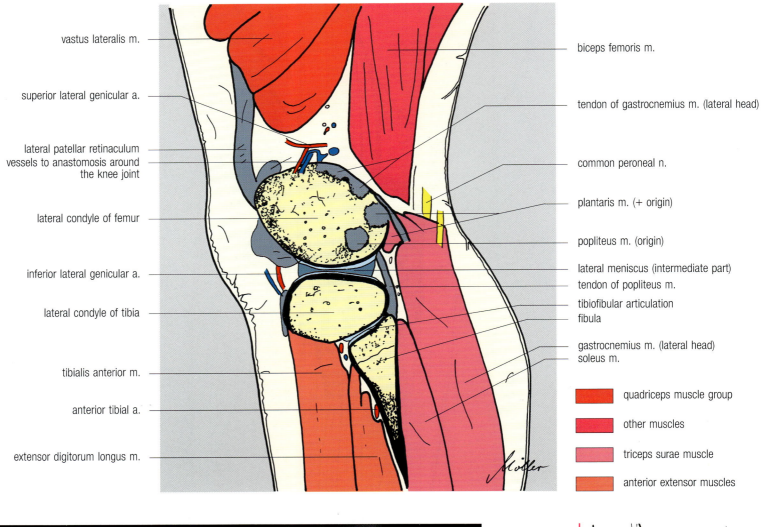

- vastus lateralis m.
- superior lateral genicular a.
- lateral patellar retinaculum vessels to anastomosis around the knee joint
- lateral condyle of femur
- inferior lateral genicular a.
- lateral condyle of tibia
- tibialis anterior m.
- anterior tibial a.
- extensor digitorum longus m.

- biceps femoris m.
- tendon of gastrocnemius m. (lateral head)
- common peroneal n.
- plantaris m. (+ origin)
- popliteus m. (origin)
- lateral meniscus (intermediate part)
- tendon of popliteus m.
- tibiofibular articulation
- fibula
- gastrocnemius m. (lateral head)
- soleus m.

- quadriceps muscle group
- other muscles
- triceps surae muscle
- anterior extensor muscles

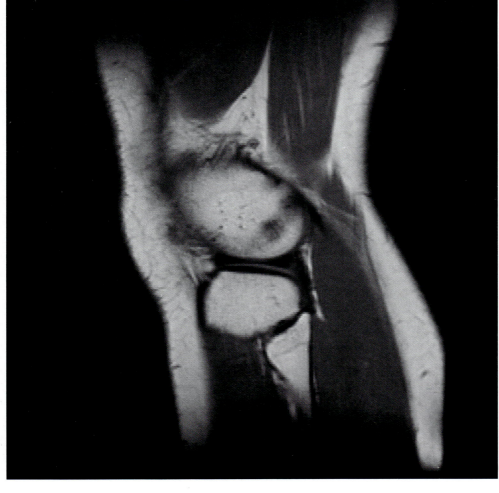

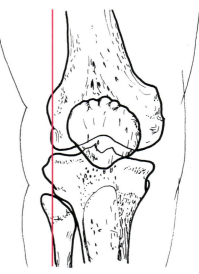

cranial
ventral dorsal
caudal

Knee – Sagittal 243

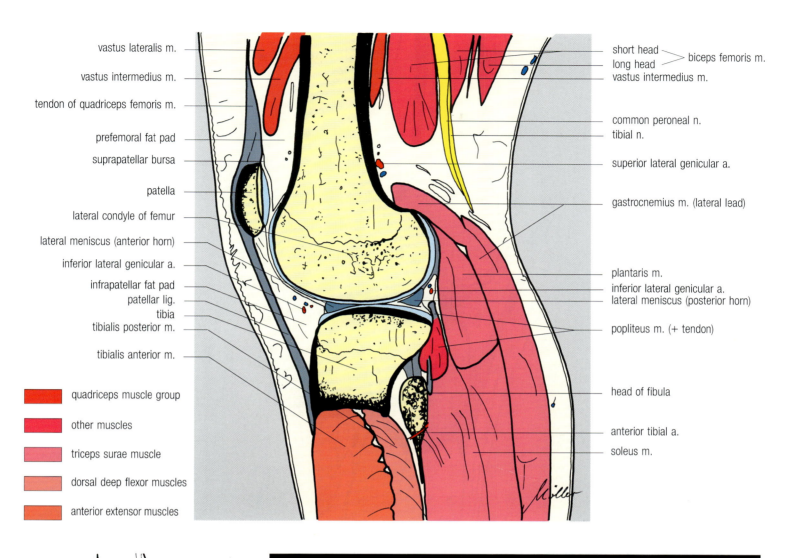

Knee – Sagittal

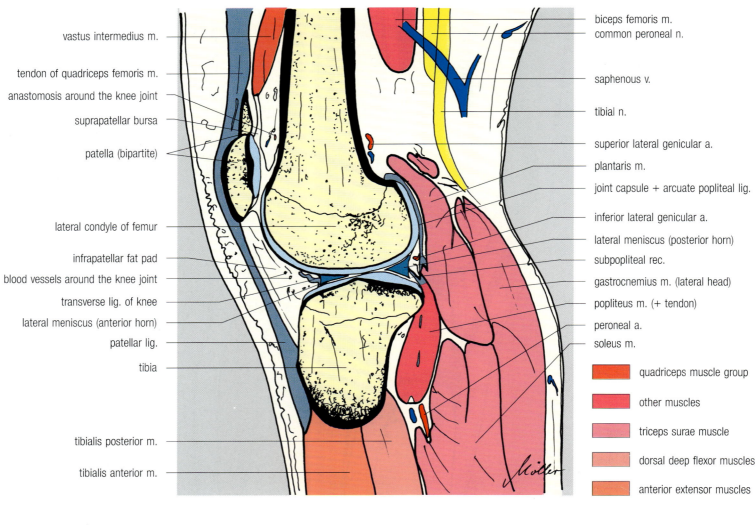

- vastus intermedius m.
- tendon of quadriceps femoris m.
- anastomosis around the knee joint
- suprapatellar bursa
- patella (bipartite)
- lateral condyle of femur
- infrapatellar fat pad
- blood vessels around the knee joint
- transverse lig. of knee
- lateral meniscus (anterior horn)
- patellar lig.
- tibia
- tibialis posterior m.
- tibialis anterior m.
- biceps femoris m.
- common peroneal n.
- saphenous v.
- tibial n.
- superior lateral genicular a.
- plantaris m.
- joint capsule + arcuate popliteal lig.
- inferior lateral genicular a.
- lateral meniscus (posterior horn)
- subpopliteal rec.
- gastrocnemius m. (lateral head)
- popliteus m. (+ tendon)
- peroneal a.
- soleus m.

- quadriceps muscle group
- other muscles
- triceps surae muscle
- dorsal deep flexor muscles
- anterior extensor muscles

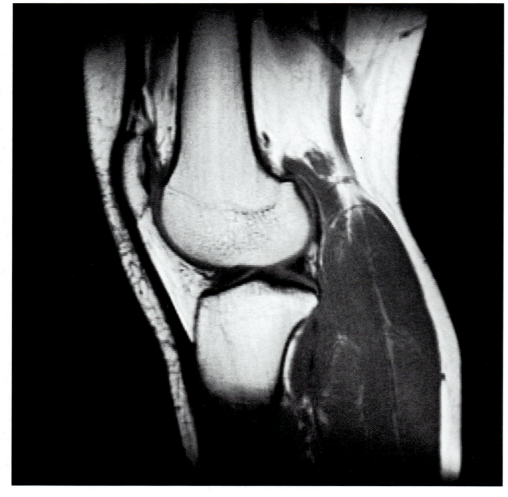

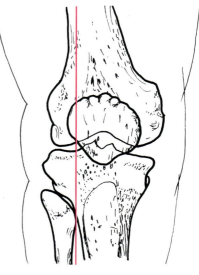

cranial / ventral / dorsal / caudal

Knee – Sagittal

245

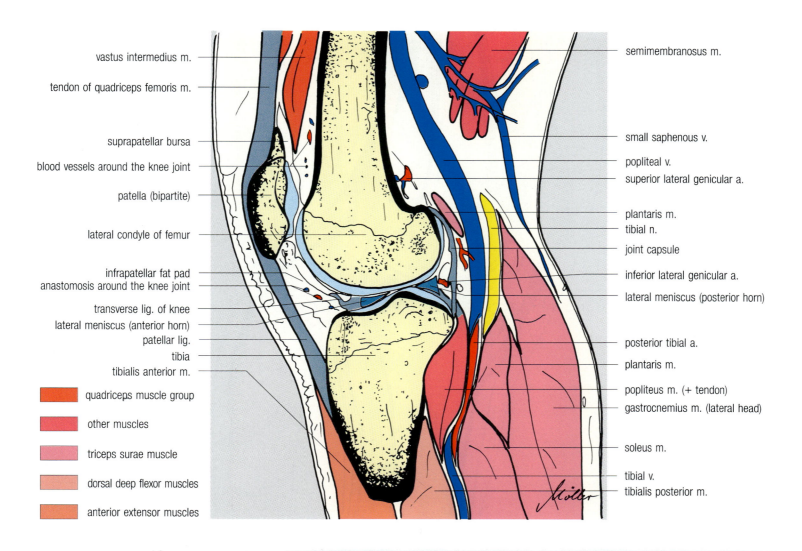

- vastus intermedius m.
- tendon of quadriceps femoris m.
- suprapatellar bursa
- blood vessels around the knee joint
- patella (bipartite)
- lateral condyle of femur
- infrapatellar fat pad
- anastomosis around the knee joint
- transverse lig. of knee
- lateral meniscus (anterior horn)
- patellar lig.
- tibia
- tibialis anterior m.
- semimembranosus m.
- small saphenous v.
- popliteal v.
- superior lateral genicular a.
- plantaris m.
- tibial n.
- joint capsule
- inferior lateral genicular a.
- lateral meniscus (posterior horn)
- posterior tibial a.
- plantaris m.
- popliteus m. (+ tendon)
- gastrocnemius m. (lateral head)
- soleus m.
- tibial v.
- tibialis posterior m.

- quadriceps muscle group
- other muscles
- triceps surae muscle
- dorsal deep flexor muscles
- anterior extensor muscles

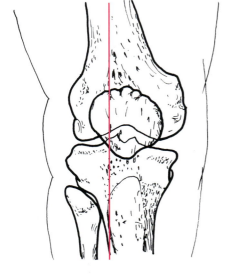

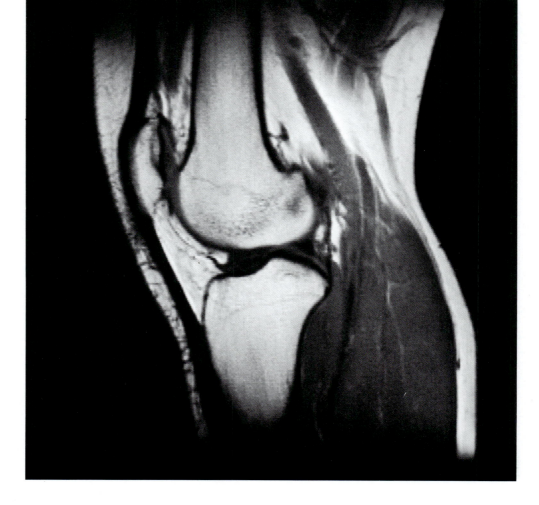

cranial
ventral — dorsal
caudal

Knee – Sagittal

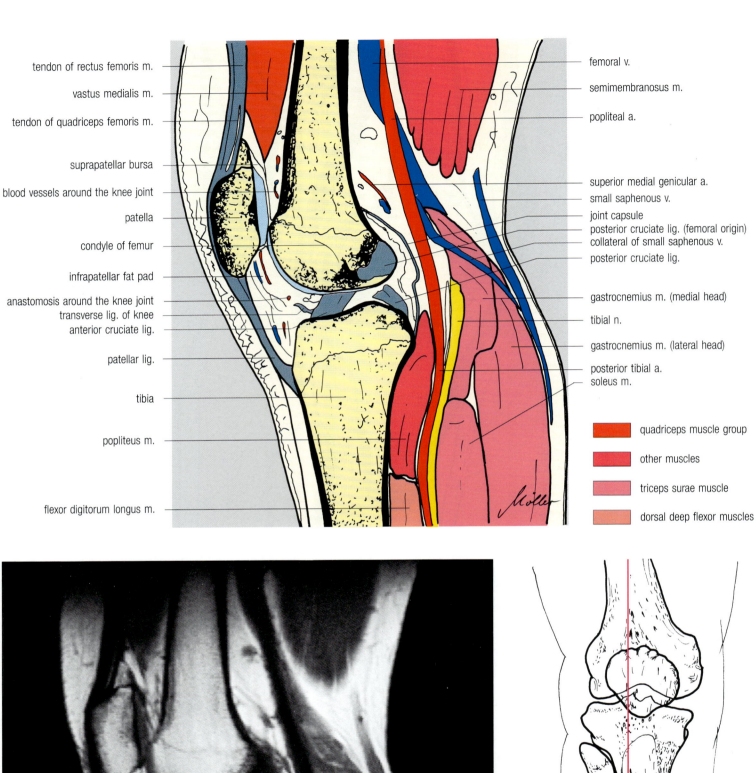
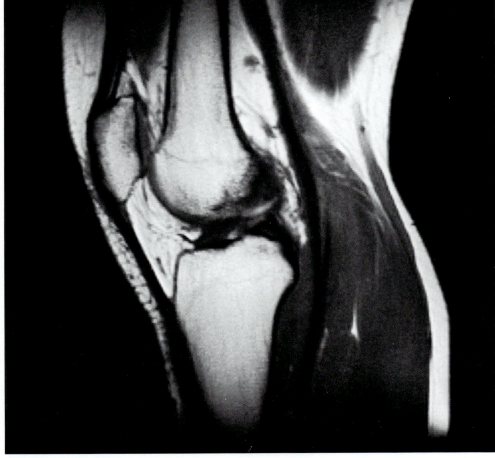
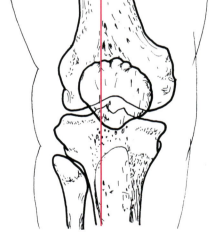

Knee – Sagittal

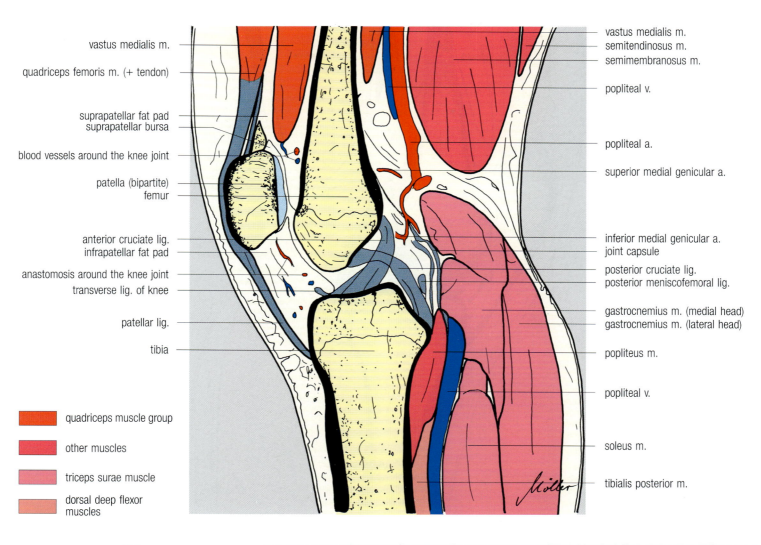

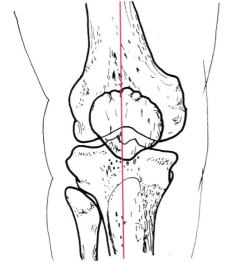

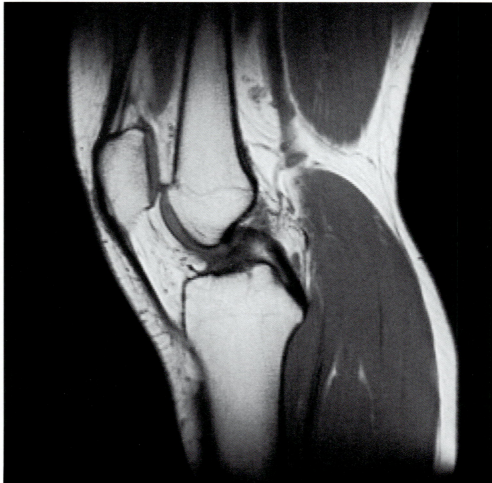

248 Knee – Sagittal

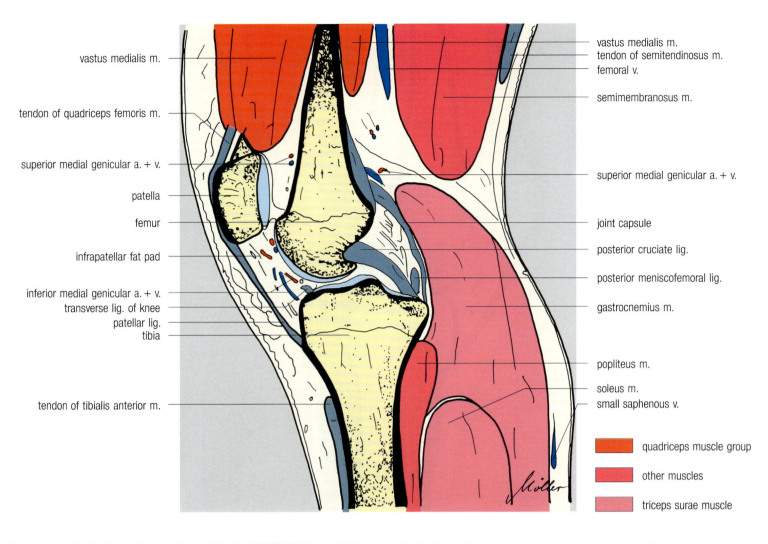

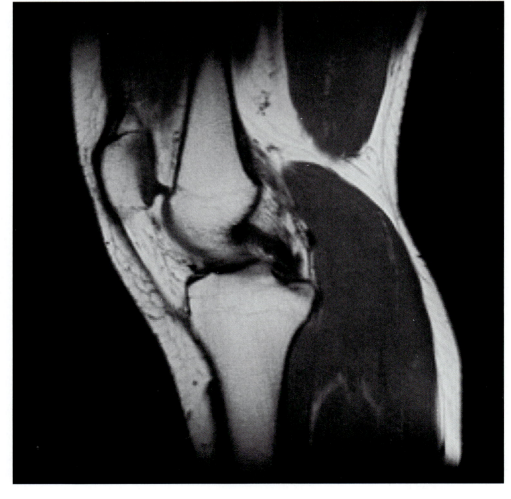

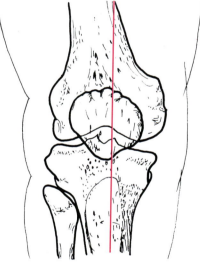

Knee – Sagittal 249

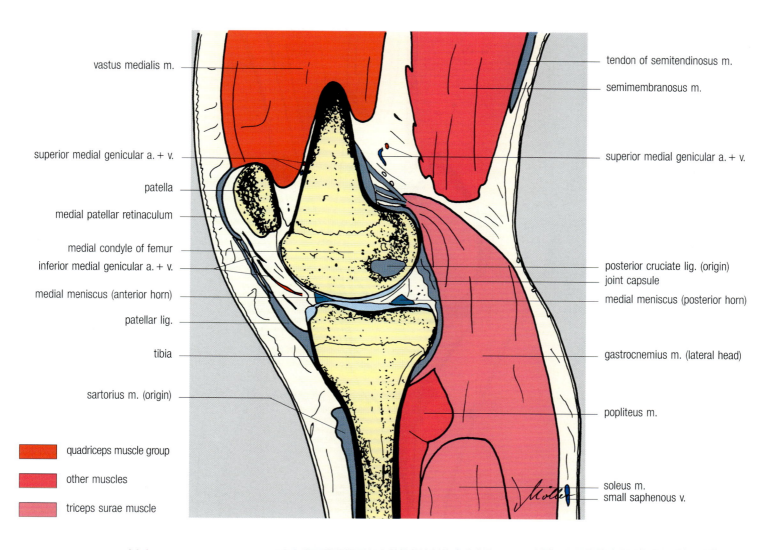

- vastus medialis m.
- superior medial genicular a. + v.
- patella
- medial patellar retinaculum
- medial condyle of femur
- inferior medial genicular a. + v.
- medial meniscus (anterior horn)
- patellar lig.
- tibia
- sartorius m. (origin)

- tendon of semitendinosus m.
- semimembranosus m.
- superior medial genicular a. + v.
- posterior cruciate lig. (origin)
- joint capsule
- medial meniscus (posterior horn)
- gastrocnemius m. (lateral head)
- popliteus m.
- soleus m.
- small saphenous v.

- quadriceps muscle group
- other muscles
- triceps surae muscle

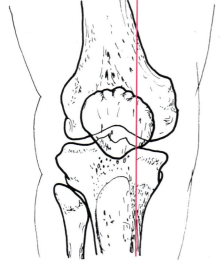

cranial
ventral — dorsal
caudal

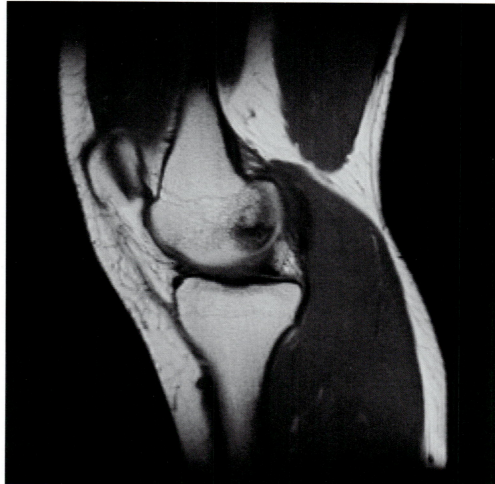

Knee – Sagittal

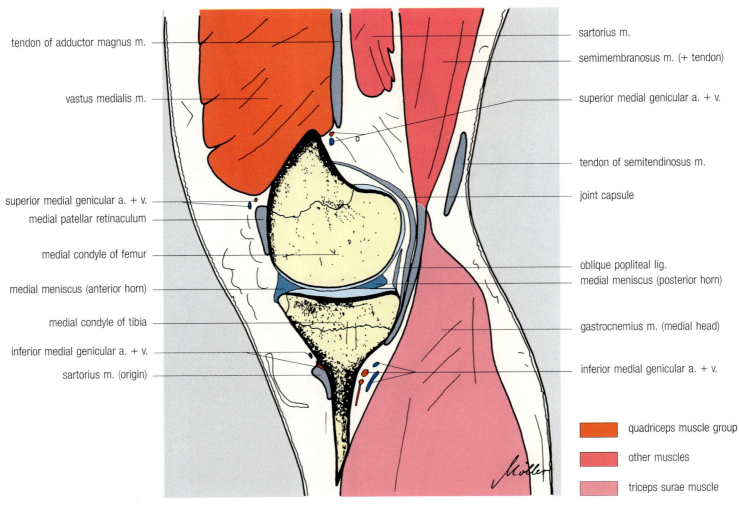

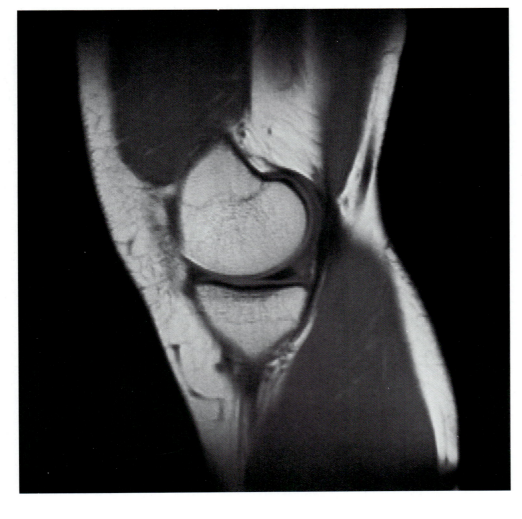

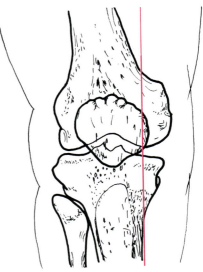

Knee – Sagittal

251

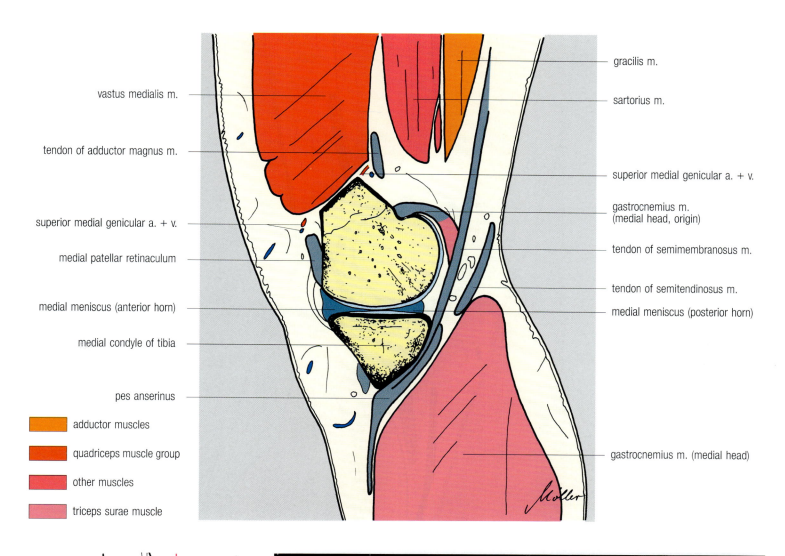

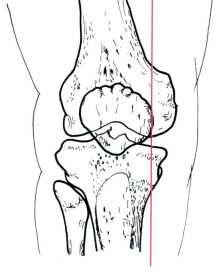

Knee – Sagittal

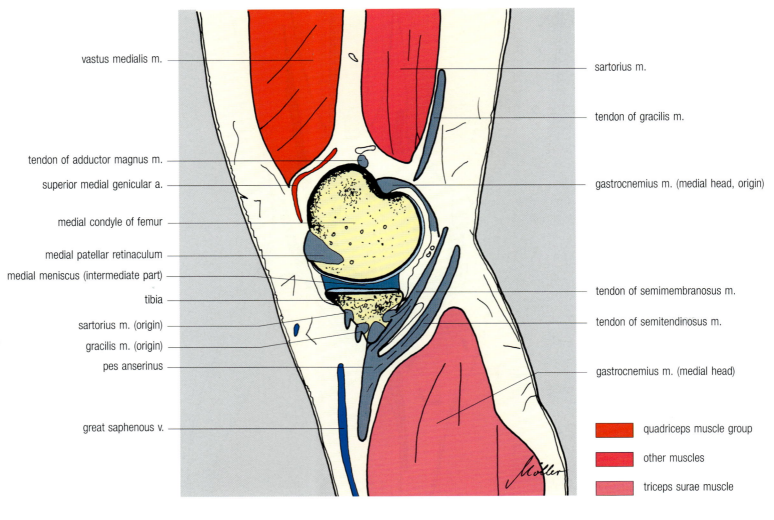

- vastus medialis m.
- tendon of adductor magnus m.
- superior medial genicular a.
- medial condyle of femur
- medial patellar retinaculum
- medial meniscus (intermediate part)
- tibia
- sartorius m. (origin)
- gracilis m. (origin)
- pes anserinus
- great saphenous v.
- sartorius m.
- tendon of gracilis m.
- gastrocnemius m. (medial head, origin)
- tendon of semimembranosus m.
- tendon of semitendinosus m.
- gastrocnemius m. (medial head)

■ quadriceps muscle group
■ other muscles
■ triceps surae muscle

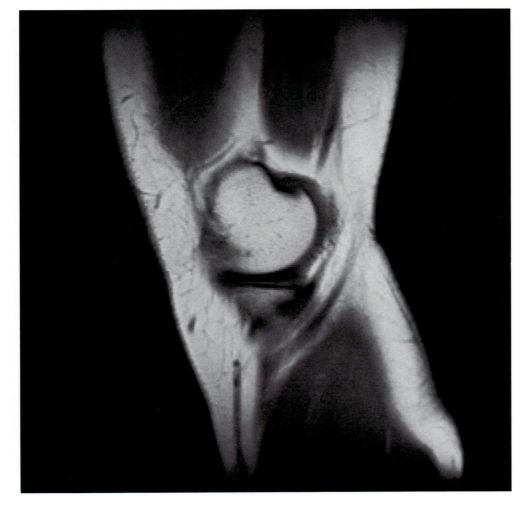

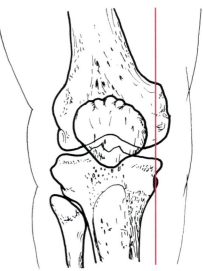

cranial
ventral   dorsal
caudal

Lower Leg

Coronal
Sagittal

Lower Leg – Coronal

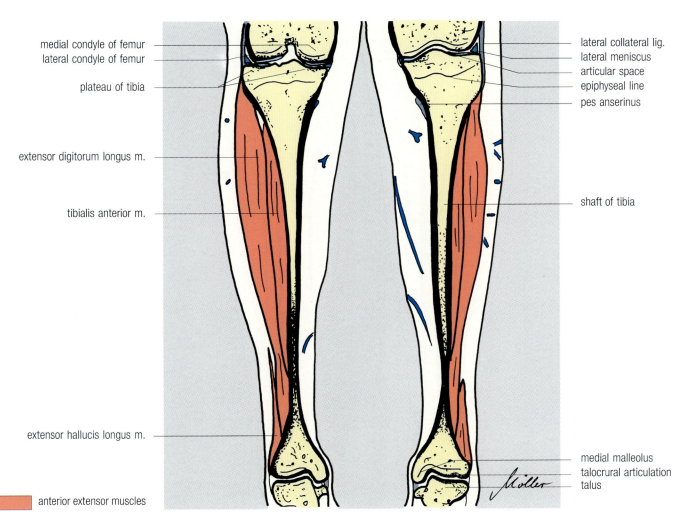
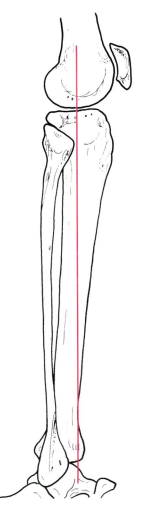
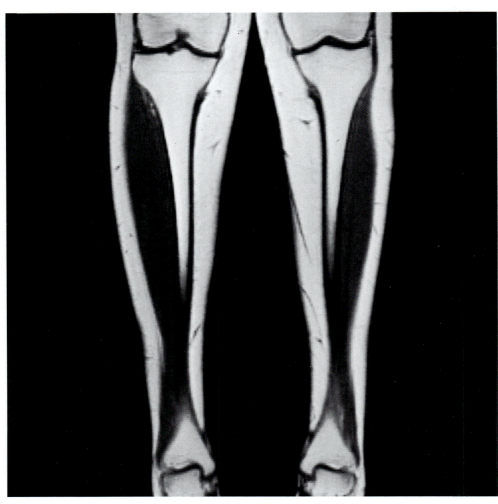

Lower Leg – Coronal

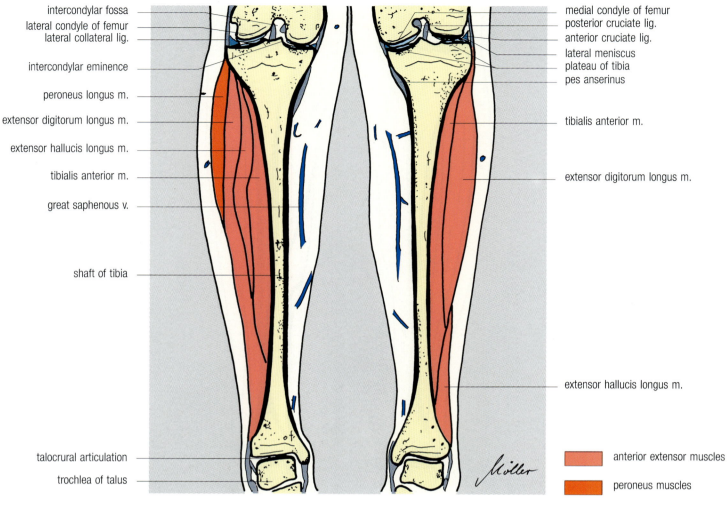
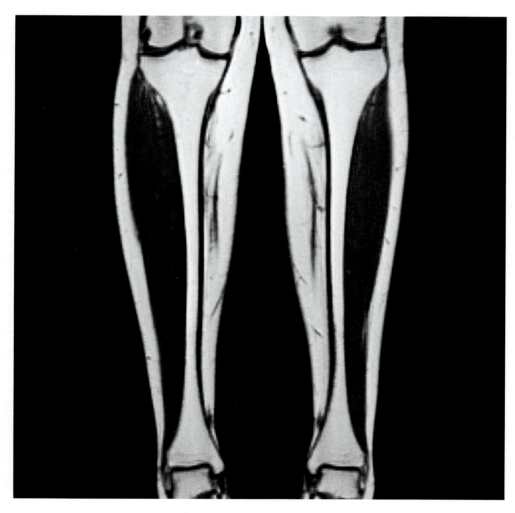
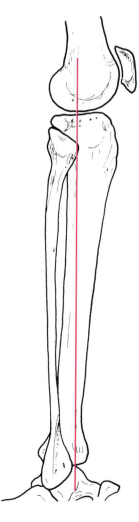

Lower Leg – Coronal

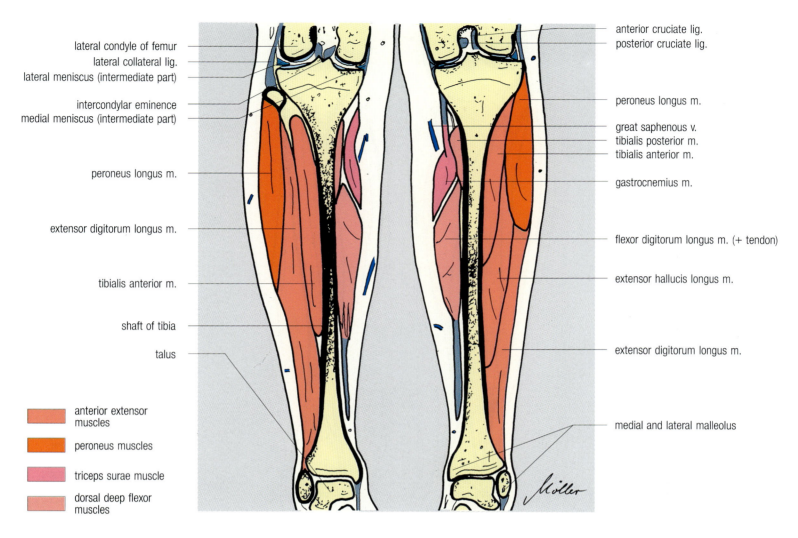

- lateral condyle of femur
- lateral collateral lig.
- lateral meniscus (intermediate part)
- intercondylar eminence
- medial meniscus (intermediate part)
- peroneus longus m.
- extensor digitorum longus m.
- tibialis anterior m.
- shaft of tibia
- talus

- anterior extensor muscles
- peroneus muscles
- triceps surae muscle
- dorsal deep flexor muscles

- anterior cruciate lig.
- posterior cruciate lig.
- peroneus longus m.
- great saphenous v.
- tibialis posterior m.
- tibialis anterior m.
- gastrocnemius m.
- flexor digitorum longus m. (+ tendon)
- extensor hallucis longus m.
- extensor digitorum longus m.
- medial and lateral malleolus

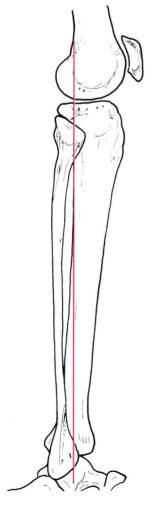

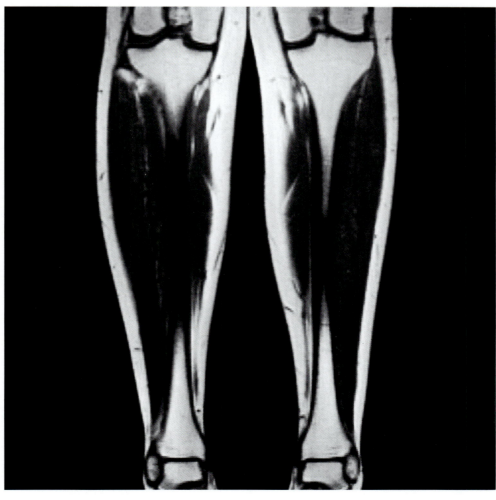

Lower Leg – Coronal

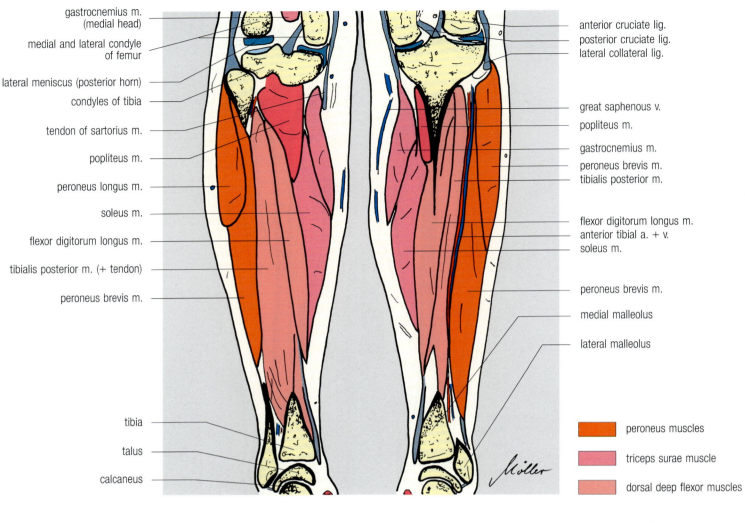

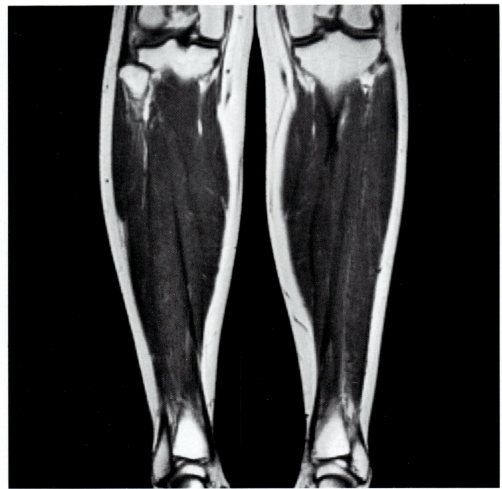

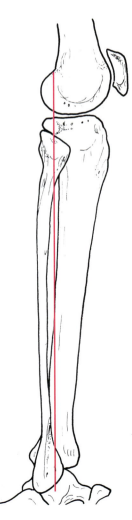

Lower Leg – Coronal 259

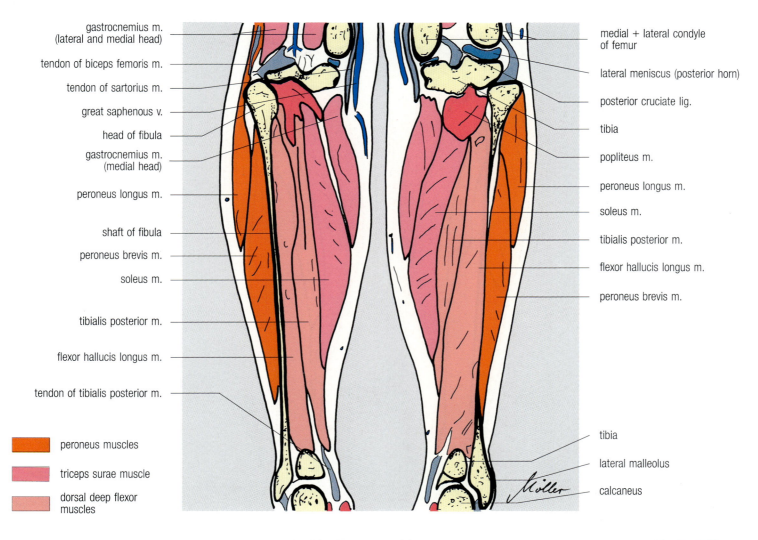

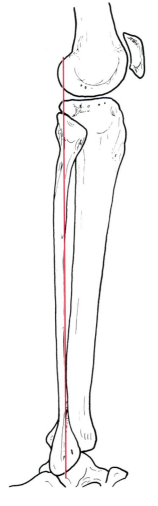
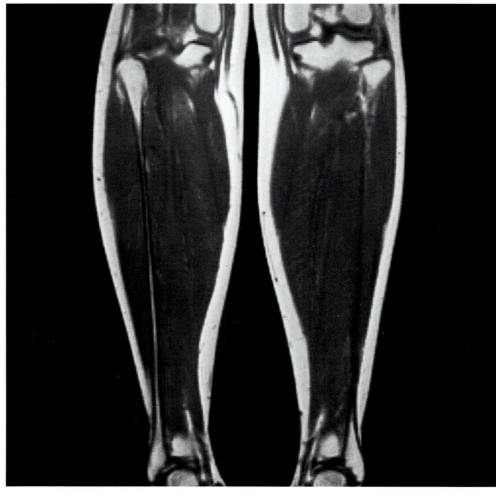

Lower Leg – Coronal

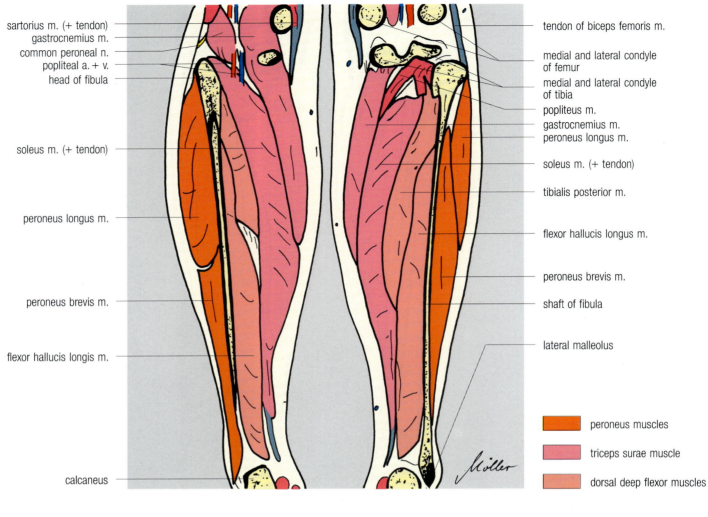
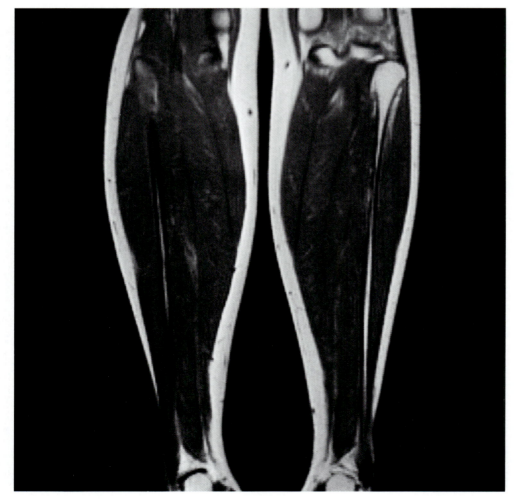
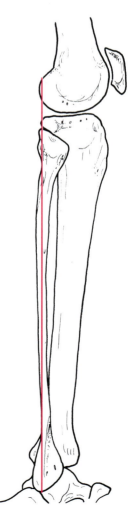

Lower Leg – Coronal

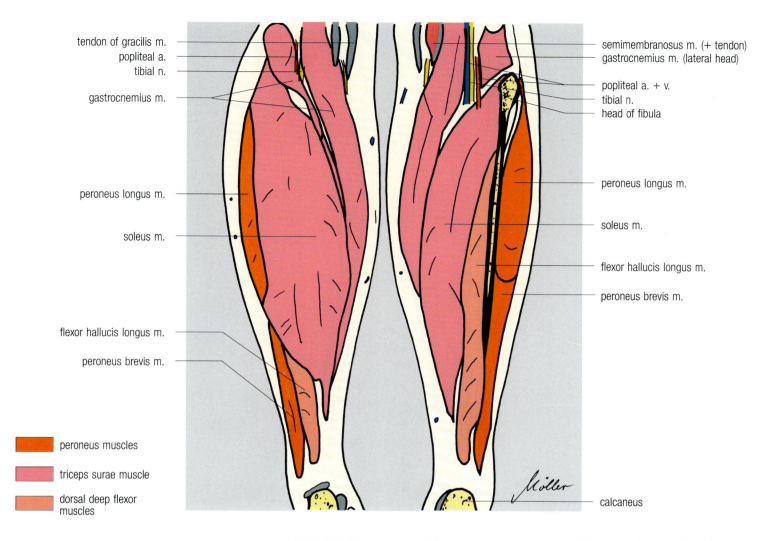

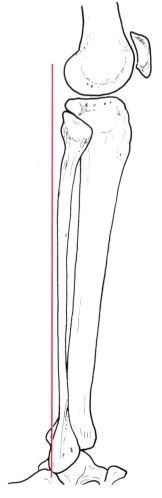

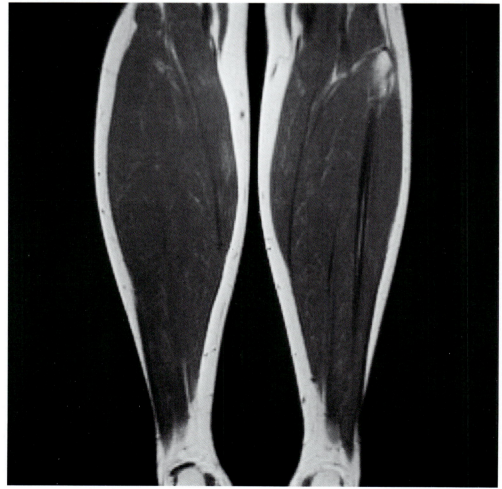

262 Lower Leg – Coronal

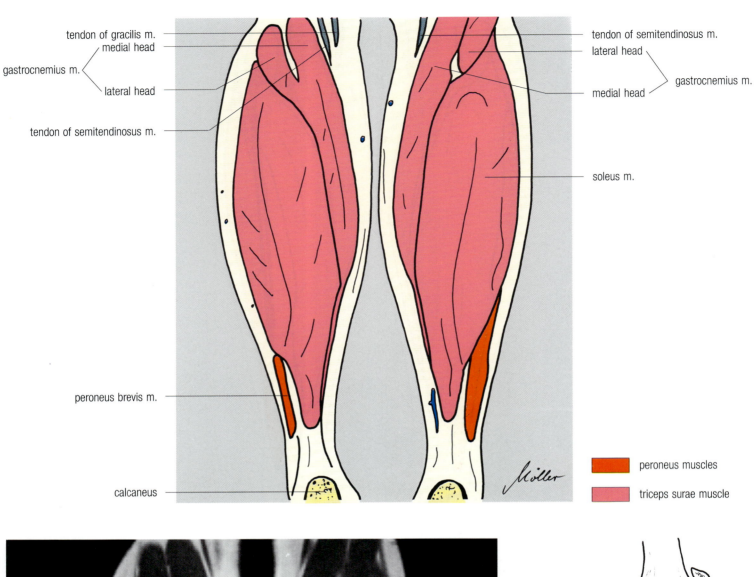

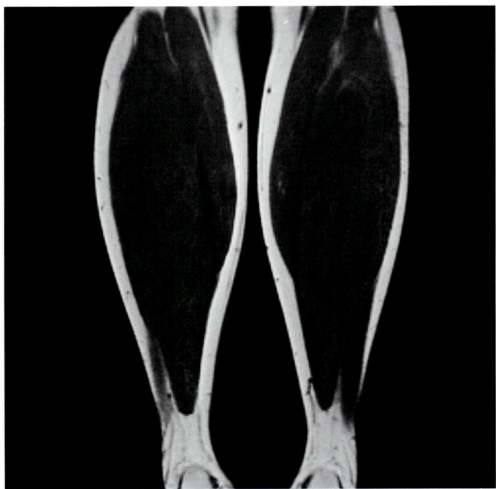
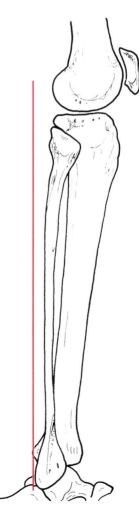

Lower Leg – Coronal 263

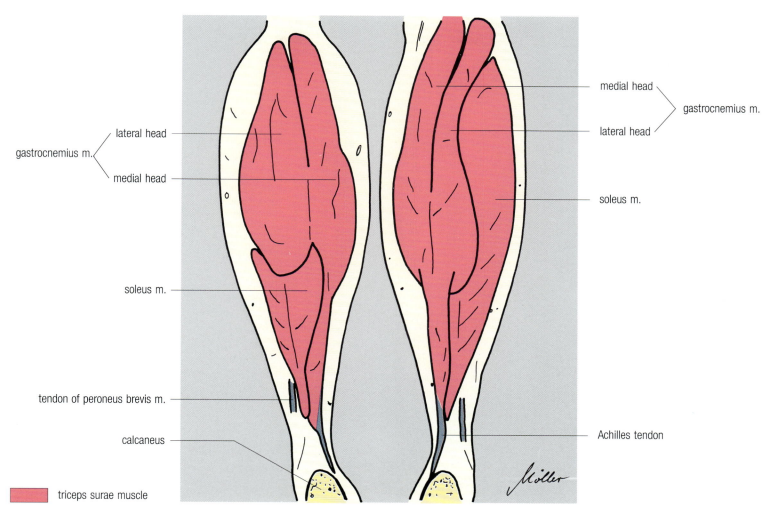

- gastrocnemius m.
  - lateral head
  - medial head
- soleus m.
- tendon of peroneus brevis m.
- calcaneus
- triceps surae muscle
- medial head
- lateral head
- gastrocnemius m.
- soleus m.
- Achilles tendon

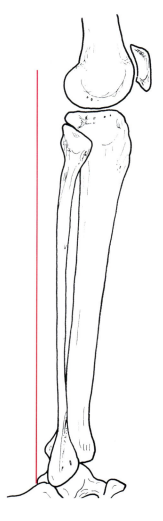

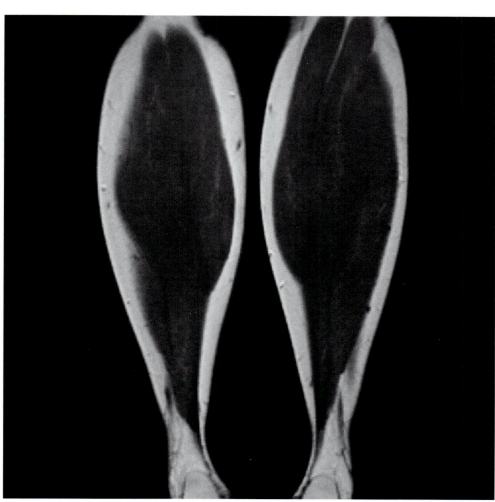

Lower Leg – Sagittal

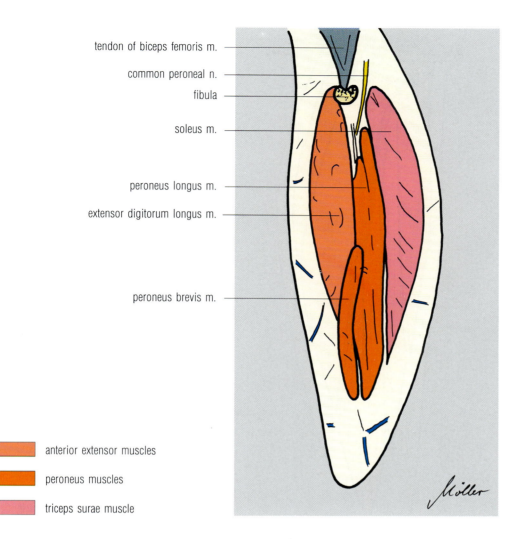

- tendon of biceps femoris m.
- common peroneal n.
- fibula
- soleus m.
- peroneus longus m.
- extensor digitorum longus m.
- peroneus brevis m.

■ anterior extensor muscles
■ peroneus muscles
■ triceps surae muscle

proximal
ventral ☐ dorsal
distal

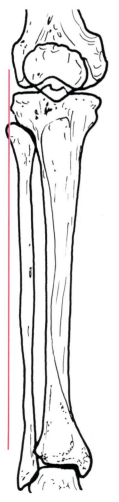
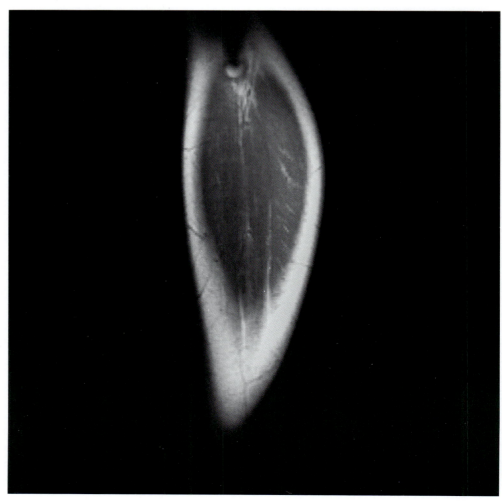

Lower Leg – Sagittal

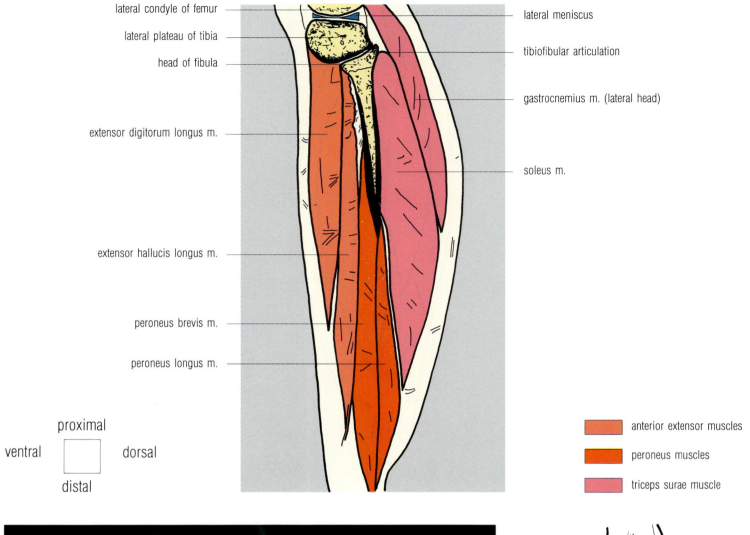

- lateral condyle of femur
- lateral plateau of tibia
- head of fibula
- extensor digitorum longus m.
- extensor hallucis longus m.
- peroneus brevis m.
- peroneus longus m.
- lateral meniscus
- tibiofibular articulation
- gastrocnemius m. (lateral head)
- soleus m.

proximal
ventral — dorsal
distal

■ anterior extensor muscles
■ peroneus muscles
■ triceps surae muscle

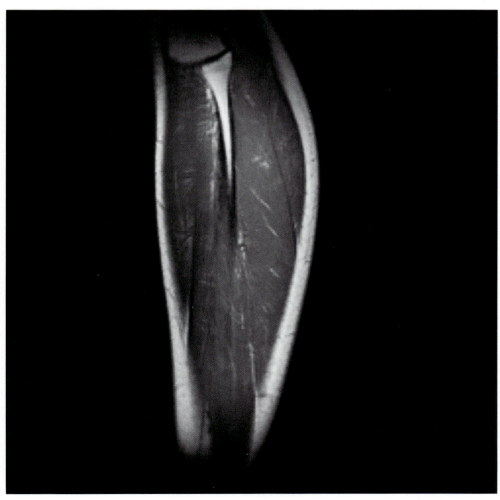
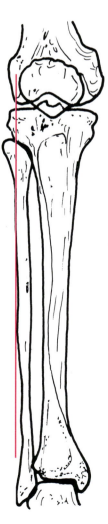

Lower Leg – Sagittal

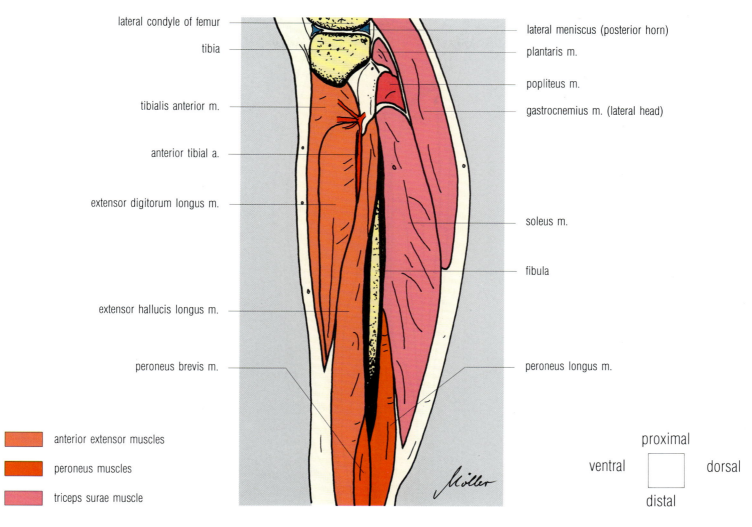

- lateral condyle of femur
- tibia
- tibialis anterior m.
- anterior tibial a.
- extensor digitorum longus m.
- extensor hallucis longus m.
- peroneus brevis m.
- lateral meniscus (posterior horn)
- plantaris m.
- popliteus m.
- gastrocnemius m. (lateral head)
- soleus m.
- fibula
- peroneus longus m.

■ anterior extensor muscles
■ peroneus muscles
■ triceps surae muscle

proximal
ventral — dorsal
distal

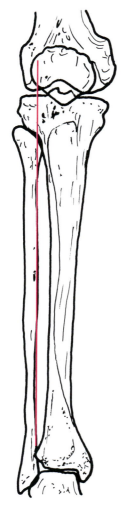
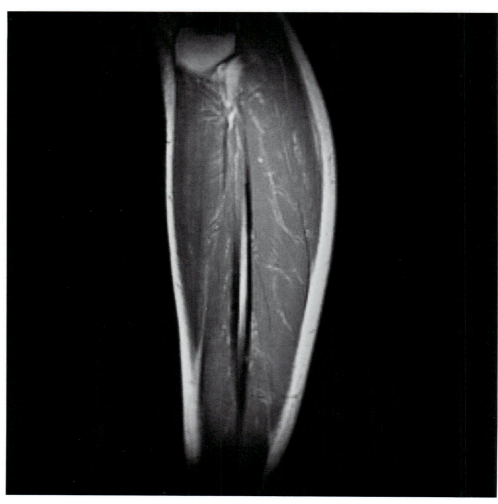

268 Lower Leg – Sagittal

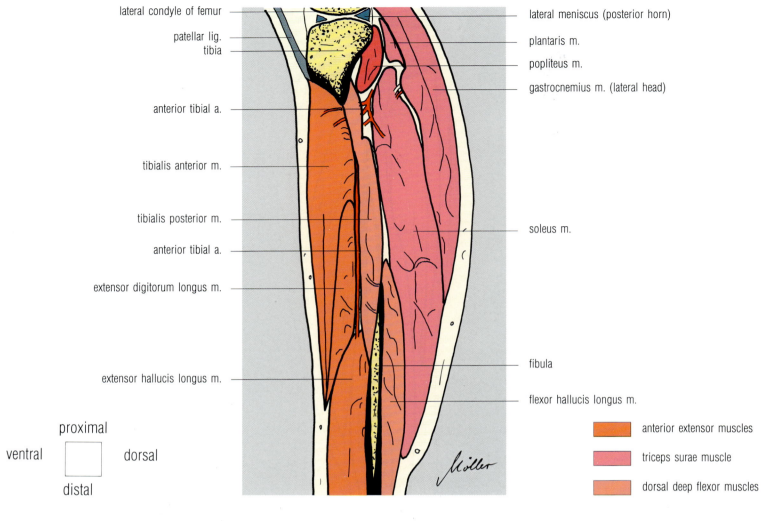

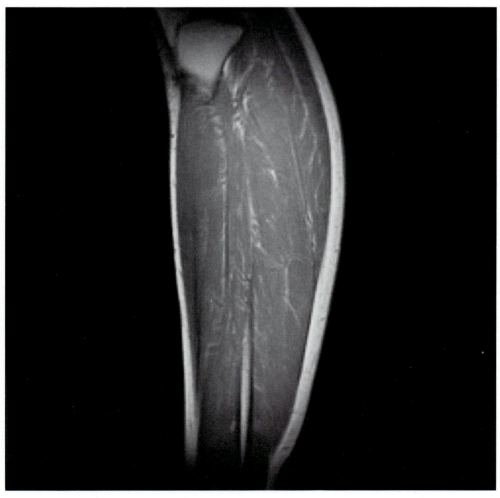
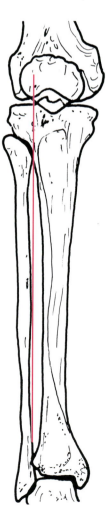

Lower Leg – Sagittal

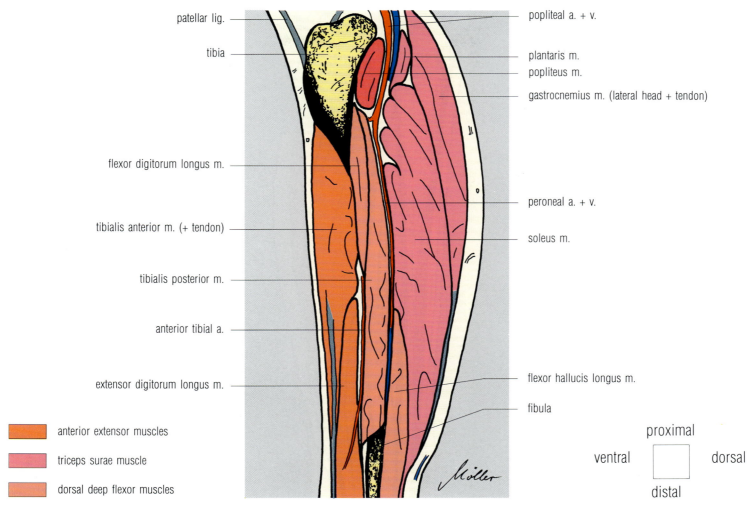

- patellar lig.
- tibia
- flexor digitorum longus m.
- tibialis anterior m. (+ tendon)
- tibialis posterior m.
- anterior tibial a.
- extensor digitorum longus m.
- popliteal a. + v.
- plantaris m.
- popliteus m.
- gastrocnemius m. (lateral head + tendon)
- peroneal a. + v.
- soleus m.
- flexor hallucis longus m.
- fibula

■ anterior extensor muscles
■ triceps surae muscle
■ dorsal deep flexor muscles

proximal
ventral — dorsal
distal

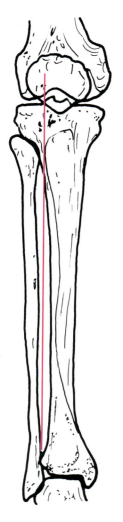

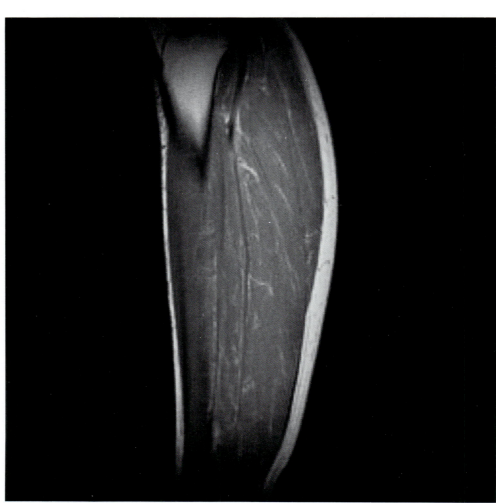

Lower Leg – Sagittal

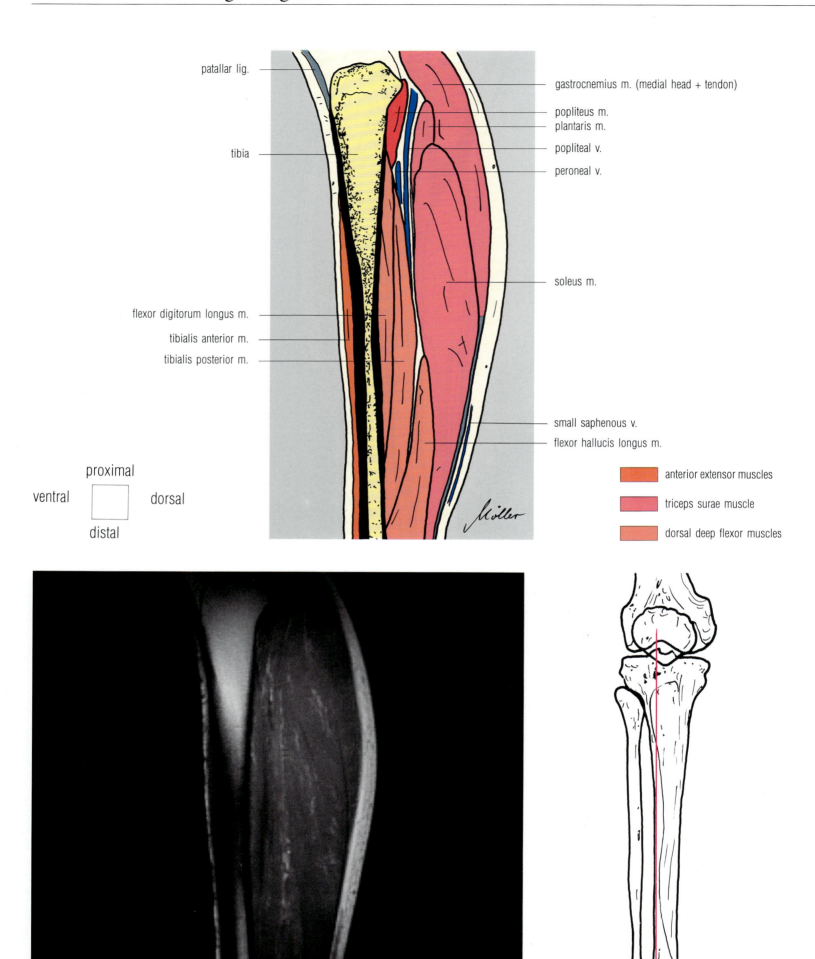

Lower Leg – Sagittal

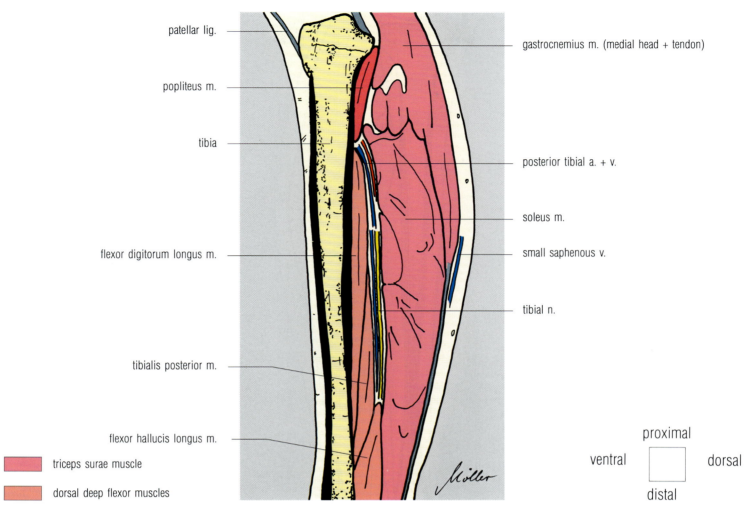
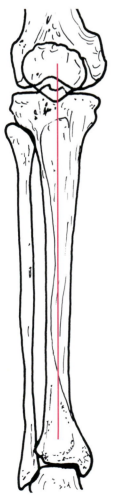
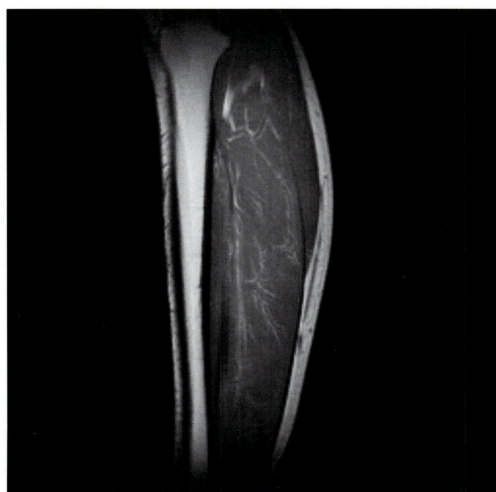

Lower Leg – Sagittal

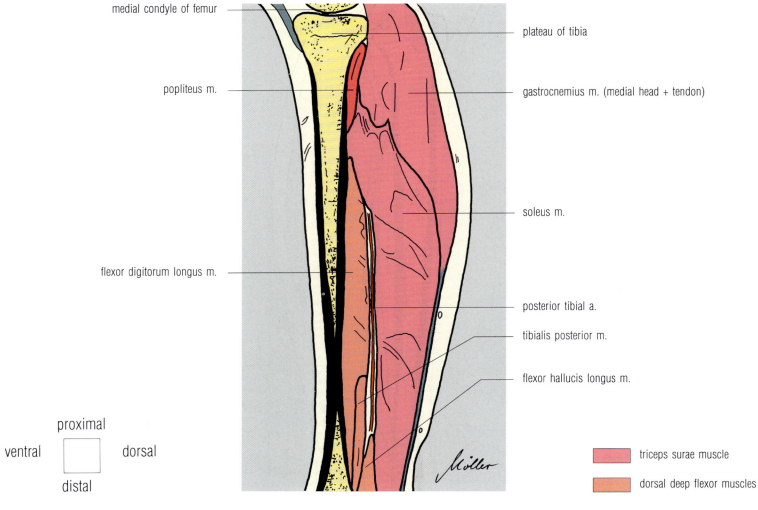

- medial condyle of femur
- popliteus m.
- flexor digitorum longus m.
- plateau of tibia
- gastrocnemius m. (medial head + tendon)
- soleus m.
- posterior tibial a.
- tibialis posterior m.
- flexor hallucis longus m.

proximal — ventral — dorsal — distal

■ triceps surae muscle
■ dorsal deep flexor muscles

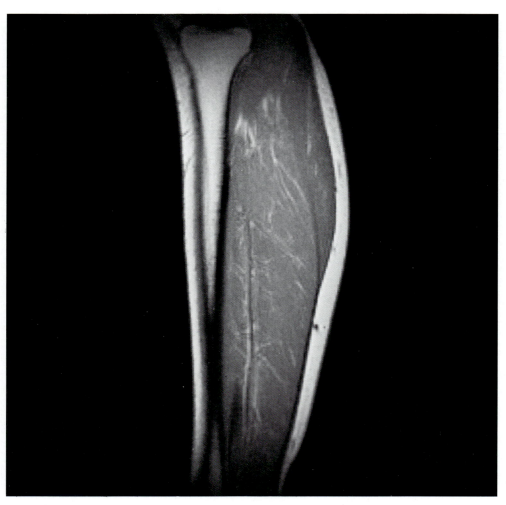

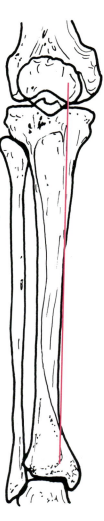

Lower Leg – Sagittal

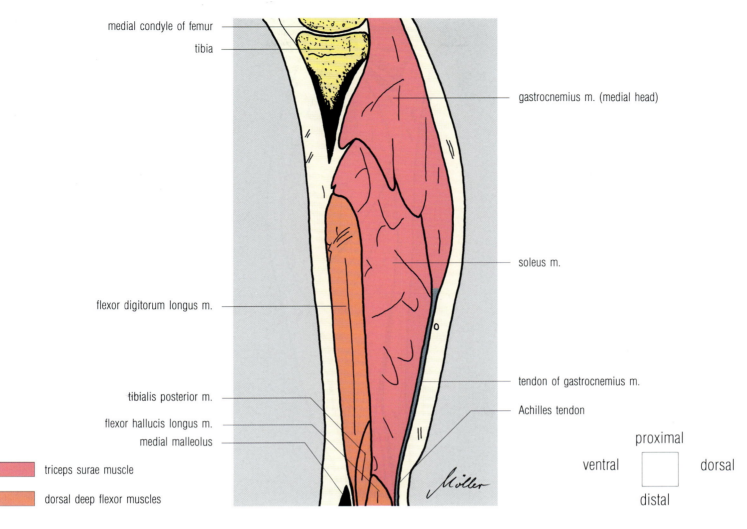

- medial condyle of femur
- tibia
- gastrocnemius m. (medial head)
- soleus m.
- flexor digitorum longus m.
- tibialis posterior m.
- flexor hallucis longus m.
- medial malleolus
- tendon of gastrocnemius m.
- Achilles tendon

■ triceps surae muscle
■ dorsal deep flexor muscles

proximal
ventral — dorsal
distal

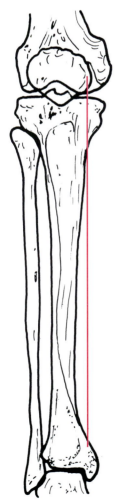
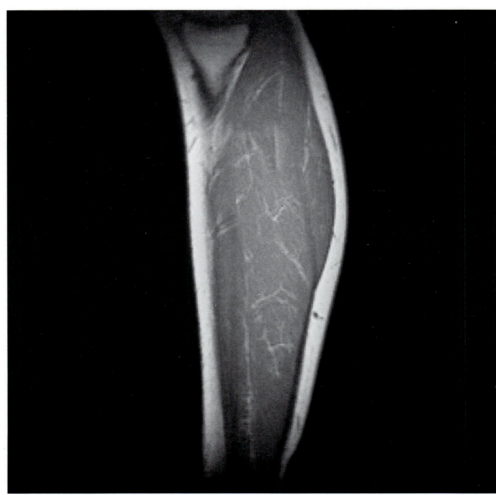

Lower Leg – Sagittal

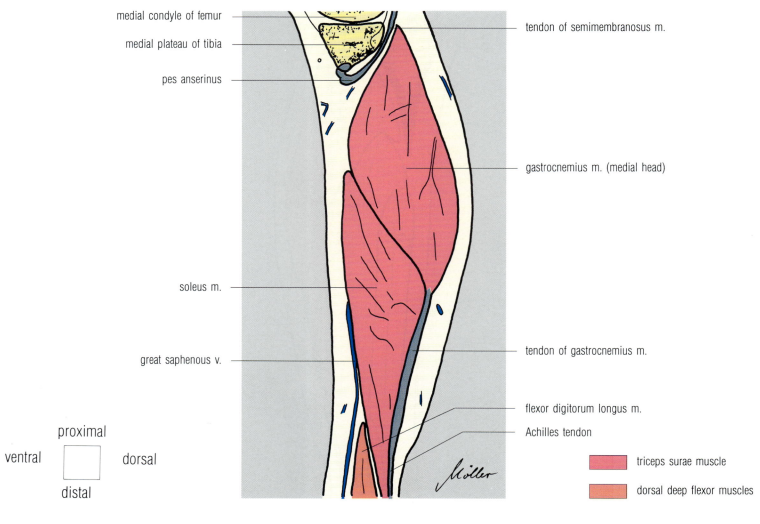

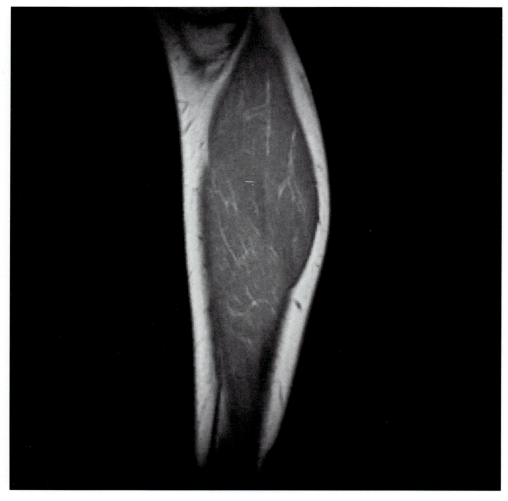
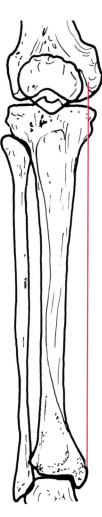

Ankle and Foot

Coronal
Sagittal

Ankle and Foot – Coronal 277

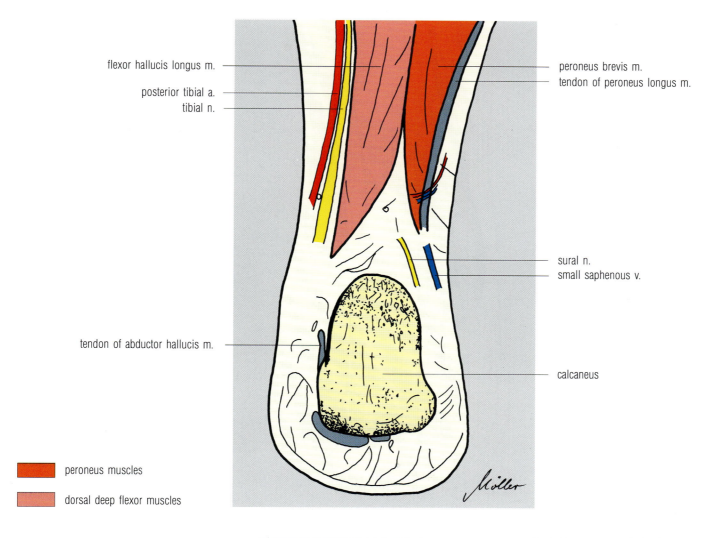

- flexor hallucis longus m.
- posterior tibial a.
- tibial n.
- peroneus brevis m.
- tendon of peroneus longus m.
- sural n.
- small saphenous v.
- tendon of abductor hallucis m.
- calcaneus

■ peroneus muscles
■ dorsal deep flexor muscles

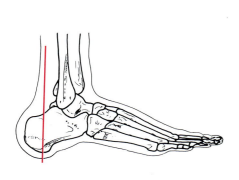

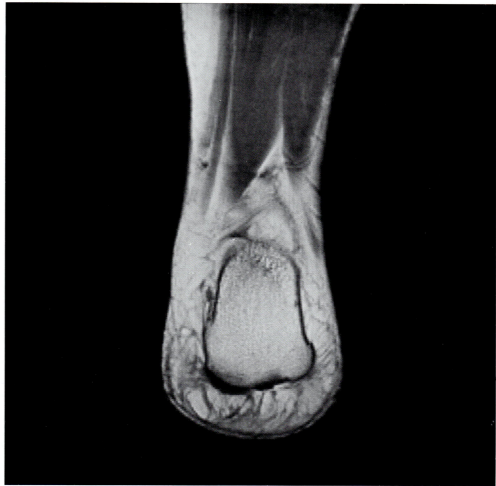

medial — proximal / distal — lateral

Ankle and Foot – Coronal

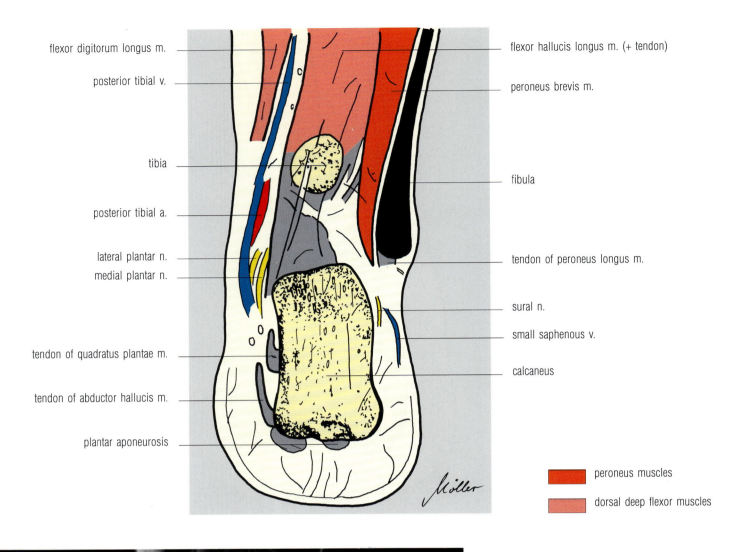

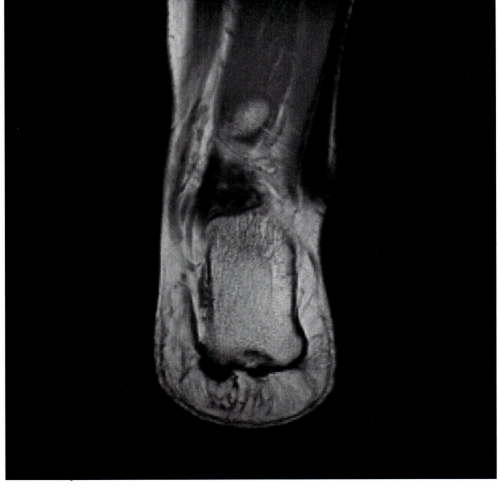

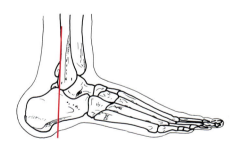

Ankle and Foot – Coronal 279

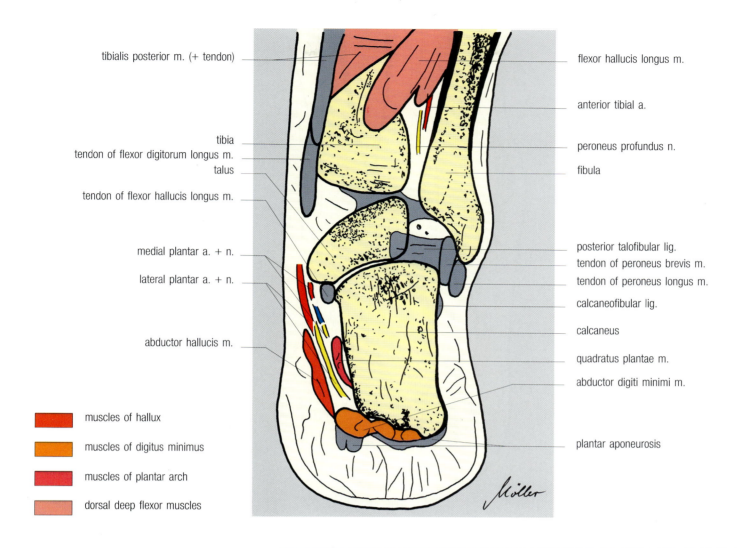

- muscles of hallux
- muscles of digitus minimus
- muscles of plantar arch
- dorsal deep flexor muscles

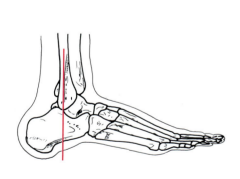

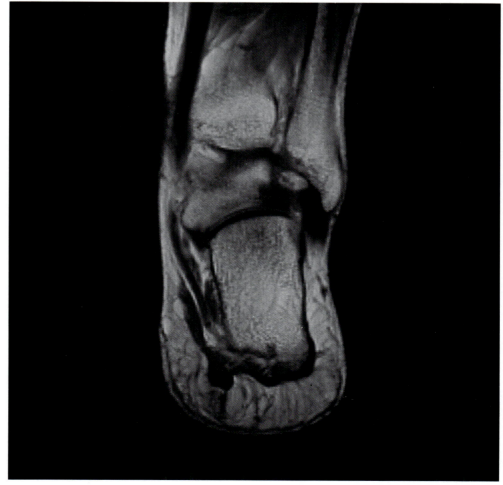

280 Ankle and Foot – Coronal

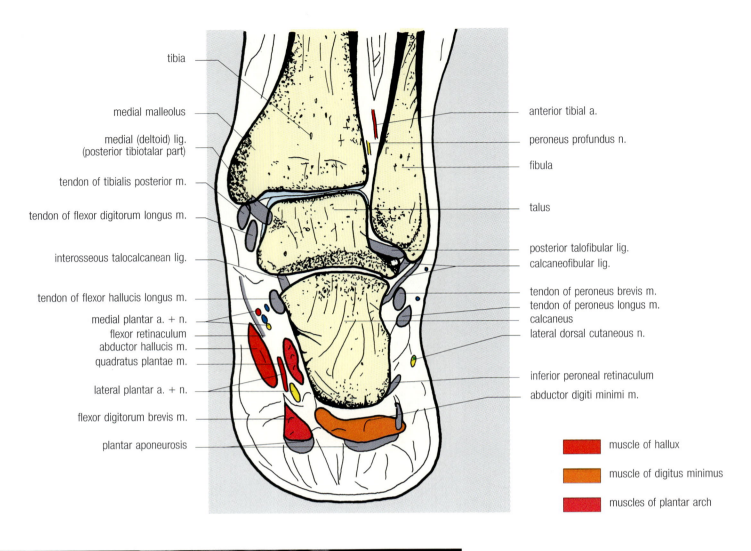

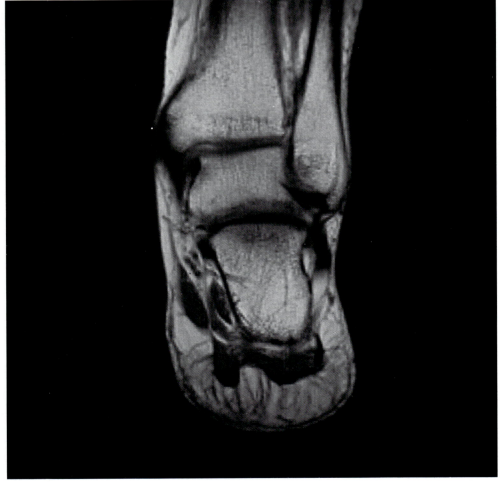

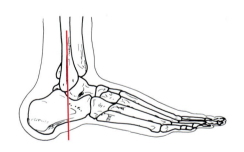

Ankle and Foot – Coronal

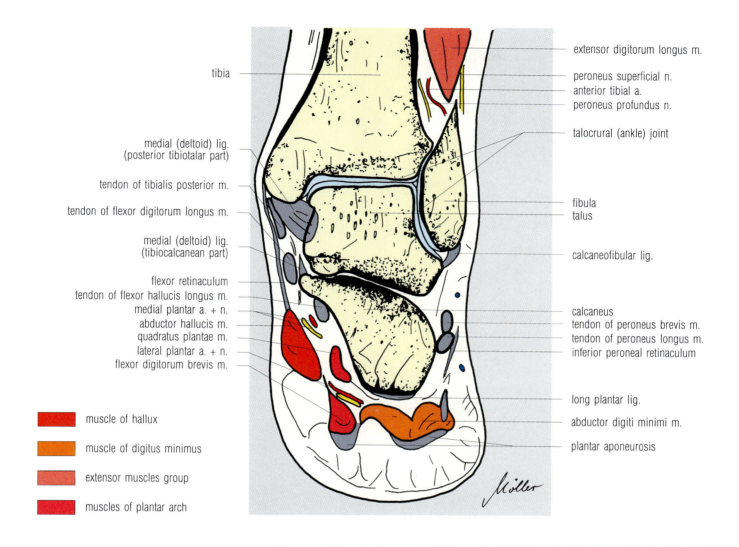
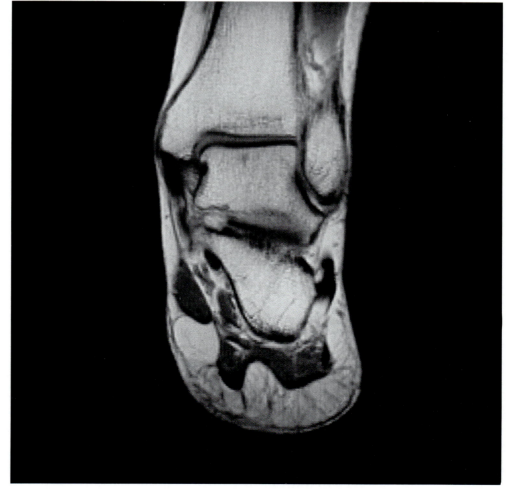
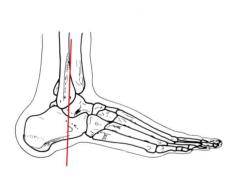

282 Ankle and Foot – Coronal

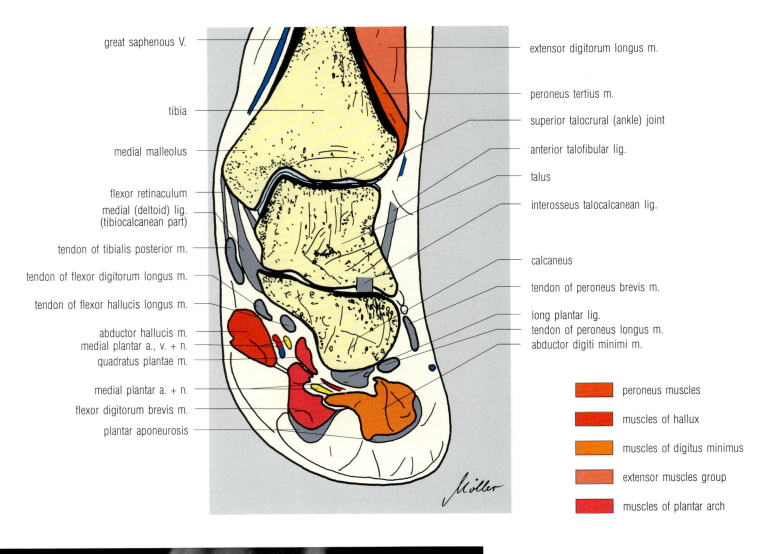

- great saphenous V.
- tibia
- medial malleolus
- flexor retinaculum
- medial (deltoid) lig. (tibiocalcanean part)
- tendon of tibialis posterior m.
- tendon of flexor digitorum longus m.
- tendon of flexor hallucis longus m.
- abductor hallucis m.
- medial plantar a., v. + n.
- quadratus plantae m.
- medial plantar a. + n.
- flexor digitorum brevis m.
- plantar aponeurosis

- extensor digitorum longus m.
- peroneus tertius m.
- superior talocrural (ankle) joint
- anterior talofibular lig.
- talus
- interosseus talocalcanean lig.
- calcaneus
- tendon of peroneus brevis m.
- long plantar lig.
- tendon of peroneus longus m.
- abductor digiti minimi m.

- peroneus muscles
- muscles of hallux
- muscles of digitus minimus
- extensor muscles group
- muscles of plantar arch

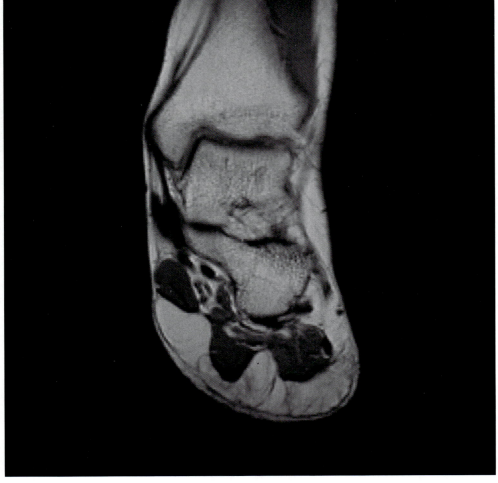

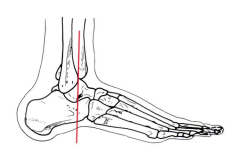

proximal
medial — lateral
distal

Ankle and Foot – Coronal

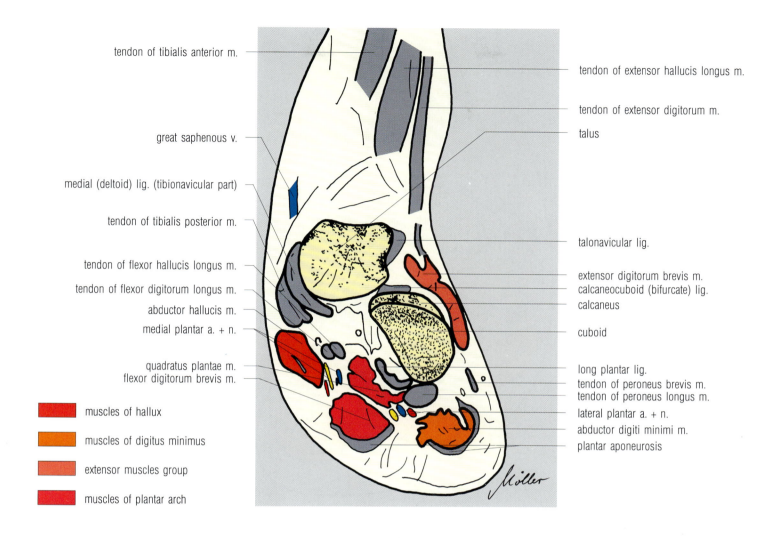

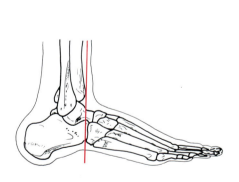

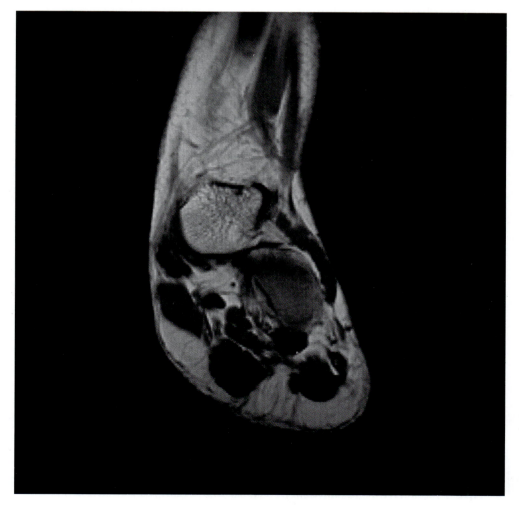

284 Ankle and Foot – Coronal

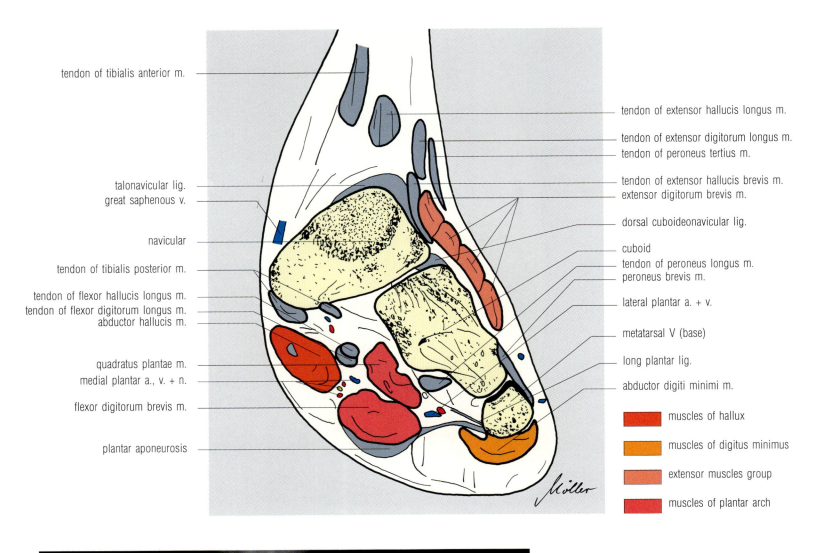
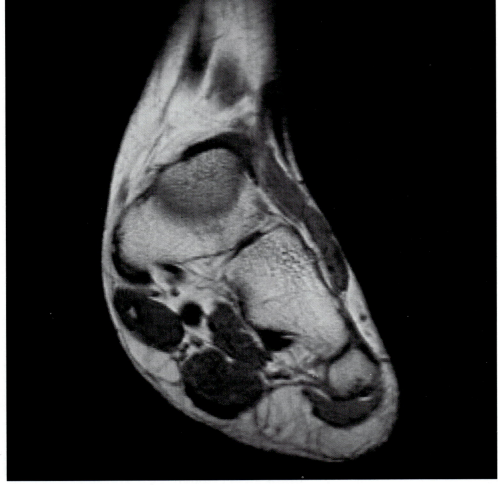
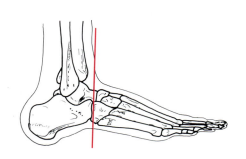

Ankle and Foot – Coronal

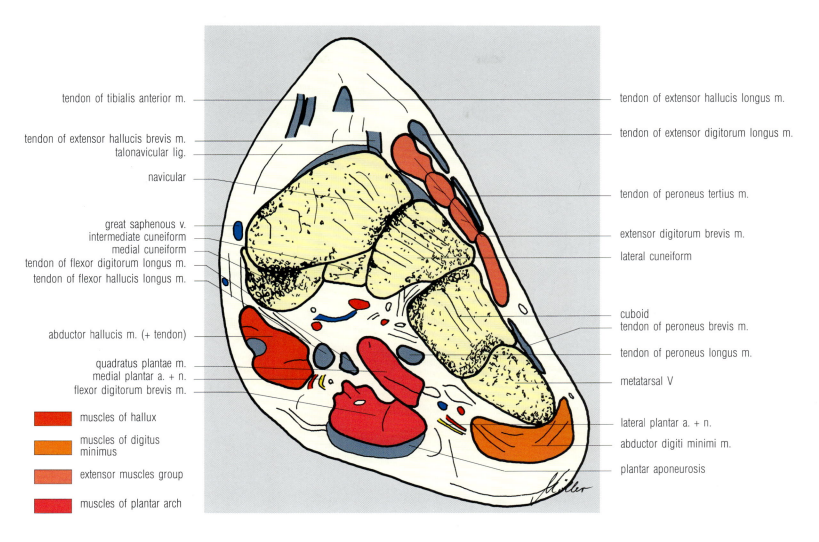

- tendon of tibialis anterior m.
- tendon of extensor hallucis brevis m.
- talonavicular lig.
- navicular
- great saphenous v.
- intermediate cuneiform
- medial cuneiform
- tendon of flexor digitorum longus m.
- tendon of flexor hallucis longus m.
- abductor hallucis m. (+ tendon)
- quadratus plantae m.
- medial plantar a. + n.
- flexor digitorum brevis m.

- tendon of extensor hallucis longus m.
- tendon of extensor digitorum longus m.
- tendon of peroneus tertius m.
- extensor digitorum brevis m.
- lateral cuneiform
- cuboid
- tendon of peroneus brevis m.
- tendon of peroneus longus m.
- metatarsal V
- lateral plantar a. + n.
- abductor digiti minimi m.
- plantar aponeurosis

■ muscles of hallux
■ muscles of digitus minimus
■ extensor muscles group
■ muscles of plantar arch

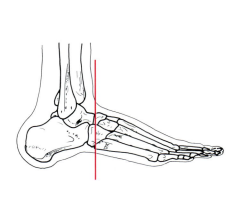

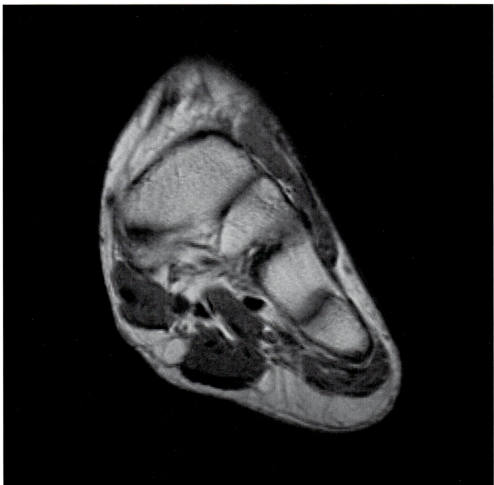

```
        dorsal
medial  □  lateral
       plantar
```

Ankle and Foot – Coronal

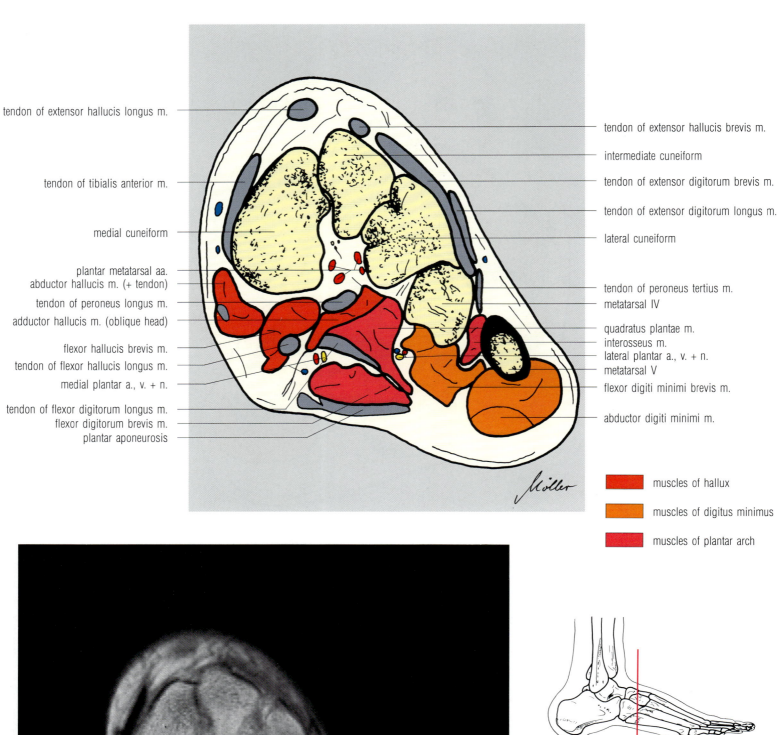

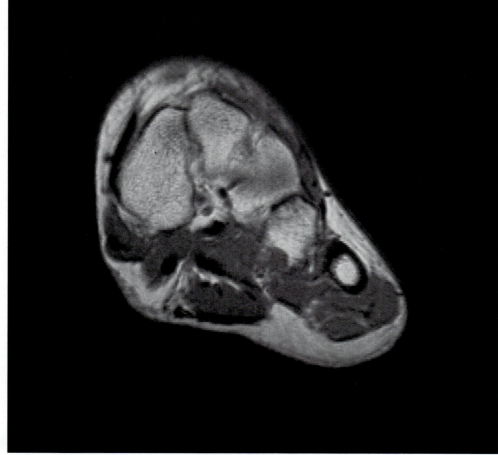

Ankle and Foot – Coronal

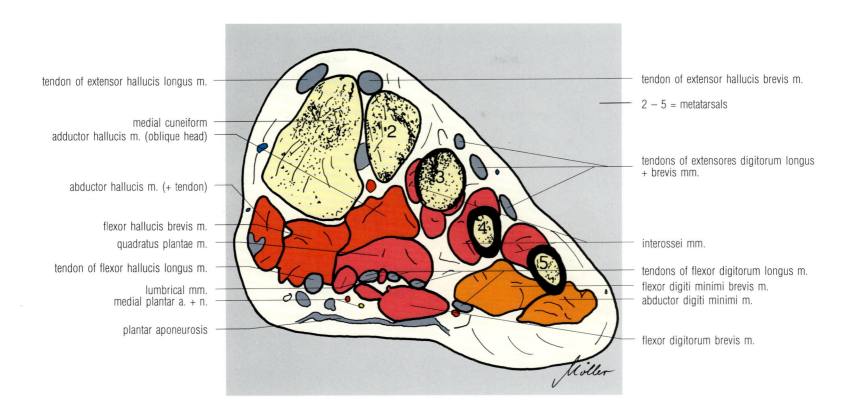

- muscles of hallux
- muscles of digitus minimus
- muscles of plantar arch

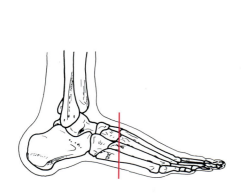

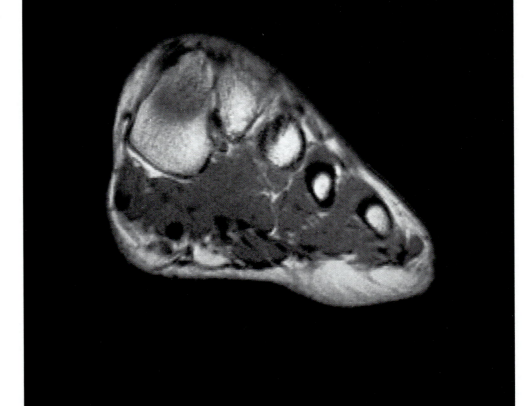

288 Ankle and Foot – Coronal

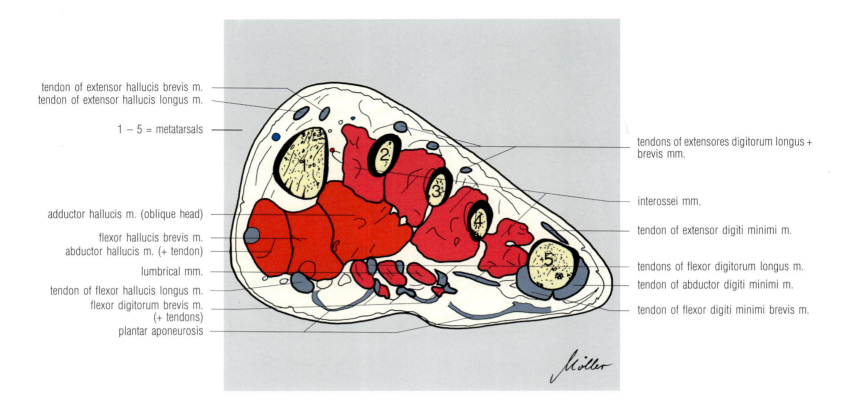

- tendon of extensor hallucis brevis m.
- tendon of extensor hallucis longus m.
- 1 – 5 = metatarsals

- adductor hallucis m. (oblique head)
- flexor hallucis brevis m.
- abductor hallucis m. (+ tendon)
- lumbrical mm.
- tendon of flexor hallucis longus m.
- flexor digitorum brevis m. (+ tendons)
- plantar aponeurosis

- tendons of extensores digitorum longus + brevis mm.
- interossei mm.
- tendon of extensor digiti minimi m.
- tendons of flexor digitorum longus m.
- tendon of abductor digiti minimi m.
- tendon of flexor digiti minimi brevis m.

■ muscles of hallux
■ muscles of plantar arch

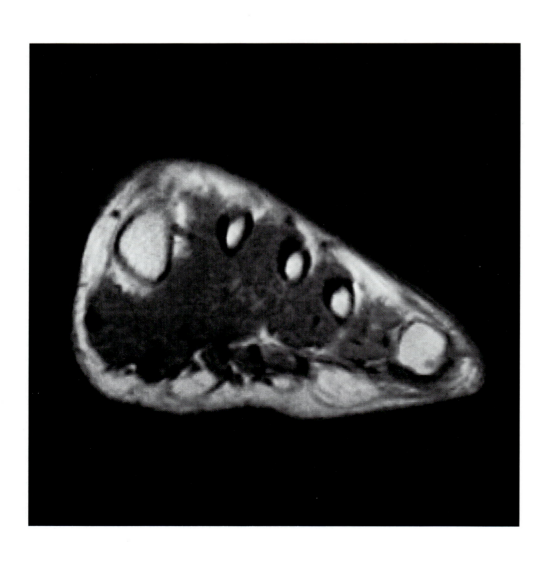

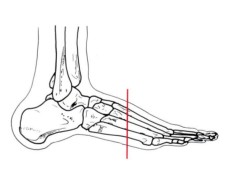

dorsal
medial — lateral
plantar

Ankle and Foot – Coronal

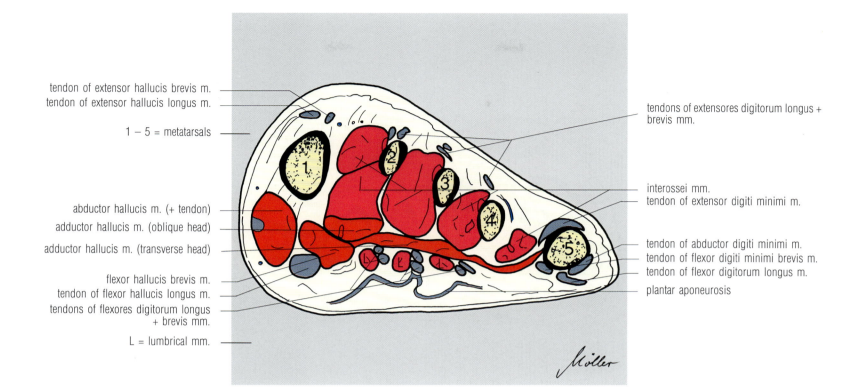

muscles of hallux

muscles of plantar arch

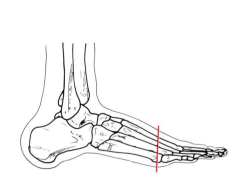

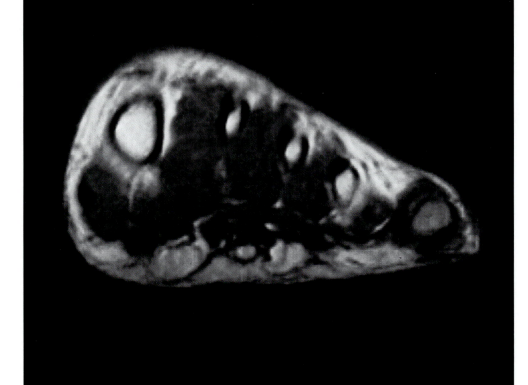

dorsal
medial · lateral
plantar

Ankle and Foot – Coronal

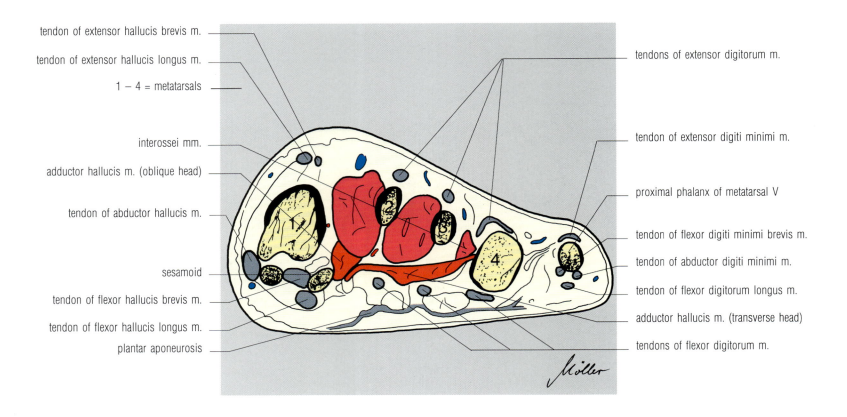

muscles of hallux
muscles of plantar arch

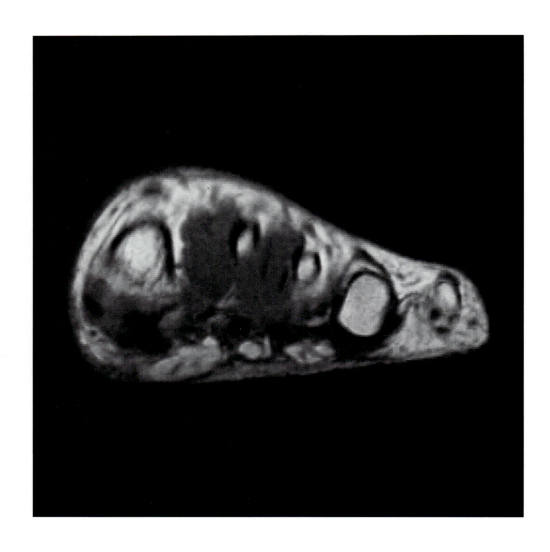

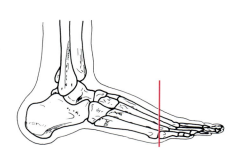

Ankle and Foot – Coronal 291

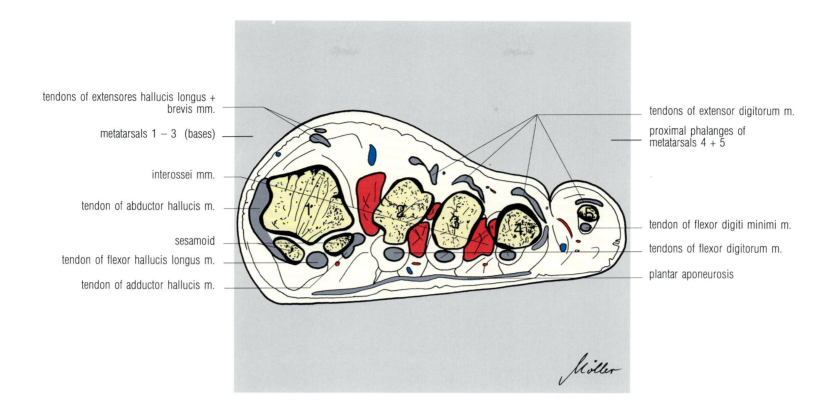

tendons of extensores hallucis longus + brevis mm.
metatarsals 1 – 3 (bases)
interossei mm.
tendon of abductor hallucis m.
sesamoid
tendon of flexor hallucis longus m.
tendon of adductor hallucis m.

tendons of extensor digitorum m.
proximal phalanges of metatarsals 4 + 5
tendon of flexor digiti minimi m.
tendons of flexor digitorum m.
plantar aponeurosis

■ muscles of plantar arch

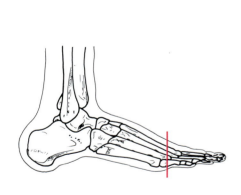

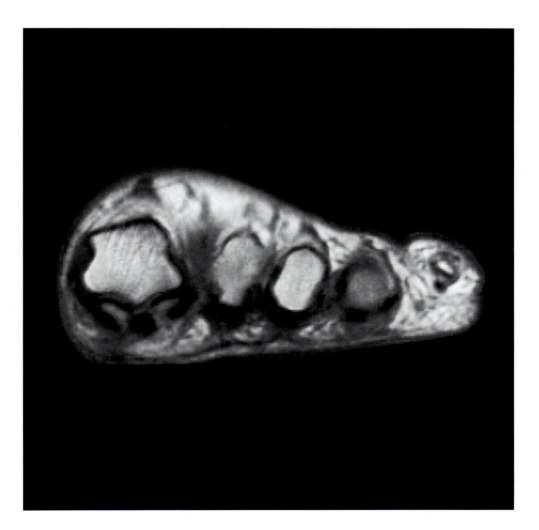

dorsal
medial   lateral
plantar

Ankle and Foot – Sagittal

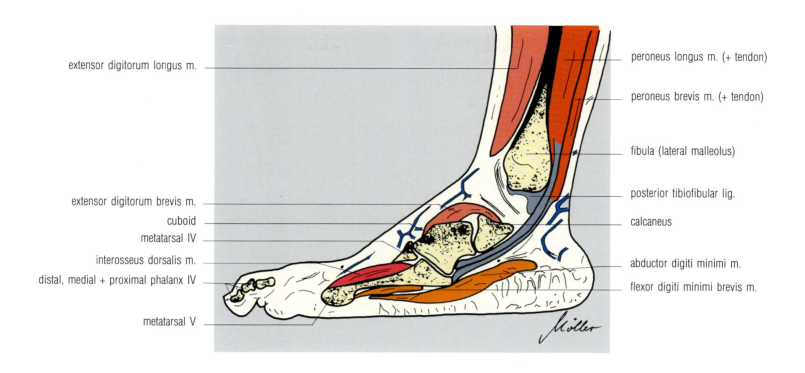

- extensor digitorum longus m.
- extensor digitorum brevis m.
- cuboid
- metatarsal IV
- interosseus dorsalis m.
- distal, medial + proximal phalanx IV
- metatarsal V
- peroneus longus m. (+ tendon)
- peroneus brevis m. (+ tendon)
- fibula (lateral malleolus)
- posterior tibiofibular lig.
- calcaneus
- abductor digiti minimi m.
- flexor digiti minimi brevis m.

- muscles of plantar arch
- muscles of digitus minimus
- extensor muscles group
- peroneus muscles

proximal / dorsal — anterior — posterior — plantar / distal

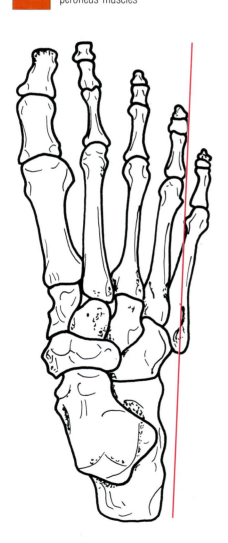
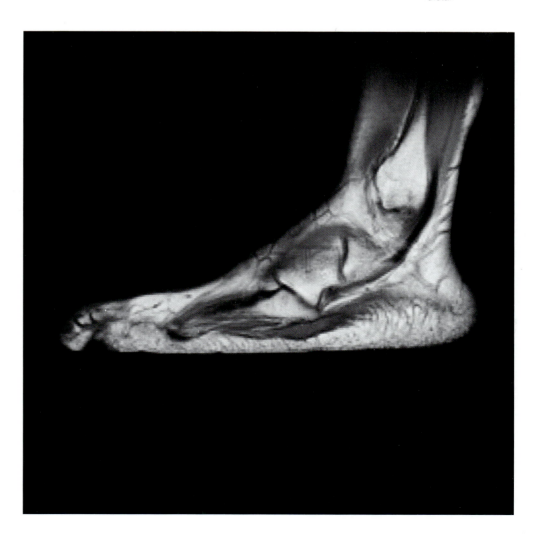

294 Ankle and Foot – Sagittal

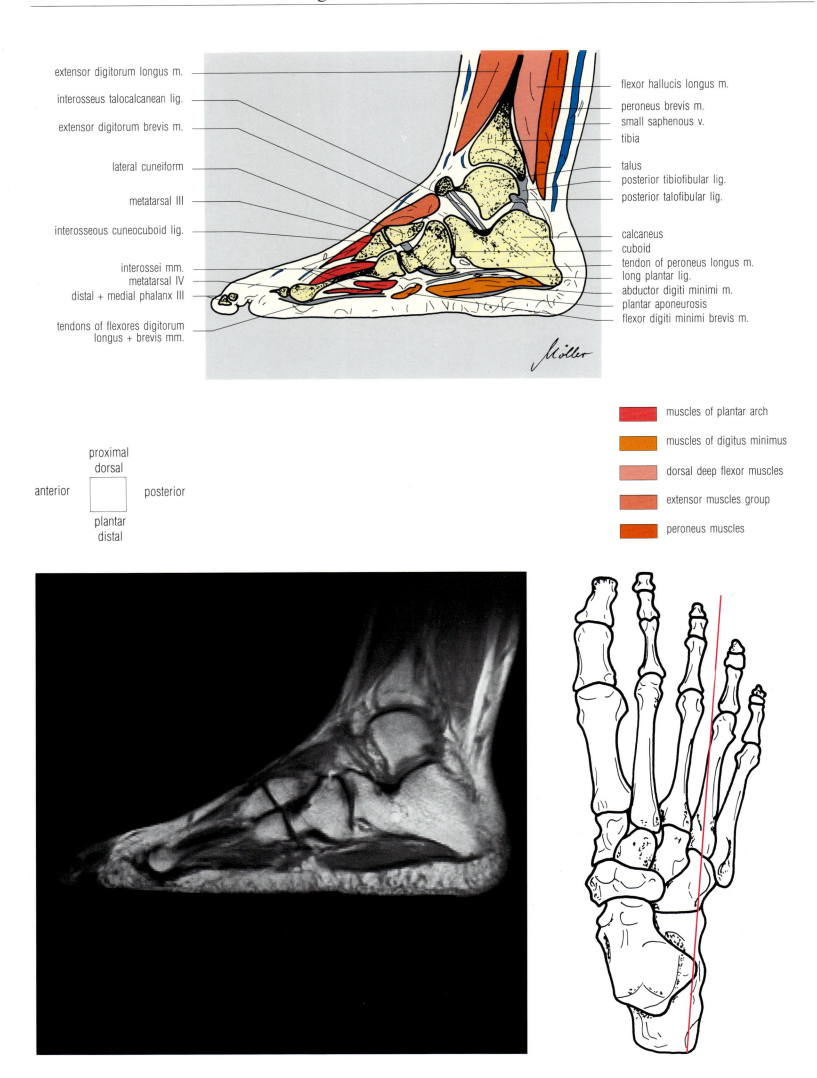

Ankle and Foot – Sagittal

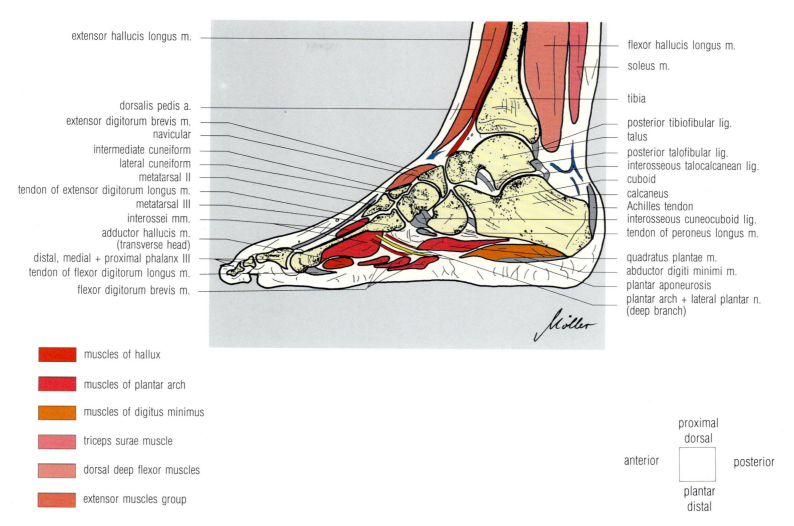

- extensor hallucis longus m.
- dorsalis pedis a.
- extensor digitorum brevis m.
- navicular
- intermediate cuneiform
- lateral cuneiform
- metatarsal II
- tendon of extensor digitorum longus m.
- metatarsal III
- interossei mm.
- adductor hallucis m. (transverse head)
- distal, medial + proximal phalanx III
- tendon of flexor digitorum longus m.
- flexor digitorum brevis m.

- flexor hallucis longus m.
- soleus m.
- tibia
- posterior tibiofibular lig.
- talus
- posterior talofibular lig.
- interosseous talocalcanean lig.
- cuboid
- calcaneus
- Achilles tendon
- interosseous cuneocuboid lig.
- tendon of peroneus longus m.
- quadratus plantae m.
- abductor digiti minimi m.
- plantar aponeurosis
- plantar arch + lateral plantar n. (deep branch)

Legend:
- muscles of hallux
- muscles of plantar arch
- muscles of digitus minimus
- triceps surae muscle
- dorsal deep flexor muscles
- extensor muscles group

Orientation: proximal/dorsal – anterior – posterior – plantar/distal

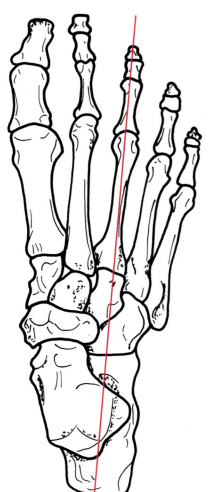

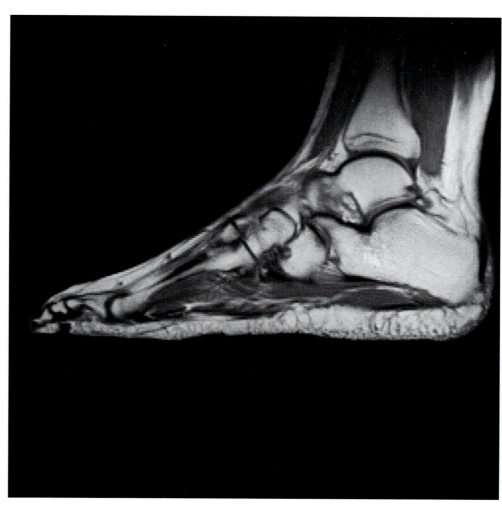

Ankle and Foot – Sagittal

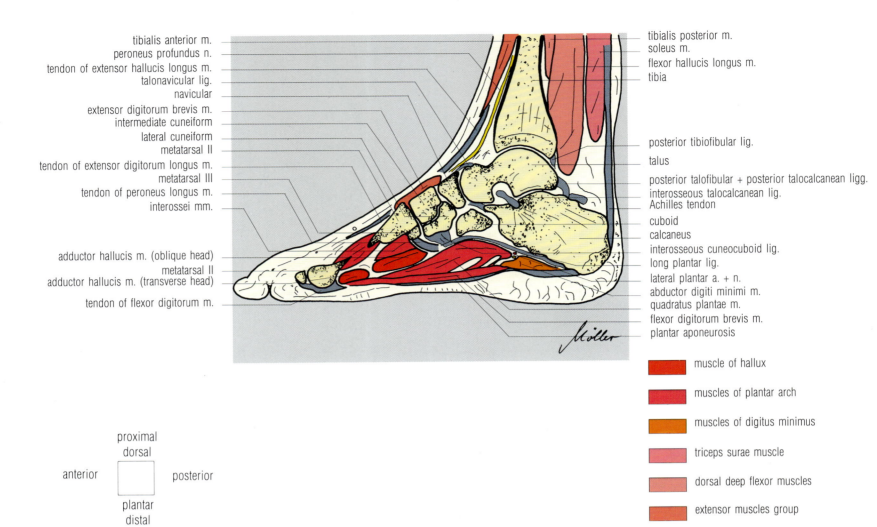

tibialis anterior m.
peroneus profundus n.
tendon of extensor hallucis longus m.
talonavicular lig.
navicular
extensor digitorum brevis m.
intermediate cuneiform
lateral cuneiform
metatarsal II
tendon of extensor digitorum longus m.
metatarsal III
tendon of peroneus longus m.
interossei mm.

adductor hallucis m. (oblique head)
metatarsal II
adductor hallucis m. (transverse head)
tendon of flexor digitorum m.

tibialis posterior m.
soleus m.
flexor hallucis longus m.
tibia

posterior tibiofibular lig.
talus
posterior talofibular + posterior talocalcanean ligg.
interosseous talocalcanean lig.
Achilles tendon
cuboid
calcaneus
interosseous cuneocuboid lig.
long plantar lig.
lateral plantar a. + n.
abductor digiti minimi m.
quadratus plantae m.
flexor digitorum brevis m.
plantar aponeurosis

- muscle of hallux
- muscles of plantar arch
- muscles of digitus minimus
- triceps surae muscle
- dorsal deep flexor muscles
- extensor muscles group

proximal / dorsal
anterior — posterior
plantar / distal

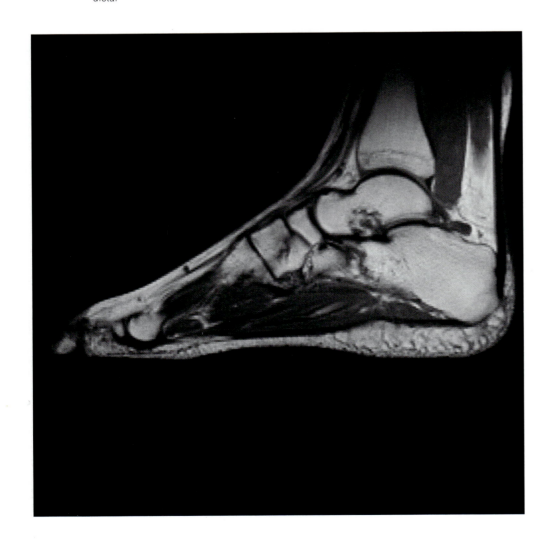

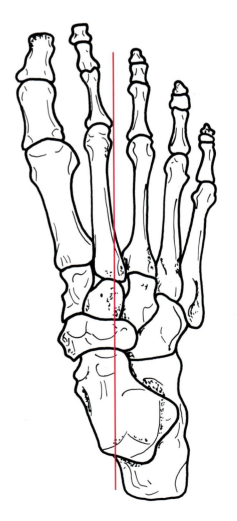

Ankle and Foot – Sagittal

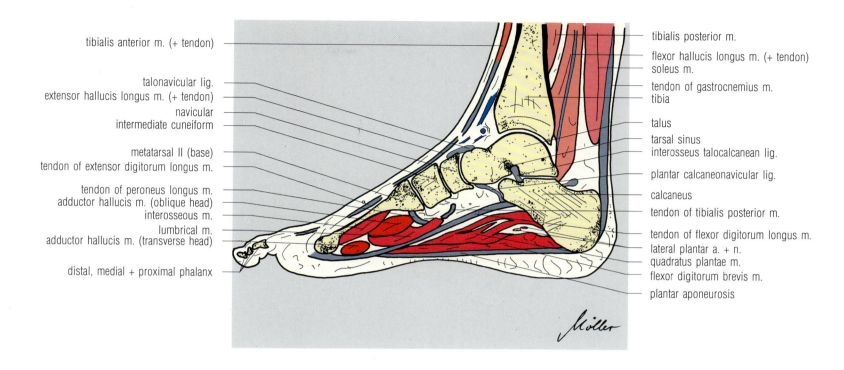

- tibialis anterior m. (+ tendon)
- talonavicular lig.
- extensor hallucis longus m. (+ tendon)
- navicular
- intermediate cuneiform
- metatarsal II (base)
- tendon of extensor digitorum longus m.
- tendon of peroneus longus m.
- adductor hallucis m. (oblique head)
- interosseous m.
- lumbrical m.
- adductor hallucis m. (transverse head)
- distal, medial + proximal phalanx

- tibialis posterior m.
- flexor hallucis longus m. (+ tendon)
- soleus m.
- tendon of gastrocnemius m.
- tibia
- talus
- tarsal sinus
- interosseus talocalcanean lig.
- plantar calcaneonavicular lig.
- calcaneus
- tendon of tibialis posterior m.
- tendon of flexor digitorum longus m.
- lateral plantar a. + n.
- quadratus plantae m.
- flexor digitorum brevis m.
- plantar aponeurosis

- muscles of hallux
- muscles of plantar arch
- triceps surae muscle
- dorsal deep flexor muscles
- extensor muscles group

proximal
dorsal

anterior   posterior

plantar
distal

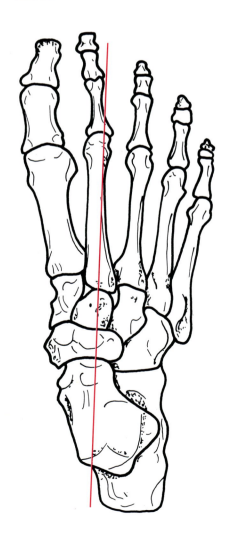

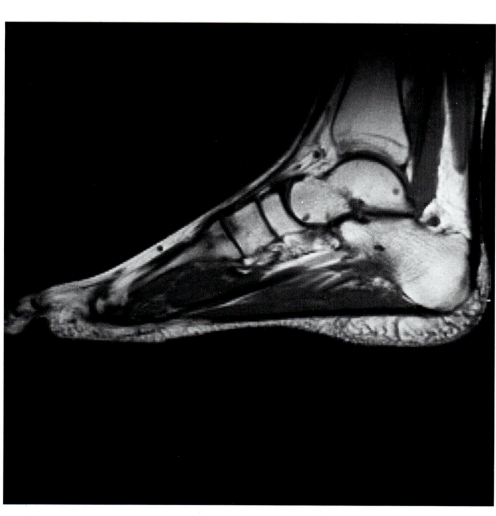

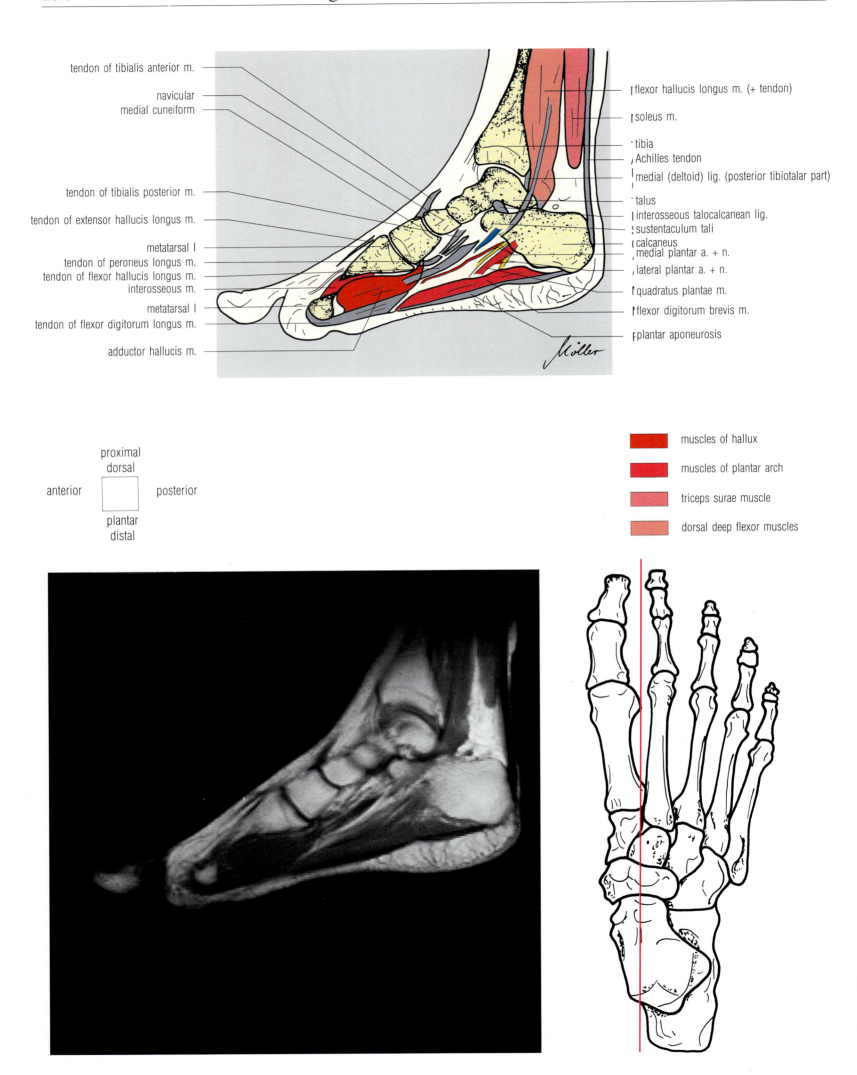

Ankle and Foot – Sagittal

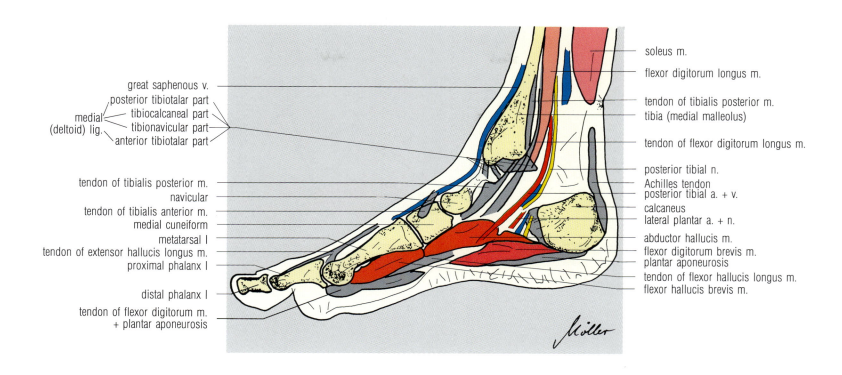

- muscles of hallux
- muscles of plantar arch
- triceps surae muscle
- dorsal deep flexor muscles

```
        proximal
         dorsal
anterior         posterior
         plantar
         distal
```

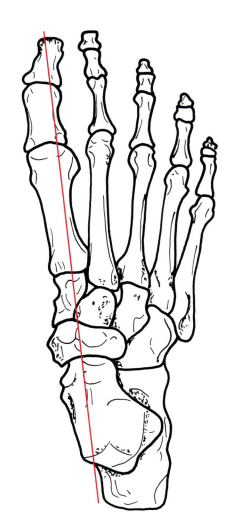
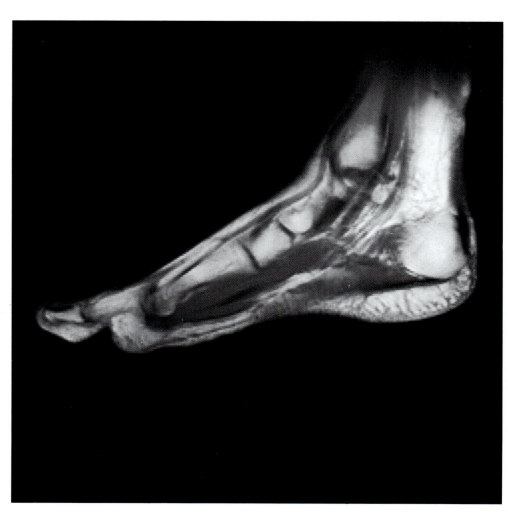

Ankle and Foot – Sagittal

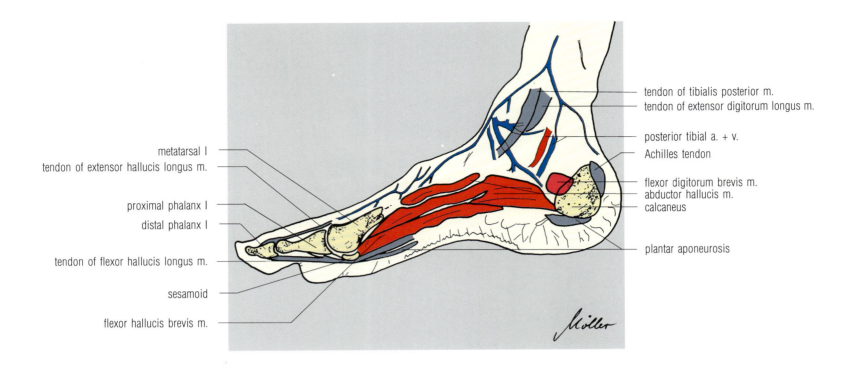

anterior — proximal/dorsal — posterior — plantar/distal

■ muscles of hallux
■ muscles of plantar arch

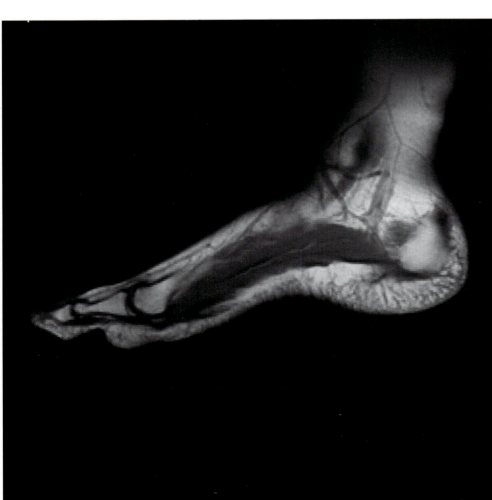
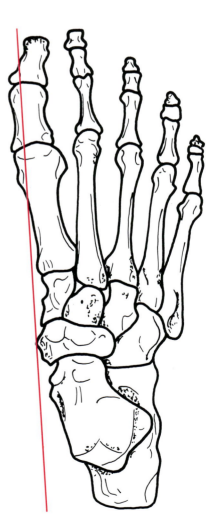

References

1. Basset, L. W., R. H. Gold, L. L. Seeger: MRI Atlas of the Musculoskeletal System. Deutscher Ärzte-Verlag, Köln (1989).
2. Cahill, D. R., M. J. Orland, C. C. Reading: Atlas of Human Cross-Sectional Anatomy. Wiley-Liss (1990).
3. Chacko, A. K., R. W. Katzberg, A. MacKay: MRI Atlas of Normal Anatomy. McGraw-Hill Inc., New York (1991).
4. El-Khoury, G. Y., R. A. Bergman, E. J. Montgomery: Sectional Anatomy by MRI/CT. Churchill, Livingstone (1990).
5. Feneis, H.: Pocket Atlas of Human Anatomy. G. Thieme Verlag, Stuttgart (1985).
6. Han, M.-C., Kim, C.-W.: Sectional Human Anatomy. Ilchokak, Seoul; Igaku-Shoin, New York-Tokio (1989).
7. Kahle, W., H. Leonhard, W. Platzer: Taschenatlas der Anatomie. G. Thieme Verlag, Stuttgart (1991).
8. Kang, H. S., D. Resnick: MRI of the Extremities: An Anatomic Atlas. W. B. Saunders Company, Philadelphia (1991).
9. Koritké, J. G., H. Sick: Atlas of Sectional Human Anatomy. Urban & Schwarzenberg, Baltimore-München (1988).
10. Meschan, I.: Synopsis of Radiologic Anatomy. W. B. Saunders Company, Philadelphia (1980).
11. Middleton, W. D., T. L. Lawson (eds.): Anatomy and MRI of the Joints. Raven Press (1989).
12. Rauber/Kopsch: Anatomie des Menschen. Lehrbuch und Atlas. (Hrsg. H. Leonhardt, B. Tillmann, G. Töndury, K. Zilles). Band I Bewegungsapparat. Thieme Verlag, Stuttgart-New York (1987).
13. Rohen, J. W.: Anatomie des Menschen. Schattauer, Stuttgart (1988).
14. Sobotta, J.: Atlas der Anatomie des Menschen. (Hrsg. J. Staubesand) Urban & Schwarzenberg, München (1988).
15. Stark, D. D., W. G. Bradley: Magnetic Resonance Imaging. Mosby, St. Louis (1992).
16. v. Hagens, G., L. J. Romrell, M. H. Ross, K. Tiedemann: The Visible Human Body. Lea & Febinger, Philadelphia, London (1991).
17. Weir, J., P. H. Abrahams: An Imaging Atlas of Human Anatomy. Wolfe, London (1992).

Subject Index

acetabulum 191f, 196
-, acetabular labrum 142, 199
- -, anterior part 140f
- -, inferior part 187–191, 197f
- -, posterior part 140f
- -, superior part 188–191, 197f, 200
-, acetabular fossa 212
-, acetabular roof 188–190, 192, 197f
-, anterior part 186
Achilles tendon 170–178, 263, 273, 295f, 298–300
acromioclavicular articulation 5
acromion 5, 49–55, 57–60, 67–72, 75–79
adductor canal 148f, 225
adductor hiatus 151, 224
anastomosis around the knee joint 244–247
ankle and foot
-, axial 171–181
-, coronal 277–291
-, sagittal 293–300
antebrachial fascia 30
arteries
-, anterior circumflex humeral a. 57–63
-, anterior interosseous a. 25–29
-, anterior tibial a. 163–171, 234, 242f, 258, 267–269, 279–281
-, arterial plexus around uterus 194
-, arterial plexus around vagina 192
-, axillary a. 7–11, 47–50, 63, 70f
-, blood vessels around the knee joint 244f, 247
-, brachial a. 12–23, 51–53, 61f, 70–72, 75, 77–79, 85, 92–94, 100–102, 109–111
-, circumflex a.
- -, of scapula 10
-, common interosseous a. 24, 102, 104
-, common plantar digital a. 180
-, deep femoral a. 195f, 207, 209–212, 225
-, dorsal digital a. 43f, 121
-, dorsalis pedis a. 295
-, external iliac a. 137f, 186
-, femoral a. 139–152, 185, 187f, 196, 205–208, 210–214, 221–223, 226
-, iliac a. 193
-, inferior gluteal a. 137, 195–198, 216
-, inferior lateral genicular a. 230f, 233, 237, 242–245
-, inferior medial genicular a. 230f, 234, 237, 247–250
-, intercostal a. 7–13
-, internal iliac a. 138, 194
- -, branches of 195
-, internal pudendal a. 137, 139
-, interosseous a. 95, 110, 112
-, interosseous recurrent a. 23

-, lateral circumflex femoral a. 144f, 187, 197–201, 207, 210, 224f
-, lateral plantar a. 176–180, 279–281, 283–286, 296–299
-, lateral thoracic a. 11–13
-, medial circumflex femoral a. 187–192, 196f, 201, 208, 211f
-, medial plantar a. 176–179, 279–287, 298
-, obturator a. 138–142, 189–193
-, palmar digital a. 43f, 125, 130
-, perforating a. 148, 150
-, peroneal a. 164–168, 244, 269
-, plantar metatarsal aa. 286
-, popliteal a. 153–163, 215, 220, 233–237, 246f, 260f, 269
-, posterior circumflex humeral a. 10, 49–55, 57–61, 68f, 75, 77–80
-, posterior interosseous a. 25–27, 29f
-, posterior interosseous recurrent a. 24
-, posterior tibial a. 164–166, 168–175, 245f, 271f, 277f, 299f
-, princeps pollicis a. 40f, 122
-, profunda brachii a. 14–20, 68, 70f, 79, 81
-, profunda femoris a. 145–148, 186–189
-, pudendal a. 140f, 216
-, radial a. 24–34, 85, 94, 99f, 112–114, 121–123, 132
- -, superficial palmar branch 34
-, radial recurrent a. 21–23
-, subscapularis a. 7–12, 49f, 53–55, 67
-, superficial femoral a. 186
-, superficial ulnar collateral a. 21f
-, superior gluteal a. 137, 195f
-, superior lateral genicular a. 152–154, 230–233, 242–245
-, superior medial genicular a. 153f, 230–233, 246–252
-, superior ulnar collateral a. 17–20, 23, 69, 91
-, suprascapular a. 5–8, 49
-, thoracodorsal a. 12
-, tibialis posterior a. 167
-, ulnar a. 24–40, 80f, 85–88, 94, 99, 100–103, 108, 110, 125, 127f
- -, deep branch 41f
axillary fossa 52, 54f
axillary recessus 51f

bicipital aponeurosis 21f
bicipital groove 7, 9f, 49
bowel loops 205
brachial plexus 7–11, 47f, 70
-, dorsal cord 48
-, lateral cord 48
-, medial cord 48
-, posterior cord 69
breast 75f

calcaneus 173–180, 258–263, 277–283, 293–300
-, tubercle 181
capitate 34–37, 119–122, 129–131
carpal canal 123
carpometacarpal articulations 122
clavicle 5, 47–50, 60–63, 69–72, 75–77
coccyx 139f
coracoid process 6, 47f, 61–63, 68–72
coronoid fossa 20
coronoid process 22f, 79, 87f, 93f, 109f
crural anterior intermuscular septum 162, 165–168
crural fascia 163
-, deep 167
cuboid 175–178, 283–285, 293–296
cuneiform
-, intermediate 174–176, 285f, 295–297
-, lateral 174–177, 285f, 294–296
-, medial 174–177, 285–287, 298f

descending colon 206
distal interphalangeal articulation 122, 129, 132
distal radioulnar articulation 120

elbow
-, axial 19–24
-, coronal 85–90
-, joint capsule 19f
-, sagittal 91–96
epiphyseal line 51–53, 192, 255

fascia lata 142, 148–151
femoropatellar articulation 154
femur 143–153, 155, 208, 212, 220f, 231f, 247f
-, cartilage 140–142, 188–190
-, condyle 246
- -, lateral 155f, 214f, 219, 233–236, 241–245, 255–260, 266–268
- -, medial 155f, 214, 223f, 233–236, 249f, 252, 255f, 258–260, 272–274
-, epiphysis 188f
-, head 139–142, 186–191, 197–199, 208–213, 225f
- -, fovea 189f, 196
-, lateral compact 210
-, neck 191, 199, 201, 209f, 224
-, shaft 201, 209–211
-, trochanter
- -, greater trochanter 141f, 191–194, 201, 209f, 212, 214, 220
- -, intertrochanteric crest 194, 213
- -, lesser trochanter 145, 194, 198–200, 213
fibula 160, 162–170, 235, 238, 242, 267–269, 278–281
-, head 161, 236f, 241, 243, 259–261, 265f

–, lateral malleolus 171f, 258–260, 293
–, shaft 259f
flexor retinaculum 33–38, 125, 129–132, 172–174, 280–282
forearm
–, axial 25–30
–, coronal 99–106
–, sagittal 107–116

glenoid cavity 49, 51–53, 63, 67f, 75
glenoid labrum
–, anterior part 7–9
–, posterior part 7–9

hamate 35–37, 119–122, 127f
–, hook 36f, 123f, 128
hip
–, axial 137–146
–, joint cavity 192, 211
–, coronal 185–194
–, sagittal 195–201
humeroradial articulation 22, 104
humeroulnar articulation 22, 104
humerus 9–18, 68f, 78f, 87–89, 93–95, 103, 105f
–, capitulum 21f, 73, 81, 86, 88f, 95, 103f, 112–116
–, epicondyle
– –, lateral 19f, 72, 96
– –, medial 19–21, 69–72, 75f, 88f, 91, 107f
–, head 6–8, 48–55, 57–62, 67–72, 75–81
–, shaft 55
–, trochlea 22, 77–80, 86–88, 92–94, 101–104, 109–111
–, tubercle
– –, greater 7, 51–54
– –, lesser 8f

iliotibial tract 143–146, 150–159, 187, 189–194, 208–210, 212f, 220, 231–233, 241
ilium 137f, 185–199, 205–213, 215–217
–, anterior superior iliac spine 200f
inferior glenoid labrum 49–52
inferior peroneal retinaculum 280f
infrapatellar fat pad 155–159, 230, 243–248
inguinal lymph node 205
intercarpal articulations 122
interosseous membrane 25–27, 29
ischiorectal fossa 144, 193f, 216f
ischiorectal tuberosity 144
ischium 139–142, 190–194, 197, 214–217
–, inferior ramus 144
–, ischial spine 140, 195
–, ischial tubercle 193–196
–, ischial tuberosity 143

knee
–, articular space 255
–, axial 155–158
–, blood vessels around the knee joint 242, 244–247
–, coronal 229–239
–, joint 242
–, joint capsule 154–158, 236, 241, 244–250
–, joint cartilage 154f, 157
–, sagittal 241–274

lateral intermuscular septum 15–18, 148
lateral patellar retinaculum 153–160, 208f, 229–231, 241f
ligaments
–, acromioclavicular lig. 50
–, anterior cruciate lig. 155–157, 220, 233–235, 246f, 256–258
–, anterior lig. of head of fibula 160
–, anterior talofibular lig. 172f, 282
–, anular lig. 22f, 86, 88, 89, 96
–, arcuate popliteal lig. 159, 236, 244
–, calcaneocuboid (bifurcate) lig. 175, 283
–, calcaneofibular lig. 173–175, 279–281
–, calcaneonavicular (bifurcate) lig. 175
–, collateral lig. 20, 43f, 121–123, 129
–, coracoacromial lig. 47–51, 58f, 61
–, coracoclavicular lig. 5f, 47, 63, 69
–, coracohumeral lig. 6, 57–60, 62
–, deltoid (medial) lig.
– –, tibionavicular part 174
– –, tibiocalcanean part 174
–, dorsal cuboideonavicular lig. 284
–, dorsal intercarpal lig. 34–36, 127–131
–, dorsal intercuneiform ligg. 175
–, dorsal metacarpal ligg. 38
–, dorsal radiocarpal lig. 32f, 129f
–, glenohumeral lig. 49, 58–60, 62
–, iliofemoral lig. 139–144, 186–191, 196f, 199f, 210
–, inguinal lig. 205
–, interosseous cuneocuboid lig. 294–296
–, interosseous talocalcanean lig. 172–176, 280, 282, 294–298
–, ischiofemoral lig. 142, 192f, 198
–, lateral collateral lig. 21, 155–159, 234–236, 241, 255–258
–, lateral fibular collateral lig. 160
–, lig. of head of femur 140f, 189–191
–, long plantar lig. 177f, 281–284, 294, 296
–, medial (deltoid) lig.
– –, anterior tibiotalar part 172, 299
– –, posterior tibiotalar part 173, 280f, 298f
– –, tibiocalcanean part 172f, 281f, 299
– –, tibionavicular part 172f, 175, 283, 299
–, medial collateral lig. 155–161, 232f
–, medial talocalcaneal lig. 174
–, meniscofemoral lig. 157
–, oblique popliteal lig. 155–160, 250
–, palmar carpometacarpal ligg. 38
–, palmar intercarpal lig. 128, 130
–, palmar metacarpal ligg. 38f
–, palmar radiocarpal lig. 31–33, 122f, 129–132
–, palmar ulnocarpal lig. 31–33, 123, 128
–, patellar lig. 154–162, 219–222, 229–231, 243–249, 268–271
–, pisohamate lig. 35f, 124, 128
–, pisometacarpal lig. 35f, 122, 124
–, plantar calcaneocuboid lig. 176
–, plantar calcaneonavicular lig. 297
–, plantar cuneonavicular lig. 176
–, posterior cruciate lig. 155–158, 220, 233–236, 246–248, 256–259
– –, femoral origin 246, 249
–, posterior lig. of head of fibula 160

–, posterior meniscofemoral lig. 236, 247f
–, posterior talocalcanean lig. 296
–, posterior talofibular lig. 172, 279f, 294–296
–, posterior tibiofibular lig. 293–296
–, radial carpal collateral lig. 121
–, radial collateral lig. 23, 88
–, radiating carpal lig. 37
–, sacrotuberal lig. 139, 195f, 217
–, sacrouterine lig. 139
–, talonavicular lig. 283–285, 296f
–, transverse lig. of knee 156f, 244–248
–, ulnar carpal collateral lig. 32f, 120, 123
–, ulnar collateral lig. 88, 91
linea aspera 148–150
lower leg
–, axial 159–170
–, coronal 255–263
–, sagittal 265–274
lumbosacral plexus 137
lunate 32–34, 110f, 119–122, 127–130
lung 48f

malleolus
–, lateral 257
–, medial 171, 255, 257f, 273, 280, 282
medial intermuscular septum 15–17
medial patellar retinaculum 153–160, 208, 229–231, 249–252
meniscus
–, lateral 255f, 266
– –, anterior horn 157, 219, 232, 243–245
– –, intermediate part 157, 233f, 241f, 257
– –, posterior horn 157, 235, 243–245, 258f, 267f
–, medial
– –, anterior horn 157, 249–251
– –, intermediate part 232f, 252, 257
– –, posterior horn 234f, 249–251
mesosalpinx 139
metacarpals 36–43, 119–125, 127–132
metacarpophalangeal articulation 122, 129, 132
metatarsals 175–181, 284–291, 293–300
muscles
–, abductor digiti minimi brevis m. 125
–, abductor digiti minimi m. 34–42, 122–124, 179–181, 279–287, 293–296
– –, tendon of 288–290
–, abductor hallucis m. 176–178, 279–284, 299f
– –, tendon of 178, 277f, 290f
–, abductor pollicis brevis m. 35–40, 123, 125, 131f
– –, origin 123
–, abductor pollicis longus m. 25–28, 102–104, 113–115
– –, tendon of 29–35, 99, 100, 116, 122–124, 132
–, adductor brevis m. 143–146, 185–191, 195f, 207–212, 225f
–, adductor hallucis m.
– –, oblique head 178–180, 286–290, 296f
– –, transverse head 180f, 289f, 295–298
–, adductor longus m. 143–149, 185–189, 195f, 206–212, 225f

Subject Index

-, adductor magnus m. 145–151, 191–198, 211–215, 217, 222–226
- -, tendon of 152–154, 250–252
-, adductor minimus m. 189–192, 211–215
-, adductor mm. 141–153, 185–200, 206–217, 222–226, 237f, 251
-, adductor pollicis m. 39–42, 124f, 131
- -, oblique head 122f, 132
- -, tendon of 38
- -, transverse head 122f, 129f
-, anconeus m. 20–24, 70, 80, 90, 95, 106, 110–114
-, anterior extensor mm. 160–172, 232–234, 241–245, 255–257, 265–270
-, biceps brachii m. 13f, 17, 49f, 60, 73, 75, 77–81, 92–96, 113f
- -, long head 11f, 15f, 18, 49, 50, 52–54, 58, 77
- -, origin 88f, 112
- -, short head 11f, 18, 49f, 59, 62, 72, 76
- -, tendon of 21f, 24, 62, 80, 85–87, 101
- - -, long head 6, 49f, 57–61, 69–71, 75–80
- - -, short head 47f, 61
-, biceps femoris m. 223–225, 233–236, 238f, 241f, 244
- -, common head of 217
- -, long head 147–152, 198, 214f, 217, 219–222, 243
- -, short head 149–153, 212–215, 219–221, 243
- -, tendon of 144, 157–160, 216, 226, 236, 241, 259f, 265
- - -, long head 145f
-, brachialis m. 14–24, 71–73, 77–81, 85–88, 92–96, 100–103, 109–116
- -, tendon of 89
-, brachioradialis m. 16–26, 71–73, 81, 85–89, 95f, 99, 100–102, 113–116
- -, tendon of 27–30
-, coccygeus m. 140
-, coracobrachialis m. 7–14, 47–52, 58, 60–63, 72, 75–78
-, deep flexor mm. 161f, 168, 244
-, deep transverse perineal m. 212–215
-, deltoid m. 6–14, 47–55, 57–63, 67–73, 75–81
- -, acromial part 5
- -, clavicular part 5
- -, spinal part 5
-, digitorum m. 44
-, dorsal deep flexor mm. 163–167, 169–172, 234f, 243, 245–247, 257–261, 268–274, 277–279, 294–299
-, dorsal interosseous m. 38–42, 119f, 128, 130–132
-, dorsal mm. of forearm 88–90
- -, deep layer 23–30, 86f, 95, 101–105, 110–116
- -, superficial layer 23–30, 96, 103–106, 109–115
-, dorsal mm. of upper arm 10–24, 53–55, 57–59, 61–63, 67–71, 75–81, 87–95
-, erector spinae m. 216f
-, extensor carpi radialis brevis m. 22–25, 71, 87, 96, 101–106, 115f
- -, tendon of 28–38, 131f
-, extensor carpi radialis longus m. 19–24, 71, 87–89, 95f, 101f, 115f

- -, tendon of 26–37, 119–121
-, extensor carpi ulnaris m. 23–25, 71, 90, 103–106, 109–112
- -, origin 96
- -, tendon of 31–37, 119, 121, 127
-, extensor digiti minimi m. 25, 105, 112
- -, tendon of 31–43, 288–290
-, extensor digitorum brevis m. 172–176, 283–285, 293–296
- -, tendon of 286–289
-, extensor digitorum longus m. 161–167, 232–234, 241f, 255–257, 265–269, 281f, 293f
-, extensor digitorum longus m. 172–176, 284–289, 295–297, 300
- -, tendon of 31–43, 119f, 128–132, 178, 283, 290f
-, extensor hallucis brevis m. 176
- -, tendon of 284–291
-, extensor hallucis longus m. 166–169, 255–257, 266–268, 295
- -, tendon of 172–177, 283–291, 296, 298–300
-, extensor indicis m. 27f, 30, 102–104, 110f
- -, tendon of 31–34
-, extensor mm. 173–176, 281–285, 293–297
-, extensor pollicis brevis m. 26f, 101, 103f, 113–115
- -, tendon of 30–35, 41, 116, 121
-, extensor pollicis longus m. 25–28, 95, 102–104, 111f
- -, tendon of 31–42, 102, 119f, 129, 132
-, extensor retinaculum m. 30–34
-, external intercostal m. 9–13
-, flexor carpi radialis m. 24–26, 76–78, 86f, 92, 99, 107–113
- -, tendon of 22f, 29–37, 124f, 132
-, flexor carpi ulnaris m. 24–26, 29, 32, 75–77, 90f, 101–104, 107
- -, humeral head 21
- -, ulnar head 21
- -, tendon of 33f, 99, 125, 127f
-, flexor digiti minimi brevis m. 288–290
-, flexor digiti longus m.
- -, tendon of 290
-, flexor digiti minimi brevis m. 38–42, 125, 179–181, 286f, 293f
-, flexor digiti minimi m.
- -, tendon of 291
-, flexor digitorum brevis m. 179–181, 280–287, 295–300
- -, tendon of 289
-, flexor digitorum longus m. 164–167, 246, 258, 269–274, 278, 299
- -, tendon of 171–181, 279–289, 295, 297–299
-, flexor digitorum m.
- -, tendon of 44, 132, 290f, 294, 296, 299
-, flexor digitorum profundus m. 23–25, 76–80, 88–94, 100–106, 108–111
- -, tendon of 22, 32–43, 42f, 123f, 127, 129f, 132
-, flexor digitorum superficialis m. 22–24, 28, 75–79, 86, 88f, 91–94, 99, 100–104, 107–110, 112–114
- -, tendon of 33–44, 125, 129, 132

-, flexor hallucis brevis m. 178, 180, 286–289, 299f
- -, lateral head 179
- -, medial head 179
- -, tendon of 290
-, flexor hallucis longus m. 166–168, 170, 259–261, 268–273, 277, 279, 294–296
- -, tendon of 173–181, 279–291, 298–300
-, flexor pollicis brevis m. 37, 39f, 123, 132
- -, deep head 36, 124
- -, tendon of deep head 38
- -, superficial head 125
-, flexor pollicis longus m. 26–29, 99, 100–102, 111–115
- -, tendon of 31–42, 122–124, 131f
-, gastrocnemius m. 235, 248, 257f, 260f
- -, lateral head 154–166, 214f, 219, 233f, 236–239, 241–247, 249, 259, 261–263, 266–268
- -, medial head 154–166, 214–216, 220–222, 233–239, 246f, 250–252, 258f, 262f, 271–274
- -, origin 251f
- -, tendon of 167–169, 241, 273f, 297
- - -, lateral head 242
- - -, medial head 270
-, gemelli mm. 199, 214f, 226
- -, tendon of 213
-, gemellus inferior m. 142, 192–196, 199
-, gemellus superior m. 141, 193–195
-, gluteus maximus m. 137–147, 193–201, 213–217, 220–226
- -, tendon of 148
-, gluteus medius m. 137–141, 185–191, 193f, 197–201, 205–209, 212–214, 220–222
- -, tendon of 143, 201
-, gluteus minimus m. 137–140, 186–189, 191–193, 197–200, 207–209
- -, tendon of 142, 192
-, gracilis m. 145–150, 159, 189–192, 210–217, 225f, 237f, 251
- -, origin 252
- -, tendon of 154–158, 160–162, 224, 233–237, 252, 261f
-, hypothenar mm. 33
-, iliacus m. 137f, 185–192, 194, 196–200, 206–211
-, iliopsoas m. 139, 141f, 144f, 185–188, 196, 198–200, 205–209, 225f
- -, tendon of 192f, 211
-, infraspinatus m. 7–11, 50, 52f, 60–63, 67f, 75–79
- -, tendon of 57f, 69, 80
-, intercostal mm. 7f, 47f, 49, 70, 72f
-, internal intercostal m. 9–13
-, interossei dorsales mm. 177f
-, interossei mm. 121–123, 179, 287–291, 294–296
-, interossei plantares m. 180
-, interosseous m. 129, 286, 297f
- -, origin 43
- -, tendon of 44, 124, 128
-, interosseus dorsalis m. 176, 293
-, interosseus plantaris m. 181
-, latissimus dorsi m. 11–13, 50–55, 60–63, 67–71, 75–79
- -, tendon of 10

–, levator ani m.   141–144, 193f, 215–217
–, lumbrical m.   41–43, 124f, 127, 130–132, 181, 287–289, 297
– –, origin   43
– –, tendon of   44, 124
–, muscles of digitus minimus   179–181, 279–287, 293–296
–, muscles of dorsal thigh
– –, origin   143
–, obliquus externus abdominis m.   199
–, obliquus internus abdominis m.   137–140, 199
–, obturator externus m.   143f, 187–193, 195–197, 209–213, 225f
– –, tendon of   193, 201, 213
–, obturator internus m.   138–144, 189–201, 210–217
– –, tendon of   141f, 192, 213
–, of forearm   70, 75–80
–, of hallux   176–181, 279, 282–290, 295–300
–, of hypothenar   34–42, 122–125, 127f
–, of metacarpus   38–43, 119–132
–, of plantar arch   176–180, 181, 279f, 281–291, 293–300
–, of shoulder   5–14, 47–55, 57–63, 67–73, 75–81
–, of thenar   35–42, 122–125, 129–132
–, of trunk   5–13, 47–51, 62f, 67–73
–, omohyoid m.   5
–, opponens digiti minimi m.   38–41, 123–125
–, opponens pollicis m.   35–41, 123–125, 131f
–, palmar interosseous m.   40–42, 127f, 132
–, palmaris brevis m.   38f
– –, tendon of   35f
–, palmaris longus m.   24f, 76, 87–89, 99–101, 107, 109f
– –, origin   21
– –, tendon of   22f, 30–35, 130
–, palmaris m.
– –, tendon of   125
–, pectineus m.   141–144, 185–191, 195–198, 206–211, 225f
– –, tendon of   192
–, pectoralis major m.   6–13, 60–63, 71–73, 75f
–, pectoralis minor m.   7–11
– –, tendon of   6, 63
–, peroneal muscles group   161–172, 232–237, 241, 256–262, 265–267, 277f, 282, 293f
–, peroneus brevis m.   165–167, 258–262, 265–267, 277f, 294
– –, tendon of   173–178, 263, 279–285
–, peroneus longus m.   161–166, 168, 232–237, 241, 256–261, 265–267
– –, tendon of   170–178, 277–286, 294–298
–, peroneus tertius m.   171, 282
– –, tendon of   173–176, 284–286
–, piriformis m.   137–140, 194–197, 214–217
– –, tendon of   141, 198–201
–, plantaris m.   155–158, 160f, 243–245, 267–270
– –, origin   242
– –, tendon of   154, 162–166, 241
–, popliteus m.   158–163, 235–237, 246–249, 258–260, 267–272

– –, origin   242
– –, tendon of   155–157, 232–236, 241f
– –, profundus m.   44
–, pronator quadratus m.   28–30, 100f, 109–113, 122f, 127–131
–, pronator teres m.   19–27, 71–73, 76–81, 85–88, 91–94, 99–103, 107–115
–, psoas m.   137f, 186–189, 195f, 207–210
–, pyramidalis m.   205
–, quadratus femoris m.   143f, 190–194, 196–201, 214f, 223–225
– –, tendon of   226
–, quadratus plantae m.   177f, 279, 280–287, 295–298
– –, tendon of   278
–, quadriceps femoris m.   247
– –, tendon of   152f, 207–209, 219–222, 229, 243–246, 248
–, quadriceps muscles group   141–153, 185–194, 197–201, 205–215, 219–225, 229–234, 241–252
–, radial muscles of forearm   16–27, 71–73, 81, 85–89, 95f, 99–106, 113–116
–, rectus abdominis m.   137–140, 195–198
– –, rectus sheath   205
–, rectus femoris m.   142–149, 186–190, 197f, 200, 205–207, 221–224
– –, origin   209
– –, tendon of   138–140, 150f, 186–190, 198, 200f, 207f, 246
–, sartorius m.   137–153, 185f, 196–201, 205–217, 224–226, 233f, 236–238, 250–252
– –, origin   249f, 252
– –, tendon of   156–158, 160f, 224, 233f, 258f
–, scalenus medius m.   6
–, semimembranosus m.   148–150, 195f, 216f, 221–226, 234–236, 238f, 245–249
– –, tendon of   144–146, 156–160, 226, 234–237, 251f, 274
–, semitendinosus m.   145–150, 194, 215, 217, 222, 224–226, 247
– –, common head   217
– –, tendon of   144, 154–162, 216, 226, 233–239, 248–252, 262
–, serratus anterior m.   5–13, 47–50, 67–73
–, soleus m.   161–170, 237–239, 241–249, 258f, 261–263, 265–274, 295–299
–, subclavius m.   5f, 70
–, subscapularis m.   6, 8–11, 48–51, 63, 67–72, 75–77
– –, tendon of   8, 48, 50, 60
–, superficial transverse perineal m. 193, 215
–, supinator m.   23–25, 73, 81, 86–90, 95, 101–105, 111–116
–, supraspinatus m.   5f, 47, 58, 60f, 63, 67f, 75–77
– –, tendon of   6, 57, 69, 71, 78–80
–, tensor fasciae latae m.   137–146, 185–189, 201, 205–208, 219–222
–, teres major m.   11f, 49–55, 57, 60–63, 67–70, 76–79
–, teres minor m.   7–11, 52–55, 58–63, 67f, 75–79
– –, tendon of   52, 57, 80

–, thigh mm.   239
–, thoracic mm.   50f
–, tibialis anterior m.   160–167, 241–245, 255–257, 267f, 270, 296
– –, tendon of   159, 170–176, 248, 283–286, 298f
–, tibialis posterior m.   161–167, 234f, 243–245, 247, 257–260, 268–273, 296f
– –, tendon of   170–176, 259, 280–284, 297–300
–, transversus abdominis m.   185f, 205f
–, trapezius m.   5f, 47–51, 62f, 67–70, 75
–, triceps brachii m.   53f, 57–59, 61–63, 67, 69, 75f, 87–89, 93–95, 109, 111, 113f
– –, lateral head   11–14, 16, 18, 54f, 68, 70, 71, 79–81
– –, long head   10–17, 55, 78–81, 91
– –, medial head   13–18, 68, 70, 78, 91
– –, origin   77f
– –, tendon of   10, 16–18, 51f, 93
–, triceps surae m.   154–170, 233–239, 241–252, 257–263, 265–274, 295–299
–, urogenital diaphragm
– –, deep transverse perineal m.   215
– –, superficial transverse perineal m.   193f, 215
–, vastus intermedius m.   145–150, 152, 189–191, 198–201, 207–212, 219–223, 243–245
–, vastus lateralis m.   143–152, 186–194, 201, 205–215, 219–223, 229f, 232–234, 241–243
– –, tendon of   153–155, 187, 229f
–, vastus medialis m.   146–153, 200f, 205–214, 223–225, 229–232, 246–252
– –, tendon of   153
–, ventral muscles of forearm   19–22, 88–94
– –, deep layer   23–32, 99–106, 108–115
– –, superficial layer   23–32, 85–87, 99–104, 107–115
–, ventral muscles of upper arm   9–24, 49–53, 58–60, 71–73, 76–81, 85–88, 92–96
–, ventral superficial flexor muscles of forearm   23–32, 85–87, 99–104, 107–115

navicular   172–175, 284f, 295–299
nerves
–, anterior interosseous n.   26–29
–, axillary n.   10, 49–55, 69
–, dorsal digital n.   33, 43f, 121
–, femoral cutaneous n.
– –, anterior branch   148
–, femoral n.   137–146, 185, 196f, 206
– –, anterior cutaneous branch   149–151
– –, branch   187
–, intercostal n.   7–13
–, lateral antebrachial cutaneous n.   20, 24–28, 30f
–, lateral dorsal cutaneous n.   280
–, lateral plantar n.   174–180, 278–281, 283, 285f, 296–299
– –, deep branch   179, 295
–, lateral sural cutaneous n.   158, 241
–, long thoracic n.   9f
–, medial antebrachial cutaneous n.   17–28, 92, 100

–, medial plantar n. 174–179, 278–287, 298
–, medial sural cutaneous n. 153–155, 160–165
–, median n. 12–40, 49–51, 61–63, 71f, 75, 77–79, 85–88, 92–94, 99–101, 109–112, 124f, 130
– –, common palmar digital nn. of 41
–, musculocutaneous n. 12–16, 71, 85
–, obturator n. 137–143, 189–192
– –, anterior branch 146
– –, posterior branch 146
–, palmar digital n. 43f, 125
–, peroneal n.
– –, common 150–162, 214–216, 220–223, 236–239, 241–244, 260, 265
– –, deep 163
–, peroneus profundus n. 164–171, 234, 279–281, 296
–, posterior antebrachial cutaneous n. 16, 19f, 22–24, 26
–, posterior interosseous n. 25–27, 29f
–, posterior tibial n. 299
–, pudendal n. 140f
–, radial n. 12–21, 49–53, 61–63, 68f, 70f, 77, 79, 81, 86, 100, 115
– –, deep branch 22–25, 85f, 88, 114f
– –, superficial branch 22–35, 95, 114
–, saphenous n. 147–150, 170f, 234–236
–, sciatic n. 139–149, 195–198, 215, 223–225
–, subscapularis n. 50, 53, 55, 57f
–, superficial peroneal n. 163–171, 281
–, superior gluteal n. 137
–, suprascapular n. 7f, 49
–, sural n. 166–171, 277f
–, tibial n. 150–169, 170, 172f, 215, 219–223, 236–239, 243–246, 261, 271, 277
–, ulnar n. 12–35, 49–53, 61–63, 68, 70f, 75–77, 89, 91, 100, 102, 105, 107, 108, 123–125, 127
– –, deep branch 36–38

obturator foramen 142
olecranon 20–22, 68–71, 77–79, 89, 92, 105f, 108–111
–, fossa 20, 71f, 88f, 94, 104
–, process 90, 93
orbicular zone 191
ovary 138, 209f

palmar aponeurosis 36–40, 129f
palmar arch 120
–, deep 35–39
patella 153f, 207–209, 219–222, 229f, 243, 246, 248f
–, bipartite 244f, 247
–, cartilage 153
–, suprapatellar bursa 153f, 230, 243–247
–, suprapatellar fat pad 152f, 229f, 247
pes anserinus 163, 232, 251f, 255f, 274
phalanx
–, distal 44, 122f, 129, 132, 179, 293–295, 297, 299f
–, medial 179, 293–295, 297
–, middle 122f, 129, 132
–, proximal 42–44, 122–124, 129, 132, 179, 291, 293, 295, 297, 299f
pisiform 33f, 109, 123–125, 127

plantar aponeurosis 181, 278–291, 294–300
plantar arch 295
portio 211f
posterior glenoid labrum 61
posterior intermuscular septum 166
–, crural 167f
prefemoral fat pad 153f, 243
proximal interphalangeal articulation 122, 129, 132
pubis 141f, 185–187, 195
–, inferior ramus 143, 189, 210–213, 214
–, superior ramus 139f, 188, 206–209
–, symphysis 205
–, tubercle 205

radiocarpal articulation 120
radius 24–32, 99–104, 110–116, 119–122, 128, 130–132
–, head 22f, 73, 81, 87–89, 95f, 105f, 111–116
–, styloid process 33
rectum 138, 142, 216f
rib 5–13, 47–49, 67–69, 72f

sacral plexus 138
sacrum 137f, 195, 212–216
–, lateral part 217
scaphoid 33–35, 114f, 119–123, 130–132
scapula 7–11, 48, 50–53, 61
–, neck 50
–, spine 5f, 50–52, 62f
sesamoid 41, 122, 124, 180, 290f, 300
shoulder
–, articular cartilage 50f, 53, 191
–, articular cavity 6, 62
–, articular surface 52
–, axial 5–12
–, coronal 47–55
–, joint 8
–, joint capsule 9, 48, 57, 60
–, sagittal
sigmoid colon 207–211, 213–215
small bowel loops 195–198, 206–214
subacromial adipose tissue 60
subacromial bursa 52f, 57–59, 72
subpopliteal rec. 244
superficial palmar arch 35
superior glenoid labrum 6, 49–51
superior peroneal retinaculum 172–175
superior radioulnar articulation 23
superior talocrural joint 282
suprapatellar bursa 153f, 230, 243–247
suprapatellar fat pad 152f, 229f, 247
sustentaculum tali 174f, 298
symphysis 186
synovial fold 36
synovial tendon sheath 31–40, 43f, 57

talocrural joint 171, 255f, 281
talus 172–174, 255, 257f, 279–283, 294–298
–, trochlea 256
tarsal sinus 297
tendon
–, of abductor digiti minimi m. 288–290
–, of abductor hallucis m. 178, 277f, 290f
–, of abductor pollicis longus m. 29–35, 99, 100, 116, 122–124, 132

–, of adductor magnus m. 152–154, 250–252
–, of adductor pollicis m. 38
–, of biceps brachii m. 21f, 24, 62, 80, 85–87, 101
– –, long head 6, 49f, 57–61, 69–71, 75–80
– –, short head 47f, 61
–, of biceps femoris m. 144, 157–160, 216, 226, 236, 241, 259f, 265
– –, long head 145f
–, of brachialis m. 89
–, of brachioradialis m. 27–30
–, of extensor carpi radialis brevis m. 28–38, 131f
–, of extensor carpi radialis longus m. 26–37, 119–121
–, of extensor carpi ulnaris m. 31–37, 119, 121, 127
–, of extensor digiti minimi m. 31–43, 288–290
–, of extensor digitorum brevis m. 286–289
–, of extensor digitorum longus m. 172–176, 284–289, 295–297, 300
–, of extensor digitorum m. 31–43, 119f, 128–132, 178, 283, 290f
–, of extensor hallucis brevis m. 284–291
–, of extensor hallucis longus m. 172–177, 283–291, 296, 298–300
–, of extensor indicis m. 31–34
–, of extensor pollicis brevis m. 30–35, 41, 116, 121
–, of extensor pollicis longus m. 31–42, 102, 119f, 129, 132
–, of flexor carpi radialis m. 22f, 29–37, 124f, 132
–, of flexor carpi ulnaris m. 33f, 99, 125, 127f
–, of flexor digiti longus m. 290
–, of flexor digiti minimi brevis m. 288–290
–, of flexor digiti minimi m. 291
–, of flexor digitorum brevis m. 289
–, of flexor digitorum longus m. 171–181, 279–289, 295, 297–299
–, of flexor digitorum m. 44, 132, 290f, 294, 296, 299
–, of flexor digitorum profundus m. 22, 32–43, 42f, 123f, 127, 129f, 132
–, of flexor digitorum superficialis m. 33–44, 125, 129, 132
–, of flexor hallucis brevis m. 290
–, of flexor hallucis longus m. 173–181, 279–291, 298–300
–, of flexor pollicis brevis m.
– –, deep head 38
–, of flexor pollicis longus m. 31–42, 122–124, 131f
–, of gastrocnemius m. 167–169, 241, 273f, 297
– –, lateral head 242
– –, medial head 270
–, of gemelli m. 213
–, of gluteus maximus m. 148
–, of gluteus medius m. 143, 201
–, of gluteus minimus m. 142, 192
–, of gracilis m. 154–158, 160–162, 224, 233–237, 252, 261f
–, of iliopsoas m. 192f, 211
–, of infraspinatus m. 57f, 69, 80

Subject Index

–, of interosseous m.   44, 124, 128
–, of latissimus dorsi m.   10
–, of lumbrical m.   44, 124
–, of obturator externus m.   193, 201, 213
–, of obturator internus m.   141f, 192, 213
–, of palmaris brevis m.   35f
–, of palmaris longus m.   22f, 30–35, 130
–, of palmaris m.   125
–, of pectineus m.   192
–, of pectoralis minor m.   6, 63
–, of peroneus brevis m.   173–178, 263, 279–285
–, of peroneus longus m.   170–178, 277–286, 294–298
–, of peroneus tertius m.   173–176, 284–286
–, of piriformis m.   141, 198–201
–, of plantaris m.   154, 162–166, 241
–, of popliteus m.   155–157, 232–236, 241f
–, of quadratus femoris m.   226
–, of quadratus plantae m.   278
–, of quadriceps femoris m.   152f, 207–209, 219–222, 229, 243–246, 248
–, of rectus femoris m.   138–140, 150f, 186–190, 198, 200f, 207f, 246
–, of sartorius m.   156–158, 160f, 224, 233f, 258f
–, of semimembranosus m.   144–146, 156–160, 226, 234–237, 251f, 274
–, of semitendinosus m.   144, 154–162, 216, 226, 233–239, 248–252, 262
–, of subscapularis m.   8, 48, 50, 60
–, of supraspinatus m.   6, 57, 69, 71, 78–80
–, of teres minor m.   52, 57, 80
–, of tibialis anterior m.   159, 170–176, 248, 283–286, 298f
–, of tibialis posterior m.   170–176, 259, 280–284, 297–300
–, of triceps brachii m.   16–18, 51f, 93
– –, lateral head   10
–, of vastus lateralis m.   153–155, 187, 229f
–, of vastus medialis m.   153
–, tendo calcaneus   170–178, 263, 273, 295f, 298–300
thigh
–, axial   147–154
–, coronal   205–217
–, sagittal   219–226
tibia   159, 161–170, 219–222, 243–249, 252, 258f, 267–271, 273, 278–282, 294–298
–, anterior margin   167
–, condyles   258
– –, intercondylar eminence   233f, 256f
– –, intercondylar fossa   156f, 234f, 256
– –, lateral condyle   158, 241f, 260
– –, medial condyle   158, 250f, 260
–, medial malleolus   299
–, plateau   160, 255f, 272
– –, lateral   232f, 235f, 266
– –, medial   232f, 235, 274
–, shaft   255–257
tibiofibular articulation   236, 242, 266
trapezium   35–37, 122–125, 132
trapezoid   35–37, 119–123, 131f
triquetral   33–35, 108, 119–123, 127f

ulna   23–31, 80, 95, 100–105, 108–111, 119–122, 127
–, styloid process   31f, 120
upper arm
–, axial   13–18
–, coronal   67–73
–, sagittal   75–81
ureter   137–142
urinary bladder   138f, 142, 185–189, 206–211
uterovaginal plexus   212, 215
uterus   138, 185f, 206–211, 213

vagina   190–192, 210, 212f
–, cave   211
–, lateral wall   211
vasto–adductor membrane   150
veins
–, accessory cephalic v.   30–35, 85
–, anterior circumflex humeral v.   57–63
–, anterior interosseous v.   25–29
–, anterior tibial v.   163–171, 234, 258
–, axillary v.   7–11, 47–50, 63, 70f
–, basilic v.   15–34, 60, 70f, 75f, 85–87, 91, 99 105, 107f, 120f
–, blood vessels around the knee joint   244f, 247
–, brachial v.   12–23, 51f, 61f, 70, 72, 75, 77, 92f, 101f, 111
–, cephalic v.   7–35, 73, 78, 80f, 85, 95, 99, 111–116, 119f
– –, accessory   103
– –, of thumb   36f
–, common interosseous v.   24, 104
–, cutaneous v.   99
–, deep femoral v.   209–212, 225
–, dorsal digital v.   43f, 119f, 130
–, dorsal subcutaneous vv.   120
–, dorsal venous arch   176
–, external iliac v.   137f, 186
–, femoral v.   139–152, 185–188, 195f, 205–207, 209–214, 221–223, 226, 246, 248
–, great saphenous v.   143–171, 185f, 206–216, 225f, 236f, 252, 256–259, 274, 282–285, 299
–, iliac v.   193
–, inferior gluteal v.   137
–, inferior lateral genicular v.   233
–, inferior medial genicular v.   234, 248–250
–, intercostal v.   7–13
–, internal iliac v.   137f, 194f
– –, branches of   195
–, internal pudendal v.   139
–, interosseous v.   95, 112
–, lateral circumflex femoral v.   144f, 197f, 201, 225
–, lateral plantar v.   284, 286
–, lateral thoracic v.   11f
–, medial circumflex femoral v.   189, 191f, 201, 211f
–, medial plantar v.   282, 284, 286
–, median cubital v.   85
–, obturator v.   138–142, 189–193
–, palmar digital v.   130
–, perforating v.   148, 150
–, peroneal v.   164–168, 269f
–, popliteal v.   153–163, 215, 233–238, 245, 247, 260f, 269f
–, posterior circumflex humeral v.   10, 54, 57–61, 68, 75, 77, 79f
–, posterior interosseous recurrent v.   24
–, posterior interosseous v.   25, 29, 30
–, posterior tibial v.   164–166, 168–171, 173–175, 271, 278, 299f
–, princeps pollicis v.   40f
–, profunda brachii v.   14–20, 70f, 79, 81
–, profunda femoris v.   145–148
–, pudendal v.   140f
–, radial v.   24–34, 94, 99, 100, 112–114, 121, 123
–, saphenous v.   244
–, small saphenous v.   154–171, 220f, 238f, 245f, 248f, 270f, 277f, 294
– –, collateral of   246
–, subcutaneous v.   30f
–, subscapularis v.   7, 9–12, 49, 54, 67
–, superficial ulnar collateral v.   21f
–, superior gluteal v.   137, 196
–, superior lateral genicular v.   153f, 231f
–, superior medial genicular v.   153f, 231f, 248–251
–, superior ulnar collateral v.   17–20, 23, 91
–, suprascapular v.   5–8
–, thoracodorsal v.   12
–, tibial v.   245
–, tibialis posterior v.   167
–, ulnar v.   24–38, 80f, 86f, 94, 99, 101, 103, 108, 125
–, venous plexus around uterus   138–140

wrist and hand
–, articular disc   32, 119–121, 127
–, axial   31–44
–, coronal   119–126
–, joint capsule   30f, 33–37
–, sagittal   127–132